T0293094

HISTORY OF FOOD AND NUTRITION TOXICOLOGY

History of Toxicology and Environmental Health Series

HISTORY OF FOOD AND NUTRITION TOXICOLOGY

Edited by

ESTHER HAUGABROOKS

Scientific and Regulatory Affairs, Risk Assessment and
Toxicology, The Coca-Cola Company,
Atlanta, GA, United States

A. WALLACE HAYES

University of South Florida College of Public Health,
Tampa, FL, United States

Series Editor

PHILIP WEXLER

Retired, National Library of Medicine (NLM),
Bethesda, MD, United States

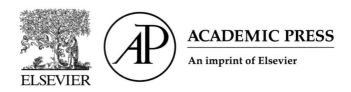

ACADEMIC PRESS

An imprint of Elsevier

ELSEVIER

Academic Press is an imprint of Elsevier
125 London Wall, London EC2Y 5AS, United Kingdom
525 B Street, Suite 1650, San Diego, CA 92101, United States
50 Hampshire Street, 5th Floor, Cambridge, MA 02139, United States
The Boulevard, Langford Lane, Kidlington, Oxford OX5 1GB, United Kingdom

Notices
Knowledge and best practice in this field are constantly changing. As new research and experience broaden our understanding, changes in research methods, professional practices, or medical treatment may become necessary.

Practitioners and researchers must always rely on their own experience and knowledge in evaluating and using any information, methods, compounds, or experiments described herein. In using such information or methods they should be mindful of their own safety and the safety of others, including parties for whom they have a professional responsibility.

To the fullest extent of the law, neither the Publisher nor the authors, contributors, or editors, assume any liability for any injury and/or damage to persons or property as a matter of products liability, negligence or otherwise, or from any use or operation of any methods, products, instructions, or ideas contained in the material herein.

ISBN: 978-0-12-821261-5

For information on all Academic Press publications
visit our website at https://www.elsevier.com/books-and-journals

Publisher: Stacy Masucci
Acquisitions Editor: Kattie Washington
Editorial Project Manager: Tracy I. Tufaga
Production Project Manager: Sajana Devasi P K
Cover Designer: Mark Rogers

Typeset by STRAIVE, India

Working together
to grow libraries in
developing countries

www.elsevier.com • www.bookaid.org

Contents

13. History of global food safety, foodborne illness, and risk assessment   **301**

Benjamin M. Liu

Contributors

Brittany Baisch
Enko Chem, Inc., Regulatory Toxicology, Mystic, CT, United States

Joseph L. Baumert
Food Allergy Research and Resource Program (FARRP), Department of Food Science and Technology, University of Nebraska, Lincoln, NE, United States

Kevin N. Boyd
The Hershey Company, Hershey, PA, United States

Roger Clemens
University of Southern California, School of Pharmacy, D.K. Kim International Center for Regulatory Science, Los Angeles, CA, United States

D. Detwiler
Northeastern University, Boston, MA, United States

Richard E. Goodman
Department of Food Science, Food Allergy Research and Resource Program, University of Nebraska-Lincoln, Lincoln, NE, United States

Esther Haugabrooks
Scientific and Regulatory Affairs, Risk Assessment and Toxicology, The Coca-Cola Company, Atlanta, GA, United States

Minerva Haugabrooks
Health and Nutrition, Lake-Sumter State College, Leesburg, FL, United States

A. Wallace Hayes
University of South Florida, College of Public Health, Tampa, FL, United States

Suzanne Hendrich
University Professor Emerita, Food Science and Human Nutrition, Iowa State University, Ames, IA, United States

Benjamin M. Liu
Division of Pathology and Laboratory Medicine, Children's National Hospital; Departments of Pediatrics, Pathology, and Microbiology, Immunology & Tropical Medicine, George Washington University School of Medicine and Health Sciences; The Center for Genetic Medicine Research, Children's National Research Institute; The District of Columbia Center for AIDS Research, Washington, DC, United States

Kelly A. Magurany
NSF International, Ann Arbor, MI, United States

Brinda Mahadevan
Brincor Associates, LLC, New Albany, OH, United States

Peter Pressman
Polyscience Consulting, Chatsworth, CA, United States

Cynthia V. Rider
Division of Translational Toxicology, National Institute of Environmental Health Sciences, Research Triangle Park, NC, United States

Lillian Smith
University of South Florida, Tampa, FL, United States

Susan C. Tilton
Environmental and Molecular Toxicology Department, Oregon State University, Corvallis, OR, United States

David Tonucci
Regulatory and Toxicology, SCiFi Foods, San Leandro, CA, United States

Series introduction

In the realm of communicating any science, history, though critical to its progress, is typically a neglected backwater. This is unfortunate, as it can easily be the most fascinating, revealing, and accessible aspect of a subject that might otherwise hold appeal for only a highly specialized technical audience. Toxicology, the science concerned with the potentially hazardous effects of chemical, biological, and certain physical agents, has yet to be the subject of a full-scale historical treatment. Overlapping with many other sciences, it both draws from and contributes to them. Chemistry, biology, and pharmacology all intersect with toxicology. While there have been chapters devoted to history in toxicology textbooks, and journal articles have filled in bits and pieces of the historical record, this new monographic series aims to further remedy the gap by offering an extensive and systematic look at the subject from antiquity to the present.

Since ancient times, men and women have sought security of all kinds. This includes identifying and making use of beneficial substances while avoiding the harmful ones, or mitigating harm already caused. Thus, food and other natural products, independently or in combination, which promoted well-being or were found to have drug-like properties and effected cures, were readily consumed, applied, or otherwise self-administered or made available to friends and family. On the other hand, agents found to cause injury or damage—what we might call *poisons* today—were personally avoided, although sometimes employed to wreak havoc upon one's enemies.

While natural substances are still of toxicological concern, synthetic and industrial chemicals now predominate as the emphasis of research. Through the years, the instinctive human need to seek safety and avoid hazard has served as an unchanging foundation for toxicology, and will be explored from many angles in this series. Although largely examining the scientific underpinnings of the field, chapters will also delve into the fascinating history of toxicology and poisons in mythology, arts, society, and culture more broadly. It is a subject that has captured our collective consciousness.

The series is intentionally broad, thus the title *History of Toxicology and Environmental Health*. Clinical and research toxicology, environmental and occupational health, risk assessment, and epidemiology, to name but a few examples, are all fair game subjects for inclusion. Volumes 1 and 2 focus on toxicology in antiquity, taken roughly to be the period up to the fall of the Roman empire and stopping short of the Middle Ages, with which period future volumes will continue. These opening volumes will explore toxicology from the perspective of some of the great civilizations of the past, including Egypt, Greece, Rome, Mesoamerica, and China. Particular substances, such as harmful botanicals, lead, cosmetics, kohl, and hallucinogens, serve as the focus of other chapters. The role of certain individuals as either victims or practitioners of toxicity (e.g., Cleopatra, Mithridates, Alexander the Great, Socrates, and Shen Nung) serves as another thrust of these volumes.

History proves that no science is static. As Nikola Tesla said, "The history of science shows that theories are perishable. With every new truth that is revealed we get a better understanding of Nature and our conceptions and views are modified."

Great research derives from great researchers who do not, and cannot, operate in a vacuum, but rely on the findings of their scientific forebears. To quote Sir Isaac Newton, "If I have seen further it is by standing on the shoulders of giants."

Welcome to this toxicological journey through time. You will surely see further and deeper and more insightfully by wafting through the waters of toxicology's history.

Philip Wexler
Retired, National Library of Medicine (NLM), Bethesda, MD,
United States

Disclaimer

The written contributions of each author were prepared in their personal capacity and do not necessarily represent the views, thoughts, and opinions of their respective employers, organization, or other affiliations.

CHAPTER 1

The interrelationships between food, nutrition, and toxicology

Esther Haugabrooks

Scientific and Regulatory Affairs, Risk Assessment and Toxicology, The Coca-Cola Company, Atlanta, GA, United States

In the beginning was food toxicology.

A simplistic definition of food toxicology is the study of adverse reactions from the consumption of food. From a creationist point of view, the principles of food toxicology are present as early as when Adam and Eve ate the fruit and were promised an adverse reaction—death (Genesis 1). From an evolutionary or survival of the fittest perspective, plants developed physical and chemical defenses that have been documented throughout the millennium to cause varied physiological effects. Subsequently, from our understanding of plants and their graded effects, we have passed down the knowledge on how to classify potential sources of foods and defined what amounts are inedible, poisonous, or nutritious.

Our observations of how food and nutrients can harm or improve health have established the overarching field of toxicology. In the same manner it was from the start of early civilization that the concepts of food toxicology were connected to our understanding of survival, nutrition, medicine, and evolution.

It is generally accepted that materials defined as food are not perceived to be toxic or may not be thought to contain toxic substances. However, foods are complex matrices comprised of thousands of chemical constituents, some of which can be problematic under varied circumstances or could prompt the development of a variety of toxicities at elevated concentrations. Thankfully, the majority of the substances found in food are not toxic when consumed in appropriate amounts and are vital to maintaining health or proper growth, otherwise called nutrients.

It may be easy to use food toxicology and nutritional toxicology as synonyms since both disciplines deal with food. However, nutritional

History of Food and Nutrition Toxicology
https://doi.org/10.1016/B978-0-12-821261-5.00022-2

toxicology is the study of how nutrients impact health, while food toxicology deals with the general principles of toxicology as it relates to substances in food or in contact with food through packaging, processing, or manufacturing.

In this chapter, we will investigate the origins of food and nutritional toxicology and overview the distinction between the fields. We will show how advancements in the field of toxicology from antiquity to the 21st century are closely related to our understanding and relationship with food.

The historical significance of the "dose makes the poison" applied to foods

It may be primarily through trial and error, not significant formal scientific evaluations that conventional wisdom developed regarding what is acceptable to eat and should be deemed food versus what could cause harm. Early civilizations identified poisonous plants and animals and utilized their extracts for warfare or hunting. As time progressed, there are documented accounts where substances like certain metals (e.g., lead, copper), arsenic, phosphorus, opium, and hemlock were used as poisons. Although some accounts are disputed, there are several famous and notable people whose deaths are attributed to poisoning: Socrates in 399 BC may have been forced to drink Hemlock (Dayan, 2009), Cleopatra is believed to have died by suicide via a poisonous snake bite in 30 BC, and Claudius (Tiberius Claudius Caesar Augustus Germanicus) died in 54 AD by either a poisonous or poisoned mushroom or by a poisoned feather used to induce vomiting (Marmion and Wiedemann, 2002).

Through documentation of poisonous substances and anecdotal stories regarding plants and their ability to provide basic sustenance, it became evident that some plants could kill while others could impart medicinal benefits. This may be one of the primary reasons the medical field and nutrition are closely linked. Throughout the centuries, as plants informed medicinal therapies and recreational pass times, the distinction between food toxicology and pharmacology became more defined. Notwithstanding, much of what we know in the field of food and nutritional toxicology is attributed to the early pioneers of toxicology.

Shennong, born Jiang Shinian (c.2695 BC), the Yan Emperor and regarded as the father of Chinese medicine, has been attributed to discovering tea potentially on a quest to discover medicinal plants for his collection of herbal remedies. It is believed he tasted over 365 herbs in his lifetime and died from an accidental overdose while trying to uncover the beneficial properties of ingested herbs or other plants. As a result, the Chinese *Materia Medica* (202 BC–220 AC) is believed to have originated from Shennong's teachings and research. There are very few written accounts of his life, thus it's not always clear what aspects of his legacy became a historical account or legend.

Hippocrates (c.460–375 BC), a Greek physician, created many connections to nutrition, medicine, and pharmacology through his written work of more than 60 texts known as the *Hippocratic Corpus (Corpus Hippocraticum)*. It may be through this work that he has been falsely attributed to saying, "let thy food be thy medicine and thy medicine be thy food," despite no account of the specific saying in any of his written works (Cardenas, 2013).

Pedanius **Dioscorides** (c.40–90 AD), a Greek physician, pharmacologist, and botanist, is known for similar work characterizing plants according to toxic or therapeutic effects. Employed as an army surgeon by the Roman emperor Nero, Dioscorides expanded the existing knowledge of medicinal herbs and minerals through his travels, which lead to *De Materia Medica* (On Medical Matters), a compilation of botany and pharmacology learnings from local medicinal herbs he encountered throughout his travels. The information from *De Materia Medica* compiled in the 1st century AD became the most extensive and reliable herbal encyclopedias available for centuries and the inspiration for many pharmacopeias.

Mangarasa (c.1350 AD), a South Indian scholar, is attributed with writing the world's first complete work dedicated to understanding Ayurveda and toxicology through pan-Indian heritage, the *Khagendra Mani Darpana* (Bhat and Udupa, 2013).

Theophrastus Bombastus Von Hohenheim, or **Paracelsus** (1493–1541), is often regarded as one of the fathers of toxicology. Known for his work as a medical scientist, physician, alchemist, and at the time, a radical philosopher in Western Europe, Paracelsus gave the field of toxicology the most quoted phrase or paraphrase, "the dose makes the poison," which can be derived from his German writings that roughly translate to

What is not poison? All things are poison, and nothing is without poison. Only the dose determines if something is not a poison.

This same attribution has been translated in a different way to read

Poison is in everything, and nothing is without poison. The dosage makes it either a poison or a remedy.

Irrespective of the preferred translation, this ideology is a valuable foundational cornerstone in food and nutritional toxicology, particularly regarding components that constitute a nutritious diet where nutritious constituents have an ideal dose that is deemed beneficial. However, when extremely high concentrations are introduced, it could produce toxic effects detrimental to the maintenance of good health.

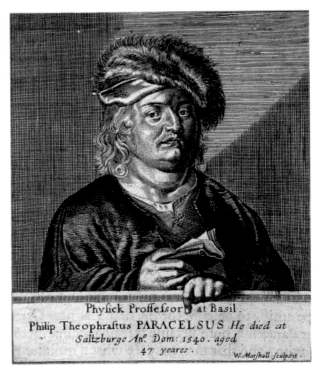

Paracelsus *(Source: Wellcome Library London. Retrieved from Michaleas et al., 2021.)*

Mathieu Joseph Bonaventure **Orfila** (1787–1853), a Spaniard, is generally regarded as the father of modern toxicology. He identified toxicology as a separate science, and in 1814 published the first textbook devoted exclusively to systematically correlating biological and chemical characteristics of poisons entitled *Traité des Poisons Tirés des Règnes Minéral, Végétal et Animal* *ou Toxicologie Générale (A treatise on poisons found in the mineral, vegetable and animal kingdoms, or, a general system of toxicology).* Orfila is attributed to being one of the first scientists in the field of toxicology to introduce animal experimentation, which was already in use for medical research. Even then, experimental methodologies that used animals as models for humans were questioned for relevance and a common critique for Orfila's application of animal models in research. Orfila primarily used canines as a model to study absorption and elimination of poisons from internal organs and the activity of antidotes (Michaleas et al., 2022).

It was during the Renaissance (14th century–17th century) and the Age of Enlightenment (17th and 18th centuries), through the contributions of scientists like Orfila, that the fundamental principles of toxicology began to develop. Much information was derived from therapeutic studies, or conversely, the use of poisons. Although poisonings are not considered scientific contributions, many women of that time made it into a career. Some popular examples are:

Giulia Tofana (died 1651) sold an arsenic concoction, Aqua Tofana, primarily to women who came to Tofana expressing interest in killing their husbands or other people death would result in personal gain.

Catherine Monvoisin (c.1640–1680), infamously known as "**La Voisin**," sold love potions and fatal poisons, also known as "inheritance powders." She became the center of the Affair of the Poisons, which was a French scandal spanning c.1677 and 1682, where some prominent and common people were accused and charged with poisoning and witchcraft.

Maria Catherina van der Linden-Swanenburg (1839–1915), "Good Mie," is believed to have poisoned over 90 people with arsenic. She was only convicted of causing the death of three people, with the intent to collect on their insurance policy or inheritance.

Good Mie and others primarily used food or beverages as their vehicle to administer the poison. This kind of food adulteration, though intentional and intended to be fatal, was not the only kind of adulteration of its time. In the 1300s, mass food production began to emerge along with common practices of food adulteration. Chemical doctoring of foods may have initially emerged to improve the appearance, stability, and profitability of foods, but without consideration of the effects on human health, food safety quickly became a major public health concern. At the beginning of the 14th century, there was very little regulatory oversight for food production, and over time some unscrupulous practices threatening public health and sometimes claiming lives surfaced.

Lead, arsenic, copper, and chrome were popular colorings. Lead was used to color candies, and red lead to color cheese. Aniline dyes, which were aniline derivatives, derived from coal tar benzene, were also used in candies, butter, and alcohol. Leaves from cherry laurels, a poisonous plant, were used in custards to impart a nutty flavor. In the 1700s adding alum (a group of hydrated double salts that usually consist of aluminum sulfate, water, and another elemental sulfate) was a popular practice among bread bakers to improve appearance and texture.

In addition to adulterating food with unsavory substances, foods were also misbranded with very little oversight. Cherry leaves were used in tea as a filler which acted as an undesired and strong laxative. Dairy cream was thickened with flour. Butter was often composed of gypsum, gelatin fat, and mashed potatoes. Beef hearts and other organ meats were canned and labeled as chicken. Oleomargarine or "bogus butter" could be made from hog fat, beef tallow, bleach, and other unlikely substances. Milk was watered down and sometimes sold with added chalk to improve the color of milk produced from diseased cows.

Cooking, salting, canning, fermentation, and chemical modifications such as the addition of preservatives are all techniques that were employed to control food safety and decrease the risk of foodborne illness. However, it wasn't enough to protect public health with no strict laws to be enforced. As food adulteration continued to threaten public health and safety, some unethical practices were used to mask spoilage or unwanted contamination. Sodium sulfates were used as meat preservatives and to induce a fresh red color despite the fact that they have been known to cause kidney damage. Yellow dye was used in butter often to mask the potential presence of foreign matter (e.g., insects, mold).

By the turn of the 19th century, there was a rapid increase in the industrial preparation and packaging of foods. Although there were some international examples of regulatory oversight for food safety, there were still many dangerous practices leading to fatalities without proper liability to merchants. In 1820, Frederick Accum (1769–1838), a German-born chemist working in London, shed a detailed spotlight on harmful food additives through his monograph entitled *A Treatise on Adulterations of Food and Culinary Poisons*. Accum is lauded for using dramatic imagery to bring attention to a grave situation that, at the time, remained largely unchecked. The first edition sold out relatively quickly after 1000 copies; the cover of the first edition and subsequent editions depicted imagery similar to a skull and bones with a caption that read:

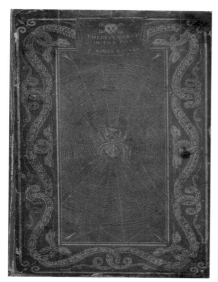
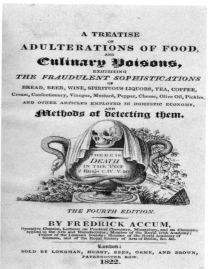

There is death in the Pot. Kings 4:40 *(1st Photo Courtesy of Science History Institute, https://digital.sciencehistory.org/works/zp38wd737; 2nd Photo title page of fourth addition from https://www.pbagalleries.com/view-auctions/catalog/id/100/lot/27089/A-Treatise-on-Adulterations-of-Food-and-Culinary-Poisons-Exhibiting-the-Fraudulent-Sophistications-of-Bread-Beer-Wine-Spiritous-Liquors-Tea-Coffee-Cream-Confectionary-Vinegar-Mustard-Pepper-Cheese-Olive-Oil-Pickles-and-Other-Articles-Employed-in-Domestic-Economy-and-Methods-of-Detecting-Them; Email: pba@pbagalleries.com.)*

The candor, passion, and eccentric methods in which Accum obtained information, coupled with the serious allegations presented in his work, made him an unliked man who, by his own account, received many threats. Despite the loyal support of some, Accum's reputation declined, and he ran into legal troubles. Shortly after the wild success of his books, Accum left Britain to return to Germany. He was one of the first effective advocates for legislative change. However, the British government did not implement meaningful legislation to protect the food supply until 1875, more than half a century after his book and over 30 years after Accum's death.

Ellen Henrietta Richards (1842–1911), a chemist and a professor at Massachusetts Institute of Technology (MIT), became interested in food chemistry during her tenure at MIT and significantly contributed to exposing the pervasive culture of food adulteration with her book *Food Materials and Their Adulterations*, published in 1885 which led to the passage of the first Pure Food and Drug Act in Massachusetts (Luma, 2021). Her contributions to food science and chemistry are largely underrated as her target demographic was women and a more general audience to teach them how to identify adulterated foods. At the core Richards was advocating to empower the public to identify food hazards to the best of their ability in an effort to mitigate risk.

Paracelsus and Orfila are broadly considered the fathers of toxicology; however, indirectly, Accum was one of the many initial pioneers in food toxicology. Similarly, **Harvey Washington Wiley** (1844–1930) is considered the father of "Pure Food." Wiley's most notable work was mainly during his tenure as the chief chemist in the Chemistry Division of the U.S. Department of Agriculture (USDA), which would later become the Bureau of Chemistry in 1901, and the Food and Drug Administration (FDA) in 1906. Wiley devised and led a notorious government experiment on human volunteers dubbed the "Poison Squad," a group of young men who in exchange for free meals agreed to eat controlled amounts of chemical preservatives like borax, formaldehyde, and benzoates in prepared meals in effort to assess their health effects after consumption.

If ever you should visit the Smithsonian Institute,
Look out that Professor Wiley doesn't make you a recruit.
He's got a lot of fellows there that tell him how they feel,
They take a batch of poison every time they eat a meal.
For breakfast they get cyanide of liver, coffin shaped,
For dinner, undertaker's pie, all trimmed with crepe;
For supper, arsenic fritters, fried in appetizing shade,
And late at night they get a prussic acid lemonade.
O, they may get over it but they'll never look the same,
That kind of bill of fare would drive most men insane.
Next week he'll give them mothballs,
a la Newburgh or else plain;
O, they may get over it but they'll never look the same.

The "Song of the Poison Squad"
Lew Dockstader's Minstrels, October 1903

It is through his life's work and advocacy that the Pure Food and Drugs Act of 1906 was passed in the US, also establishing what we know as the US FDA. The Pure Food and Drugs Act is considered the first comprehensive US law addressing food safety, prohibiting adulteration, and misbranding of food and drugs in interstate commerce. The Pure Food and Drugs Act demonstrated substantial progress but was not perfect and later amended by the Federal Food, Drug, and Cosmetic Act of 1938. The same year the Pure Food and Drug Act was passed, the Federal Meat

Inspection Act of 1906 was also passed, specifically prohibiting the sale of alternated or misbranded meat and meat products intended for food. The act also ensured that meat was slaughtered and processed under sanitary conditions.

The passage of the Federal Meat Inspection Act is attributed in part to Wiley but also to the advocacy of **Upton Sinclair** (1878–1968), a writer and non-scientist who in 1906 published his graphic political fiction, *The Jungle*. The novel depicts the unsanitary practices and conditions of the meat industry. Although a fictitious novel, *The Jungle* was an unfortunate example of art imitating life as America was already acquainted with the embalmed beef scandal where US troops were fed low-quality, heavily adulterated beef during the Spanish-American War of 1898.

> There was never the least attention paid to what was cut up for sausage; there would come all the way back from Europe old sausage that had been rejected, and that was moldy and white—it would be dosed with borax and glycerine, and dumped into the hoppers, and made over again for home consumption. There would be meat that had tumbled out on the floor, in the dirt and sawdust, where the workers had tramped and spit uncounted billions of consumption germs. There would be meat stored in great piles in rooms; and the water from leaky roofs would drip over it, and thousands of rats would race about on it. It was too dark in these storage places to see well, but a man could run his hand over these piles of meat and sweep off handfuls of the dried dung of rats.

Excerpt from Chapter 14 of *The Jungle* by Upton Sinclair

As the field of toxicology moved out of predominate observational stages, scientists like **René Truhaut** (1909–1994), a French toxicologist, became more refined in evaluating toxic reactions and mechanisms. Truhaut devoted most of his research to understating carcinogenic substances in environmental products and foodstuffs. He supported novel toxicological methodologies and through his innovative spirit was the originator of the concept Acceptable Daily Intake (ADI). Truhaut was also part of a small founding group of individuals who created the vision for the establishment of the Joint FAO/WHO Expert Committee on Food Additives (Anon., 1994).

Toxicology: Food and nutrition

Toxicology, by and of itself, is a rather large branch of science that primarily studies the deleterious effects of substances on living systems. Under the umbrella of toxicology are many subdisciplines such as forensics, environmental science, and food science that quantify and qualify chemical interactions, mechanisms of action, and graded effects. In general, toxicology follows an effect or mechanism after exposure to a hazard. Common hazards are chemical substances such as drugs, poisons, toxicants, toxins, pesticides, and colorants. Other types of hazards that are not considered chemical hazards, like physical and biological hazards, are also covered in the overarching field of toxicology. However, physical hazards are generally not a predominant concern in food or nutritional toxicology, outside of specific choking hazards and/or foreign materials that may be unintentionally introduced into foods. Biological hazards such as pathogenic bacteria and viruses are a main concern in food toxicology as they often produce chemical substances that are toxic to humans.

Chemical substances can come from natural or anthropogenic sources and produce varied effects primarily thorough associated physicochemical properties. Thus chemical substances can be grouped based on intended use (e.g., industrial chemicals), risk of adverse effects (e.g., mutagen), or chemical origin (e.g., toxins). In most branches of toxicology, chemical substances known to cause harm or adverse effects are generally called toxicants. Toxins, however, are a specific class of toxicants that are classified as an organic substance, particularly a small molecule, peptide, or conjugated protein that originates from metabolic activities of living cells or organisms (e.g., plants, animals, or microorganisms), see Table 1. Mycotoxins, like aflatoxin, are secondary metabolites of fungi and are classified as toxins based on their origin of a living organism the same as grayanotoxins (mad honey), solanine, or urushiol (poison ivy, poison oak, and poison sumac, raw cashews), which are of plant origin.

The term toxin was coined by Ludwig Brieger (1849–1919) from his work with infectious diseases, particularly typhoid fever, in contaminated food or waterborne illness caused by bacterial toxins (Brieger, 1887 as cited by Nasiripourdori et al., 2011). Under classifications of toxicants, some of the descriptors for chemical substances can be used interchangeably; for example, pesticides can also be considered poison if not used as intended and some toxins have been used as drugs (Peigneur and Tytgat, 2018).

Food and nutritional toxicology are cross-disciplinary fields that are not only considered branches of toxicology but may also intersect with other classical disciplines such as food science and pharmacology. Many other disciplines have lent important contributions to food and nutritional toxicology, such as microbiology, immunology, environmental sciences, molecular biology, behavior sciences, and epidemiology.

Table 1 Toxins are substances that originate from living organisms. Examples of toxins that can be found in human food sources.

Toxin	Origin	Source	Mechanism
Aquatic biotoxins			
Brevetoxins	Algae	Found in some shellfish but produced by *Karenia brevis*, a type of dinoflagellate (algae).	Brevetoxins cause neurological shellfish poisoning due to uncontrolled sodium influx into nerve cells from open voltage-gated sodium channels.
Ciguatoxins	Algae	A lipophilic toxin found in some fish (e.g., black grouper, king mackerel), produced by *Gambierdiscus toxicus*, a type of dinoflagellate (algae).	Ciguatoxins are high-affinity agonists on voltage-gated sodium receptors causing: Ciguatera Fish Poisoning or Ciguatera
Okadaic Acid	Algae	A lipophilic, polyether toxin produced by various dinoflagellates.	Known to inhibit serine/threonine protein phosphatases which play a role in essential cellular processes such as cellular growth, division, and death by dephosphorylation. Ingestion of okadaic acid can lead to the condition Diarrhetic Shellfish Poisoning.
Saxitoxin	Algae or Bacteria	Produced by marine algae, specifically certain dinoflagellates or freshwater cyanobacteria (also called blue-green algae although not scientifically classified as algae), which can accumulate in planktivorous invertebrates and crustaceans.	Saxitoxin is a neurotoxin that causes Paralytic Shellfish Poisoning by acting as an antagonist and blocking voltage-gated sodium channels, which will result in paralysis, respiratory failure, or death if left untreated.
Tetrodotoxin	Animal	One of the most potent neurotoxins that is most widely known to be found in certain puffer fish, although it has been found in other animal species.	Tetrodotoxin is a direct-acting toxin that inhibits voltage-gated sodium channels in nerve cells, which can lead to asphyxiation via respiratory paralysis.

Continued

Table 1 Toxins are substances that originate from living organisms. Examples of toxins that can be found in human food sources—cont'd

Toxin	Origin	Source	Mechanism
Botulinum	Bacteria	A neurotoxic protein produced by *Clostridium botulinum*.	Botulinum has Zn-protease activity and inhibits neurotransmitter acetylcholine by hydrolyzing the fusion proteins that assist in exocytosis of acetylcholine in cholinergic neurons (e.g., motor neurons), causing paralysis or botulism.
Cyanogenic Glycosides	Plant	Phytotoxins, meaning toxins produced by plants (e.g., cassava, bamboo shoots, sorghum, cocoyam, stone fruits) that are amino acid–derived aglycones.	Improper processing of edible plants containing cyanogenic glycosides can cause the release of hydrogen cyanide from spontaneous degradation or hydrolysis of the glycosidic linkage. Significant amounts can lead to acute cyanide poisoning or irreversible neurological condition. Low concentrations can interfere with dietary iodine metabolism leading to iodine deficiency that promotes goiters or hypothyroidism.
Furocoumarins	Plant	Organic compounds that are phytotoxins synthesized by edible plants like parsnips, celery roots, and citrus as defense molecules.	Furocoumarins are phototoxins that can cause serious skin reactions, such as skin inflammation when exposed to light due to photoactivation, which converts furocoumarins into an excited and highly reactive triplet state. Furocoumarins inhibit DNA synthesis and repair by entering the cell, intercalating with the DNA, and forming DNA adducts and cross-links when activated by UV.
Grayanotoxins	Plant	A diterpene, a polyhydroxylated cyclic hydrocarbon, produced in the leaves and flowers of plants of the Ericaceae family, which can end up in nectar or other secondary products of plants.	Grayanotoxin intoxication or Mad Honey Disease from contaminated honey (Jansen et al., 2012) occurs because of grayanotoxin binding to open voltage-dependent sodium channels preventing them from closing or becoming inactive. This heightened state of depolarization can lead to nausea, vomiting, and dizziness as minor symptoms or hypotension, bradycardia, and atrioventricular block (Ozhan et al., 2004).

Hypoglycin A	Plant	A water-soluble, cholestatic hepatotoxin found in higher concentrations of the seed and rind of unripe Ackee fruit.	Ingestion of hypoglycin A can cause gastrointestinal (GI) distress and microvesicular steatosis or "Jamaican Vomiting Sickness" and induces severe hypoglycemia. The primary method of toxicity is believed to be through the inhibition of fatty acid oxidation (Barceloux, 2009).
Lectins	Plant	Proteins found in vegetables and raw beans (i.e., before drying or processing). Phytohemagglutinins (PHA) from raw or undercooked kidney bean (*Phaseolus vulgaris*) seeds are plant lectins.	Improper preparation of foods with lectins can cause GI tract distress such as nausea, vomiting, and diarrhea. Lectins bind to carbohydrates and selectively bind to cell wall glycoproteins, with an affinity for the surface of gut epithelial cells, which may potently inhibit plasma membrane repair (Miyake et al., 2007) although exact mechanism of lectin poisoning is not currently known.
Microcystins	Bacteria	Produced by certain freshwater cyanobacteria (e.g., Microcystis) or blue–green algae.	Microcystis covalently bond to and inhibit protein phosphatases and can cause liver damage and pansteatitis.
Muscimol and Muscarine	Fungus	Wild mushroom toxins: Muscimol is psychoactive isoxazole found primarily in *Amanita muscaria* mushrooms. Muscarine can be found in trace amounts in *Amanita muscaria* although more common in Inocybe and Clitocybe mushroom species.	Muscimol is an analog of GABA and a potent GABA$_A$ receptor agonist. Tachycardia, bradycardia, and hypertension may occur from muscimol poisoning and death in rare cases. Muscarine mimics the neurotransmitter acetylcholine (agonist) in the muscarinic part of the cholinergic (parasympathetic) nervous system by continuous impulses or uncontrolled receptor hyperstimulation or muscarine poisoning
Mycotoxins	Fungus	Produced by mold on dry grains, cereals, fruits, nuts, and spices. Common mycotoxins of food safety concern are Aflatoxins, Beauvericin, Citrinin, Deoxynivalenol (DON), Ergot alkaloids, Fumonisins, Ochratoxins, Patulin, and Zearalenone.	Mycotoxins can cause a variety of adverse health effects, such as renal damage and cancer, and pose a serious health threat to humans and animals (Hussein and Brasel, 2001).

Continued

Table 1 Toxins are substances that originate from living organisms. Examples of toxins that can be found in human food sources—cont'd

Toxin	Origin	Source	Mechanism
Pyrrolizidine Alkaloids	Plant	Are produced in many plants, mainly in the Boraginaceae, Asteraceae, *and* Fabaceae families.	Pyrrolizidine alkaloids are metabolized in the parenchymal cells into pyrroles which act on hepatocytes and blood vessels in the liver or lungs by damaging hepatic sinusoidal and endothelial cells.
Solanine	Plant	A glycoalkaloid poison found in species of the nightshade family within the genus *Solanum*, such as the potato (*Solanum tuberosum*), the tomato, and eggplant.	Solanine interacts with potassium channels on mitochondrial membranes decreasing membrane potential and altering intestinal permeability, which is believed to lead to gastrointestinal distress.
Staphylococcal Enterotoxin B	Bacteria	Produced by the gram-positive coccus bacterium *Staphylococcus aureus*, which can proliferate in unrefrigerated meats or contaminated dairy and bakery products.	Staphylococcal enterotoxin B (SEB) is the most potent staphylococcal enterotoxin that causes infections outside food poising, although ingestion can lead to multiorgan system failure and death in extreme cases. Adverse effects can also occur through the immune system by stimulation of cytokine release and inflammation.

The primary focus of food toxicology is on toxicants, including toxins, present in food; whereas, nutritional toxicology focuses on the interactions between toxicants and dietary components that may have acute or chronic health effects at varied doses. Before overviewing some of the current applications of both fields, it is important to understand the basic principles of each and the connections between food and nutritional toxicology.

Food toxicology basics

Congruent with toxicologists in other fields, food toxicologists study the adverse effects of substances found specifically in food. Under the principles of toxicology, experimental models or epidemiological data are applied to understand the dose–response of hazards in foods and other potentially damaging effects of food substances on living organisms. The types of models that can be used span from in vitro (e.g., cell or tissue cultures, organoids), computational modeling (in silico), to animal models. Most empirical learnings have been from single chemical exposures in controlled environments; however, particularly within food matrixes there is a growing demand to generate information regarding how toxicology modeling can be expanded to complex mixtures. For instance, the threshold of toxicological concern (TTC), a widely known predictive risk assessment tool used to establish a human exposure threshold value for chemical substances that may have detailed chemistry and exposure information but little to no toxicity information, is gaining application for chemically complex matrices within foods (Rennen et al., 2011). The utility of TTC addresses how to establish a low probability of appreciable risk to human health while reducing reliance on single chemical animal studies that struggle to keep up with innovation and are resource intensive. Notwithstanding, single chemical studies have added tremendous knowledge to the field of food toxicology and are needed to quantify hazards from individual ingredients or food components.

The concept that the dose makes the poison has already been introduced; therefore, the idea that all components in food—inherent or otherwise—are toxicants should not be foreign. However, if all components in food are toxicants, the concept of toxicants in foods begins to lose its meaning. In addition, if we generally regard food as safe, referencing all its components as toxicants would most definitely become confusing—as it does—when considering what foods are truly safe to consume. This is why understanding the general principles of toxicology in context of exposure, hazard, and risk is essential in food toxicology.

Fundamental principles of toxicology are characterizing the hazard, understanding the route of entry (oral, dermal, inhalation), establishing an appropriate dose-response, then quantifying the risk. Hazard identification is the first step in a classical risk assessment; however, even if a classical risk assessment is not conducted, hazard identification or classification is important to determine how a substance is toxic and to what severity. In other words, a hazard explains an adverse response under defined circumstances. Does the hazard have the potential to cause acute and/or chronic effects? If so, at what dose? Does changing the route of entry affect toxicity? After careful characterization using quantifiable information concerning the specific hazard, hazards are often ranked or classified by the potential severity of adverse effects.

In food toxicology the main route of entry is oral, therefore what is a hazard via the oral route might not be a concern via inhalation, or vice versa. Diacetyl, generally used as a flavoring agent, was recognized as safe for human (oral) consumption but can lead to an irreversible and rare condition called bronchiolitis obliterans or popcorn lung from occupational inhalation exposure (Kreiss et al., 2002). Popcorn lung is generally not a concern for consumer exposure (Egilman and Schilling, 2012); however, there was one notable lawsuit where the plaintiff won a settlement for chronic inhalation exposure where they claimed to have eaten the minimum of 2–3 microwaveable bags of popcorn a day for over 10 years. This is an example of how diacetyl could be a hazard in food that contributes to a rare condition under highly specific circumstances and brings to bear that the mere presence of a hazard may or may not necessarily be sufficient to produce an adverse outcome.

The safety of a potential ingredient in a food is established based on the intended use and use level of that ingredient. The intended use of an ingredient should include the dose, the purpose or technical effect, and the potentially exposed population (e.g., adults, babies). To rank or quantify acceptable exposure, reference values are generated from hazard and dose-response information (Hayes and Kobets, 2023).

The **Estimated Daily Intake (EDI)** is based on likely exposure in context to daily intake (I) of the food source(s) that the substance is used in and the concentration (C) of the substance in the food(s).

$$EDI = (C)(I)$$

Another reference value is the **Acceptable Daily Intake (ADI)**, which is an exposure amount of a substance with no appreciable health risk over a lifetime. ADIs are conservative estimates derived from toxicology studies:

$$ADI = NOAEL \div SF$$

where the NOAEL is the No-Observed-Adverse-Effect Level or the highest dose from a toxicology study that does not produce an adverse effect. SF is a safety factor or an uncertainty factor that accounts for species differences and other sources of variability. In general, when assessing the safety of an additive, risk assessors rely on evidence that a food additive is safe for the intended use where the EDI < ADI. Concerning contaminates, the term **Tolerable Daily Intake (TDI)** is used, which uses the same calculation as ADI. A provisional tolerable daily intake (PTDI) is used for contaminates that may accumulate and are not rapidly cleared from the body (Herrman and Younes, 1999).

Since both ADIs and TDIs are estimates for lifetime exposures, short-term exposures that marginally exceed these values may not be of appreciable concern. Tolerable intakes can also be expressed as weekly or monthly threshold values, tolerable weekly intake (TWI) or tolerable monthly intake (TMI), respectively. For the calculation of ADI and tolerable intakes, the NOAEL or the LOAEL is used as a point of departure (POD) for estimating safe exposure levels. A POD is an experimental or observational value that should be used to establish a safe intake if it can be scientifically justified and when supported by other toxicology data (FAO/WHO, 2009).

After quantification of the hazard, it is appropriate to understand risk. Risk is the probability that an adverse reaction will occur, considering the following equation:

$$Risk = Hazard \times Exposure$$

No substantive conversation about risk should be made without disclosing appropriate exposure scenarios associated with the defined hazard. In other words, the use of the term risk in food toxicology should factor in how likely it is for a defined set of circumstances to lead to an adverse outcome. Therefore risk can be ranked from low to high and the mere presence of a hazard without consideration of the dose or amount of exposure cannot appropriately rank risk.

Toxicants in foods
Most foods or items deemed suitable for foods are rarely straightforward and are usually comprised of more than a single component. Even foods that are perceived to be relatively simple, such as watermelon composed of $\geq 90\%$ water, intrinsically have many different chemicals (see Table 2).

Table 2 Select chemical components in watermelon.

	Chemical components in watermelon
Macronutrients	Water, carbohydrates, protein, fiber, lipids,
Minerals	K, Ca, Mg, Cu, Zn, Fe
Antioxidants	
Flavonoids	Rutin
Carotenoids	Lycopene, cryptoxanthin, β-carotene, zeaxanthin, lutein
Vitamins	niacin, vitamin A, vitamin C or ascorbic acid
Citrulline	
Predominate fatty acids in seeds:	Linoleic acid, oleic, palmitic, and stearic acids
Minor fatty acids in seeds:	Linolenic, palmitoleic, and myristic acids
Other seed constituents:	Alkaloid, cardiac glycosides, oxalate, phytate, saponin

Table compiled from Ibrahim et al. (2021), Imen et al. (2011), Albishri et al. (2013), and Araoye and Otutu (2016).

Photo from https://www.freepik.com/free-photo/slice-watermelon-white--background_20978830. htm#query=watermelon&position=0&from_view=keyword.

News articles, social media, and consumer blogs suggest the public usually struggles with the idea that foods even without any added chemicals still contain chemicals. At the core, anything made up of atoms that form elements can be considered a chemical. Water (CAS-No. 7732-18-5), also known as dihydrogen oxide or oxidane, is one of the most abundant and pervasive chemicals on Earth. While water is a chemical, the public will not categorize it as such and largely perceives "natural" substances to be devoid of harm. The use of the term "chemicals" within the general population has generated a strict and often misleading connotation of something artificial with impending danger. This concept is substantiated by research conducted on a public cohort in the Netherlands revealing the majority believed "most chemical substances are harmful for health" (Jansen et al., 2020).

Although inherent constituents of food are chemicals, other words that may also confer a benefit are used for major constituents, such as macronutrient, micronutrient, mineral, phytochemical.

In addition to nutrients, naturally occurring toxicants, and other inherent food constituents, foods can contain chemicals such as:

Food additives	Heavy metals (e.g., arsenic, cadmium, mercury, or lead)
Color additives	
Pesticide residues	Unintentional contaminants
Packing materials	Biological contaminants
Processing aids	Environmental contaminants
Radioactive elements	Heat formed by products

Food additives are probably considered one of the main contributors to toxicants in foods. In this introductory chapter, the term food additives will be presented broadly as any substances that can be added to food. However, note, the term food additive may have its own regulatory definition based on region or function, and therefore different types of substances added to food are termed and potentially regulated differently.

In the broadest characterization, food additives are substances added to food. In the United States, food additives are substances regulated under the Food Additives Amendment that are added directly or indirectly to food, previously sanctioned additives, substances considered Generally Recognized as Safe (GRAS), color additives, and flavoring ingredients or substances used in conjunction with flavors. All food additives are intended to serve a purpose whether the purpose was intended in the preparation process or in the final product. There are many examples where food additives serve dual functions or technical effects; for example, a substance that is an antioxidant can also be considered a preservative. The safety of food additives is determined by intended use, including factors such as chemical composition, manufacturing processes, concentration in a final food product, and technical effect.

In theory, food additives can be broken into two main categories: direct and indirect food additives (see Table 3). To overgeneralize the concept further, a direct food additive is any substance added for a specific purpose in a final food or food product. Generally, direct food additives are usually identified in the ingredient label. Indirect food additives are substances that may become part of the food from manufacturing, packaging, or storage processes; however, they may serve no technical effect in finished product and may be inadvertently found in trace amounts of the final product. For regulatory purposes, indirect food additives in the US are also classified as food contact substances—substances from materials that come into direct contact with the final food and that may migrate to the final food product. In Table 3, the only examples of indirect additives are food contact substances. It is important to note that indirect substances can also be broadly applied to pesticides (e.g., organochlorines, carbamates), veterinary drug (e.g., synthetic hormones, antibiotics) residues, and radioactive elements (e.g., gamma and X-rays) when found in small and legally permissible quantities. In 1995 based on a *de minimis* principle, the U.S. Food and Drug Administration (FDA) introduced the Threshold of Regulation for indirect food additives or food contact substances (21 C.F.R. §170.39), which

Table 3 General food additives categorization and examples.

Category	Primary examples	Secondary examples
Direct additives	Sensory agents or organoleptic modifiers	Colorants	Allure Red
			Annatto
			Paprika oleoresin
			Sunset yellow
		Flavors and flavor enhancers	Natural seasonings, extracts, and flavorings
			Pickling agents
			Spices
			Synthetic flavor and extracts
		Sweeteners	Nonnutritive sweetener
			Nutritive sweetener
		Texturizers	Dough strengtheners
			Emulsifier
			Leavening agents
			Stabilizers and thickeners
	Nutritional additives	Nutrients or dietary supplements	Beta-carotene
			Calcium
			Vitamin B12 (cobalamin)
			Zinc
	Processing agent	Anticaking agent	Aluminum silicate
		Antifoaming agent	Oleic acid
		Bleaching agent	Benzoyl peroxide
		Enzymes	Bromelain
		Humectants	Glycerin
		Neutralizing or pH controlling agent	Adipic acid
		Sequestrants	Disodium EDTA
		Solvents	Diethylene glycol monoethyl ether

Category	Subcategory	Type / component	Examples or list reference
Preservatives		Antioxidant	Propyl gallate, Sulfur dioxide, Tocopherols
		Antimicrobial	Potassium metabisulfite, Sodium benzoate
		Antibrowning	
		Synthetic preservatives	
		Pesticides	Fumigants, Fungicides, Herbicides
Indirect additives or food contact substances[a]	Adhesives and coatings	Adhesives	See list in 21 CFR 175.105
		Pressure-sensitive adhesives	See list in 21 CFR 175.125
		Components of coatings	See list in 21 CFR 175.210–390
	Adjuvants	Animal glue	See list in 21 CFR 178.3010–3120, 3450
		Esters of stearic and palmitic acids	
	Paper and paperboard components	Acrylamide–acrylic acid resins	See list in 21 CFR 176
		Alkyl ketene dimers	
		Chelating agents	
		Slimicides	
	Polymers and plastics	Polyolefins, polyesters, polystyrene, polyamides, etc.	See list in 21 CFR 177
	Production aids	Antioxidants and stabilizers for polymers	See list in 21 CFR 178.2010–2650
		Anticorrosive agents	See list in 21 CFR 178.3125–3400
		Antistatic and/or antifogging agents	
		Clarifying agents for polymers	
		Colorants for polymers	
		Corrosion inhibitors	
		Surface-active agents	
	Sanitizers	Sanitizing solutions	See list in 21 CFR 178.1010

a Substances permitted in use in the following categories.

Adapted from 21 CFR Parts 170–178, 181–186, Güngörmüş, C., Kılıç, A., 2012. The safety assessment of food additives by reproductive and developmental toxicity studies. Food Additive. doi:10.5772/30787; Davidson, P.M., Singh, R.P., 2018. Food additive. Encyclopedia Britannica, Vol. 3. https://www.britannica.com/topic/food-additive.

exempts substances migrating from packaging into food at levels below a threshold of 0.5 ppb from being listed as food additives. When found above the tolerance prescribed for indirect additives, they are reclassified and may be binned as contaminants.

Food additives or substances inherent in food can lead to several adverse effects or toxic responses such as allergic reactions, nonallergic food hypersensitivity, and food intolerance. Food allergies are an immune-mediated response, typically an immunoglobulin E (IgE) response to a specific protein in a food even in small quantities. Some of the most common food allergens and their associated proteins are as follows:

Milk	Casein, whey
Eggs	Ovalbumin, ovomucoid
Peanuts	Ara proteins
Tree nuts	Albumins, vicilins, globulins
Soybean	Glycinin and beta-conglycinin
Wheat	Gliadin, prolamins, gluten
Fish	Parvalbumins
Sesame	Albumins, globulin proteins
Shellfish	Tropomyosin

Adapted from Valenta, R., Hochwallner, H., Linhart, B., Pahr, S., 2015. Food allergies: the basics. Gastroenterology 148 (6), 1120–1131.e4. doi:10.1053/j.gastro.2015.02.006. Epub 2015 Feb 11; PMID: 25680669; PMCID: PMC4414527.

Food intolerances are not as well documented as food allergies, but one of the most well known food intolerance, lactose intolerance, has likely been a common condition for thousands of years (Silanikove et al., 2015). Food intolerances arise from the body's inability to digest or metabolize specific foods or their components. Other frequently observed food intolerances are gluten and histamine intolerance. Some metabolic responses can be considered food intolerance, including a phenylalanine hydroxylase deficiency, which is a hereditary condition impairing the body's ability to metabolize phenylalanine.

Food poisoning is another adverse reaction that occurs when a person consumes food that is contaminated with harmful bacteria, viruses, or toxins. Notable examples of food poisoning include the outbreak of typhoid fever in the early 1900s, which is speculated to be caused by contaminated clams (Marineli et al., 2013) or contaminated water in Long Island, NY. Typhoid fever is caused by a virulence factor of *Salmonella typhi*, called typhoid toxin.

Another example is the various outbreak of botulism in the United States, mainly caused by contaminated canned foods (Sobel et al., 2004). Botulism is also caused by toxins produced in *Clostridium botulinum*. While microbial contamination poses a significant risk to food safety, there are other toxic substances in foods that can threaten public health. For example, metals like methylmercury can be found in seafood. Industrial pollutants, such as dioxins and polychlorinated biphenyls (PCBs), can enter the food supply through waste or manufacturing by-products. Additionally, toxic substances can form in food during cooking, such as heterocyclic amines, acrylamides, and furans, which can over time cause unintended adverse reactions from exposure through the diet.

Nutritional toxicology

Nutritional toxicology is a branch of toxicology and nutrition that studies toxicants in the diet and their effects on nutrients, nutritional processes, or the effects of nutrients and nutritional metabolism on toxicants (Hathcock, 1982). Nutritional toxicology builds upon the fundamentals of food toxicology but can be expanded as a method to protect against hazards through the modulation of diet or nutritional makeup. Therefore, as a caveat of food toxicology with many overlapping principles, nutritional toxicology remains focused on the nutritional components of food, the effects of nutritional intake, the interaction of toxicants with nutrients, and the protective effects of diet against adverse effects of toxicants.

Eating a balanced diet is an important factor for optimal health but understanding the impact of dietary interactions aids in the proper maintenance to ensure a balanced diet based on health conditions among other variables. Responses to chemical hazards in foods or even natural constituents in foods can vary by gender, age, genetics, and as previously mentioned health status.

Natural constituents in foods, like vitamins (A and D), when out of dietary balance can cause deficiencies or toxicities that can severally impact health. Likewise, when toxicants are consumed in excess they can alter nutrient intake, digestion, ADME, activation, and function. Being mindful of food sources, components, and quantities can help mitigate inappropriate exposures to harmful substances in food.

As previously discussed, foods are comprised of many chemicals, not all of which increase nutritional value. The main goals of nutritional toxicology are to prevent activation of toxic mechanisms of action and to treat or avoid negative impacts from the diet.

The food toxicology section overviewed conceptualizing risk and hazard and implied a relationship to dose-response. A dose-response is a key principle in toxicology that grades an effect (response), typically an adverse response, against the extent or amount of exposure (dose). Nutritional toxicology provides the opportunity to provide granularity with respect to understanding risk and sometimes benefit in the context of a dose-response. It is through nutrition that we grossly accept that some amount of a chemical when ingested can be deemed insufficient to cause obvious adverse effects, yet there is a dose for any substance that is deleterious. For example, water intake is essential for life. The exact amount of water a person should consume varies based on factors such as weight, temperature, and physical activity.

The National Academy of Sciences (NAS) recommends a daily adequate intake of water for healthy women and men between the age of 19 and 30 years to be approximately 74 fluid oz. and 101 fluid oz., respectively (IOM, 2005). It is in this general range of water intake that is considered optimal. Considering specific water needs in relation to a dose-response for water, intakes that are too low or too high are problematic. Humans should not consume the bare minimum of water as this could lead to dehydration and other adverse health effects (Sawka et al., 2005). Conversely, extremely excessive water intake can lead to a condition called hyponatremia, or water intoxication, resulting in confusion, disorientation, nausea, vomiting, coma, and ultimately death (Farrell and Bower, 2003; Yamashiro et al., 2013; Rangan et al., 2021). Embodying the teachings of Paracelsus, it is imperative to remember that anything has the potential to be toxic if consumed in excess of a dose that is considered to be without acute or chronic effects.

The sigmoidal (S-shaped) dose-response curve is the classic and most common dose-response curve in toxicology (Fig. 1A), where the x-axis is a semilog or logarithm scale of the dose with an often steep slope in the middle and the appearance of a plateau in the response at the tail ends of the curve. It is generally accepted that most toxicants fit a sigmoidal dose-response curve; at low concentration, there is little to no observable effect; as the concentration increases the percentage of the response becomes more pronounced until there is a maximum level where increases to the dose may only marginally change the response, if at all. As nutrients are essential to support optimal health, low concentrations can produce adverse reactions, thus essential nutrients do not fit an S-shaped curve but rather fit a U-shaped curve where the response is an adverse

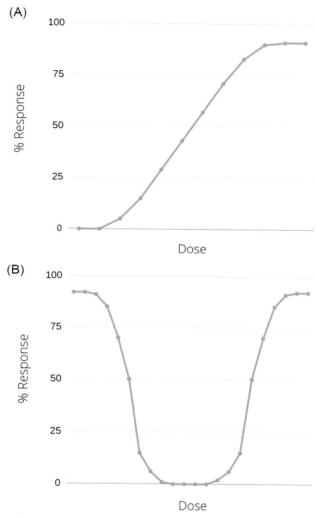

Fig. 1 Classical dose-response curves.

effect at concentrations leading to nutrient deficiencies and high doses will cause an increase in the percentage of the response. Whereas, doses in the middle of the curve where nutrient content is considered appropriate will produce a minimal response. This phenomenon generally produces a U-shaped curve (Fig. 1B). The U-shaped dose-response model can also be characterized as a low-dose stimulation and a high-dose inhibition or non-monotonic dose-response or hermetic curve (Calabrese, 2003).

Current applications and regulatory use

Data gathered under the disciplines of both food and nutritional toxicology can be used to inform regulatory decisions to protect public health through ingredient and product safety.

Through scientific investigation, the overall aim of toxicologists is to understand the intrinsic properties of hazards, their damaging effects on living organisms, and to thoroughly characterize hazardous exposures. Methodologies or various models used to evaluate hazards are becoming more sophisticated which can span from computational modeling, cell and tissue cultures in vitro, and refined animal models (e.g., rodents) to clinical trials. Most of the learnings from experimental methodologies have been from single chemicals; however, the field of toxicology, particularly under food and nutritional toxicology, is most useful when knowledge is expanded to complex mixtures or matrices. Modernized toxicology has not only provided more tools but has driven the need to appreciate methods that can determine what occurs down to the molecular level.

The process of growing, creating, manufacturing, or preserving food products, even simple products like a fresh apple, can involve the use of chemicals that may not innately be found in the product. Apples specifically rely on the use of pesticides pre- and postharvest to control pests and reduce spoilage from molds. Food–grade wax is often added to improve the visual appeal of the apple while awaiting sale in the produce aisle. Food products like frozen foods often rely on food additives and manufacturing aids to generate stable and tasty dishes. Whether it is processed or fresh food, regulations take care to set legal tolerances for additives, maximum residue limits for pesticides, and permissible levels for toxicants or contaminants.

Examples of regulatory bodies

French Agency for Food, Environmental and Occupational Health & Safety (ANSES)
Health Canada and Canadian Food Inspection Agency (CFIA)
European Food Safety Authority (EFSA)
US Food and Drug Agency, Center for Food Safety and Applied Nutrition (CFSAN)
Food Standards Australia New Zealand (FSANZ)

Other organizations

Codex Alimentarius Commission: Established by Food and Agriculture Organization of the United Nations (FAO) and the World Health Organization (WHO), the Codex Alimentarius Commission develops harmonized international food standards, guidelines, and codes of practice that national regulations can use to protect consumer health while promoting fair practices in the food safety.

FEMA: The trade association, Flavor and Extract Manufacturers Association (FEMA), has established expert panels that evaluate and make independent conclusions on the generally recognized as safe (GRAS) status of flavoring substances.

JECFA: The Joint Expert Committee on Food Additives (JECFA) is an international expert scientific committee that is administered jointly by the Food and Agriculture Organization of the United Nations (FAO) and the World Health Organization (WHO).

The current era provides easy access to information. Thus increased consumer awareness to diet and food production has mounted heightened concerns for a food supply that suits dietary preferences and can be appropriate for individualized health concerns. The global demand for safe and nutritious food that can be tailored to consumers' needs creates the necessity for the role of toxicology to evaluate food safety, interactions, and appropriate intake.

Though small in comparison to other branches of toxicology, food and nutritional toxicology is still rapidly evolving. The fields of food and nutritional toxicology are expected to continue advancing including the areas of analytical techniques, molecular biology, and bioinformatics. Innovations in food additives, pesticides, food packing materials, and food processing equipment will continue to drive an improved understanding of hazard identification and quantification of potential toxicological effects. The future of nutritional toxicology is likely to focus on developing personalized nutrition interventions based on individual genetic and metabolic profiles. Merging interdisciplinary studies with big data will help fill data gaps that are challenging to obtain through single chemical studies and other traditional methods.

While society has benefited from the many contributions made to further our understanding of the selection of safe foods and nutritious diets, the practitioners of food and nutritional toxicology are still some of the unsung heroes. However, our understanding of historical contributions in conjunction with future advancements will continue to ensure a safe and healthy food supply.

The aim of this introductory chapter on the History of Food and Nutritional Toxicology was to provide an overview of the origins of these fields that have become more sophisticated in understanding the various factors that components of foods and food production can play a role in toxicity. In the upcoming chapters, we will explore specific hazards, such as toxicants or nutritional components, as well as chemical contaminants associated with the diet. We will explore the significance of risk assessment and the regulatory framework that has provided the foundation for safety evaluations, including topics such as the history of genetic modification or bioengineered foods. Additionally, we will analyze historical case studies that highlight the specific toxicological effects of food components, the methods used to evaluate food toxicity, and the regulatory frameworks that oversee food safety.

Although Confucius (551–479 BC), a Chinese philosopher, did not make any notable contributions to the fields of toxicology or nutrition, his teachings on ethics and harmony can be repurposed for how we understand the balance of what makes a poison or nutritious food, as well as how we generate appropriate methodologies to understand what doses are safe or harmful. Therefore, as you continue through this book, remember the saying famously attributed to Confucius:

Study the past if you would define the future.

Glossary

Adequate intake (AI) An experimentally derived intake level of a nutrient that is recommended to meet general nutritional needs essential to support all members of a defined healthy population.

Agonists A chemical compound that competitively binds to a receptor in lieu of its usual ligand and activates the receptor.

Antagonists A chemical that binds to receptors without activating it but still prevents the binding of other ligands inhibiting the functionality of the receptor.

Atom The smallest unit of matter with distinct chemical properties made up of neutrons, protons, and electrons. Hydrogen, carbon, and oxygen are examples of atoms that can be used as building blocks for substances or molecules. For example, water is made up of three atoms: 2 hydrogen atoms and 1 oxygen atom. Glucose is made up of 24 atoms: 6 carbon, 12 hydrogen, and 6 oxygen.

Chemical A chemical is composed of different atoms that are bound together (e.g., covalent, ionic) to make up a chemical compound with varied physicochemical properties. Chemicals are usually referred to as artificial or synthesized substances, although they can also be extracted or concentrated natural substances as well.

Element Substances made up of one type of atom.

Hazard A substance, place, thing, or situation that is a source of danger, harm, or any deleterious effect. It is a hazard even if it poses a risk of any magnitude (low or high risk) for harm.

LOAEL A Lowest-Observed-Adverse-Effect-Level (LOAEL) is the lowest dose from a series of doses in a dose-response study or toxicological study at which there was an observed toxic or adverse effect in the treated experimental unit. Can also be exchanged for the term Lowest-Observed-Effect-Level (LOEL).

NOAEL A No-Observed-Adverse-Effect-Level (NOAEL) is the highest dose from a series of doses in a dose-response study or toxicological study at which there is no observed toxic or adverse response in the treated experimental unit. Can also be exchanged for the term No-Observed-Effect-Level (NOEL).

Toxicant A hazardous or toxic chemical substance that is artificially produced or naturally occurring.

Toxin A hazardous or toxic chemical substance that is produced by a living organism, that is, a fungi, bacteria, plant, or animal. Not to be used as a synonym for toxicant, a toxin is a toxicant, but not all toxicants are toxins.

References

Albishri, H.M., Almaghrabi, O.A., Moussa, T.A., 2013. Characterization and chemical composition of fatty acids content of watermelon and muskmelon cultivars in Saudi Arabia using gas chromatography/mass spectroscopy. Pharmacogn. Mag. 9 (33), 58–66. https://doi.org/10.4103/0973-1296.108142.

Anon., 1994. Obituary: René truhaut. Food Addit. Contam. 11 (5), 537. https://doi.org/10.1080/02652039409374254.

Araoye, K.T., Otutu, O.L., 2016. Phytochemical composition and radical scavenging activities of watermelon (*Citrullus lanatus*) seed constituents. Croat. J. Food Sci. Technol. 8, 83–89. https://doi.org/10.17508/CJFST.2016.8.2.07.

Barceloux, D.G., 2009. Akee fruit and Jamaican vomiting sickness (Blighia sapida Köenig). Dis. Mon. 55 (6), 318–326. https://doi.org/10.1016/j.disamonth.2009.03.002.

Bhat, S., Udupa, K., 2013. Taxonomical outlines of bio–diversity of Karnataka in a 14th century Kannada toxicology text Khagendra Mani Darpana. Asian Pac. J. Trop. Biomed. 3 (8), 668–672.

Brieger, L., 1887. Zur Kenntniss der Aetiologie des Wundstarrkrampfes nebst Bemerkungen über das Choleraroth. Dtsch. Med. Wochenschr. 13, 303–305.

Calabrese, E.J., 2003. The maturing of hormesis as a credible dose-response model. Nonlinearity Biol. Toxicol. Med. 1 (3), 319–343. https://doi.org/10.1080/15401420390249934.

Cardenas, D., 2013. Let not thy food be confused with thy medicine: the Hippocratic misquotation. e-SPEN J. 8 (6), e260–e262.

Dayan, A.D., 2009. What killed Socrates? Toxicological considerations and questions. Postgrad. Med. J. 85 (999), 34–37. https://doi.org/10.1136/pgmj.2008.074922 (PMID: 19240286).

Egilman, D.S., Schilling, J.H., 2012. Bronchiolitis obliterans and consumer exposure to butter-flavored microwave popcorn: a case series. Int. J. Occup. Environ. Health 18 (1), 29–42. https://doi.org/10.1179/1077352512Z.0000000005.

FAO/WHO, 2009. Principles and Methods for the Risk Assessment of Chemicals in Food. Environmental Health Criteria. 240 World Health Organization. Note: ch 5 updated in 2020 https://www.who.int/publications/i/item/9789241572408.

Farrell, D.J., Bower, L., 2003. Fatal water intoxication. J. Clin. Pathol. 56 (10), 803–804. https://doi.org/10.1136/jcp.56.10.803-a.

Hathcock, J., 1982. Nutritional Toxicology v1—Needs Citation. https://www.elsevier.com/books/nutritional-toxicology-v1/hathcock/978-0-12-332601-0.

Hayes, A.W., Kobets, T., 2023. 7th Edition of Hayes' Principles and Methods of Toxicology. CRC Press, London.

Herrman, J.L., Younes, M., 1999. Background to the ADI/TDI/PTWI. Regul. Toxicol. Pharmacol. 30 (2 Pt 2), S109–S113. https://doi.org/10.1006/rtph.1999.1335. 10597623.

Hussein, H.S., Brasel, J.M., 2001. Toxicity, metabolism, and impact of mycotoxins on humans and animals. Toxicology 167 (2), 101–134. https://doi.org/10.1016/s0300-483x(01)00471-1. 11567776.

Ibrahim, S., Ali, N.A., Abd El Hakeem, B.S., Hakeem, A., Abdegadir, A.M., Sulieman, A.M.E., 2021. Proximae chemical composition of watermelon (*Citrullus vulgaris*). Plant Cell Biotechnol. Mol. Biol. 22, 114–121.

Imen, T., Hdider, C., Lenucci, M.S., Riadh, I., Jebari, H., Dalessandro, G., 2011. Bioactive compounds and antioxidant activities of different watermelon (*Citrullus lanatus* (Thunb.) Mansfeld) cultivars as affected by fruit sampling area. J. Food Compos. Anal. 24, 307–314. https://doi.org/10.1016/j.jfca.2010.06.005.

Institute of Medicine (IOM), 2005. Water. In: Dietary Reference Intakes for Water, Potassium, Sodium, Chloride, and Sulfate. The National Academies Press, Washington, DC, pp. 73–185, https://doi.org/10.17226/10925 (Chapter 4).

Jansen, S.A., Kleerekooper, I., Hofman, Z.L., Kappen, I.F., Stary-Weinzinger, A., van der Heyden, M.A., 2012. Grayanotoxin poisoning: 'mad honey disease' and beyond. Cardiovasc. Toxicol. 12 (3), 208–215. https://doi.org/10.1007/s12012-012-9162-2.

Jansen, T., Claassen, L., van Kamp, I., Timmermans, D.R.M., 2020. 'All chemical substances are harmful.' public appraisal of uncertain risks of food additives and contaminants. Food Chem. Toxicol. 136, 110959. https://doi.org/10.1016/j.fct.2019.110959.

Kreiss, K., Gomaa, A., Kullman, G., Fedan, K., Simoes, E.J., Enright, P.L., 2002. Clinical bronchiolitis obliterans in workers at a microwave-popcorn plant. N. Engl. J. Med. 347 (5), 330–338. https://doi.org/10.1056/NEJMoa020300. 12151470.

Luma, M., 2021. Women in toxicology in the United States. Toxicol. Res. 10 (4), 902–910. https://doi.org/10.1093/toxres/tfab075.

Marineli, F., Tsoucalas, G., Karamanou, M., Androutsos, G., 2013. Mary Mallon (1869-1938) and the history of typhoid fever. Ann. Gastroenterol. 26 (2), 132–134.

Marmion, V.J., Wiedemann, T.E., 2002. The death of Claudius. J. R. Soc. Med. 95 (5), 260–261. https://doi.org/10.1177/014107680209500515.

Michaleas, S.N., Laios, K., Tsoucalas, G., Androutsos, G., 2021. Theophrastus Bombastus Von Hohenheim (Paracelsus) (1493–1541): the eminent physician and pioneer of toxicology. Toxicol. Rep. 8, 411–414. https://doi.org/10.1016/j.toxrep.2021.02.012.

Michaleas, S.N., Veskoukis, A.S., Samonis, G., Pantos, C., Androutsos, G., Karamanou, M., 2022. Mathieu Joseph Bonaventure Orfila (1787-1853): the founder of modern toxicology. Maedica 17 (2), 532–537. https://doi.org/10.26574/maedica.2022.17.2.532.

Miyake, K., Tanaka, T., McNeil, P.L., 2007. Lectin-based food poisoning: a new mechanism of protein toxicity. PLoS One 2 (8), e687. https://doi.org/10.1371/journal.pone.0000687. 17668065. PMCID: PMC1933252.

Nasiripourdori, A., Taly, V., Grutter, T., Taly, A., 2011. From toxins targeting ligand gated ion channels to therapeutic molecules. Toxins 3 (3), 260–293. https://doi.org/10.3390/toxins3030260.

Ozhan, H., Akdemir, R., Yazici, M., Gündüz, H., Duran, S., Uyan, C., 2004. Cardiac emergencies caused by honey ingestion: a single Centre experience. Emerg. Med. J. 21 (6), 742–744.

Peigneur, S., Tytgat, J., 2018. Toxins in drug discovery and pharmacology. Toxins (Basel) 10 (3), 126. https://doi.org/10.3390/toxins10030126.

Rangan, G.K., Dorani, N., Zhang, M.M., Abu-Zarour, L., Lau, H.C., Munt, A., Chandra, A.N., Saravanabavan, S., Rangan, A., Zhang, J.Q.J., Howell, M., Wong, A.T., 2021. Clinical characteristics and outcomes of hyponatraemia associated with oral water intake in adults: a systematic review. BMJ Open 11 (12), e046539. https://doi.org/10.1136/bmjopen-2020-046539.

Rennen, M.A.J., Koster, S., Krul, C.A.M., Houben, G.F., 2011. Application of the threshold of toxicological concern (TTC) concept to the safety assessment of chemically complex food matrices. Food Chem. Toxicol. 49 (4), 933–940. https://doi.org/10.1016/j.fct.2010.12.017.

Sawka, M.N., Cheuvront, S.N., Carter, R., 2005. Human water needs. Nutr. Rev. 63, S30–S39. https://doi.org/10.1111/j.1753-4887.2005.tb00152.x.

Silanikove, N., Leitner, G., Merin, U., 2015. The interrelationships between lactose intolerance and the modern dairy industry: global perspectives in evolutional and historical backgrounds. Nutrients 7 (9), 7312–7331. https://doi.org/10.3390/nu7095340.

Sobel, J., Tucker, N., Sulka, A., McLaughlin, J., Maslanka, S., 2004. Foodborne botulism in the United States, 1990-2000. Emerg. Infect. Dis. 10 (9), 1606–1611. https://doi.org/10.3201/eid1009.030745.

Yamashiro, M., Hasegawa, H., Matsuda, A., Kinoshita, M., Matsumura, O., Isoda, K., Mitarai, T., 2013. A case of water intoxication with prolonged hyponatremia caused by excessive water drinking and secondary SIADH. Case Rep. Nephrol. Urol. 3 (2), 147–152. https://doi.org/10.1159/000357667.

CHAPTER 2

Inherent toxicants

Suzanne Hendrich
University Professor Emerita, Food Science and Human Nutrition, Iowa State University,
Ames, IA, United States

Inherent foodborne toxicants are harmful substances naturally present in foods, including the toxic constituents of plants (phytotoxins), foodborne mycotoxins (fungal toxins), and phycotoxins (algal toxins, often occurring in seafood species). Foodborne bacterial toxins may also be included in this list, but will not be discussed in this chapter and are more appropriate to a history of foodborne bacterial illnesses. Nutrients may also be toxic in cases of overconsumption, following Paracelsus' concept that the dose makes the poison. Overconsumption of calories when this results in obesity is linked to severe human diseases, especially type 2 diabetes (Bray et al., 2018). Overconsumption of ethanol, likewise, is linked to cirrhosis (Roerecke et al., 2019) and teratogenic and mentally disabling fetal alcohol syndrome (Mattson et al., 2019).

This account of the history of inherent toxicants in foods shall be limited to reports of scientific experiments on these substances, with an acknowledgment that traditional knowledge and practices of peoples throughout human history and prehistory must have included knowledge of how to avoid or mitigate such toxicants. Perhaps the early human discovery of cooking was a crucial enabler of human civilization as we know it, because the foundational foods, staples of agriculturally based human population groups, grains, and legumes, were often inedible unless cooked, at least in part because of the antinutritional protease, amylase, and lipase inhibitor proteins inherent in these foods (Samtiya et al., 2020). Such protein inhibitors substantially prevent digestion of energy-yielding macronutrients and have traditionally required heat processing, such as roasting, baking, steaming, or boiling, to be inactivated (Avilés-Gaxiola et al., 2018). Records of antitoxic cultural food practices deserve respectful consideration but are beyond the scope of this review.

Inherent food toxicities may be acute, from a single exposure, or occur after longer-term exposures, ranging from subchronic, defined experimentally as periods of several months, to chronic, which may extend throughout the lifespan of the test organism. Generally, the more acute the toxicity, the greater the potency of the compound, i.e., the more minuscule the dose required for the harm. Most phytotoxins (cyanogenic glycosides, the toxalbumin ricin, and solanine) and phycotoxins (ciguatera, scombroid toxicosis, saxitoxin, tetrodotoxin) are best known for their acute toxicity. Mycotoxins including selected toxic mushroom proteins are also usually limited to acute toxicity, but several are carcinogenic (aflatoxin B1, fumonisin B1, ochratoxin A), which takes years to develop in humans.

Probing the recent history of foodborne poisonings, most often occurring acutely, is facilitated by the Annual Reports of the US Poison Control Centers, produced since 1983 by the 55 American Association of Poison Control Centers (AAPCC) (https://poisonhelp.hrsa.gov/poison-centers). These reports provide insight into the ill effects of oral exposures to plant toxins, minerals and vitamins, dietary supplements, nonspecific adverse reactions to foods, and adverse reactions to specific foods, such as capsicum-containing peppers and mushrooms. Botanical dietary supplements were added to this report in 2004 (Watson et al., 2005) and seafood toxins in 2009 (Bronstein et al., 2009). Deaths from these food-related substances have been extremely rare. Mushrooms and nonspecific adverse reactions to foods accounted on average for approximately 33 and 34 cases, respectively, of the major reported adverse reactions (requiring hospitalization and producing significant illness). There have been no reported major adverse reactions for Capsicum peppers from 2005 to the present. Mushroom poisonings fluctuated a bit but showed no obvious trend over the same time. Major adverse nonspecific reactions to food have decreased since 2005, with cases fluctuating between 50 and 100/year between 1993 and 2004, declining to 10 or fewer cases/year in the more recent reports. This downward trend interestingly coincided with the adoption of the US Food and Drug Administration 2005 Food Code, which advanced food safety practices. A similar organization, the ASPCA Animal Poison Control Center (APCC), reports information on poisoning in companion animals (https://www.aspca.org/pet-care/animal-poison-control).

Plant toxins in foods

Toxins are present in a variety of plants and when consumed can be harmful to human health. Plant toxins are chemically diverse (Hajslova et al., 2004) but are usually metabolites produced to defend against various host predators. These secondary metabolites are often species specific resulting in a particular plant characteristic, e.g., colors and flavors. Examples include lectins in kidney beans; cyanogenic glycosides in apricot seed, bamboo shoots, cassava (Padmaja, 1995), and flaxseeds; glycoalkaloids in potatoes; 4'-methoxypyridoxine in ginkgo seeds; colchicine in fresh lily flowers; and muscarine in some wild mushrooms. Information on plant toxins is detailed in Hayes' *Principles and Methods of Toxicology*, Chapter 19, Plant and Animal Toxins.

Poisoning caused by plant toxins mainly occurs in one of the following circumstances: (1) Consumption of plants not intended for human consumption, for example, consumption of wild mushrooms or giant elephant ears mistaken as edible plants. Both contain toxins not easily destroyed by cooking. (2) Consumption without proper processing: Green beans and cyanogenic plants such as bitter apricot seeds can cause food poisoning when eaten in sufficient amounts and raw but are safe when thoroughly cooked in boiling water. (3) Consumption where the toxin is not destroyed by cooking or processing: Since these toxins are heat stable, food poisoning can occur even when the greened or sprouted potatoes, source of the glycoalkaloids (GAs), solanine and chaconine, are thoroughly cooked. In general, whether poisoning will occur depends on the amount of the plant ingested, the level of toxins present, and the susceptibility of the individual. The level of toxins present in a plant can vary widely according to the species, growth conditions, region of the plant, and geographical factors. Different toxins may cause different symptoms ranging from mild gastrointestinal symptoms to severe central nervous system symptoms (Zahnley, 1984; Rietjens et al., 2005). The discovery of fire for cooking made it possible for grains and legumes to become staples of the human diet.

In other cases, the notoriety of the toxin comes from its extreme or unusual effects. For example, ricin, a lectin, is a potent toxin isolated from the seeds of the castor oil plant, *Ricinus communis*. The mouse IP LD_{50} of ricin is approximately 22 mg/kg but is far less toxic by oral exposure. An estimated lethal oral dose in humans is approximately 1 mg/kg (Audi et al., 2005). Ricin has been involved in numerous incidents as an agent of biochemical terrorism. Although ricin intoxication is an uncommon medical condition, a case of ricin poisoning occurred in a 42-year-old Saudi male who ingested an herbal mixture containing ricin bean powder and subsequently died following cardiac arrest (Assin, 2012). Glycyrrhizin (glycyrrhizic acid or glycyrrhizinic acid) is one of the sweet-tasting constituents of *Glycyrrhiza glabra* (licorice) root. Glycyrrhizic acid inhibits 11-hydroxysteroid dehydrogenase, which causes acute mineralocorticoid excess, reported in rare cases to cause extreme hypertension after ingesting hundreds of grams of licorice candy (Essers et al., 1998).

From the AAPCC database, among many plant toxins, three foodborne plant toxins have been tracked from 1983 to 2019 (Fig. 1). Fatalities were extremely rare. Major adverse effects were also rare, with no obvious trend over time. Solanine accounted for slightly more poisonings than either cyanogenic glycosides or oxalates. For that reason, solanine and related GAs will be used as examples of plant toxins for our historical investigation.

Solanine was first isolated in 1820 from black nightshade berries and named for the plant genus, *Solanum* (Desfosses, 1820). Edible *Solanum* species include tomatoes, eggplant, and potatoes, with most reports of food toxicity from solanine and the closely related chaconine (Fig. 2) in potatoes (*Solanum tuberosum*), presumably because potatoes are a staple of many diets. The toxic effect of GAs is most typically gastrointestinal distress (Friedman, 2006). Potato GAs can be diminished by as much as 50% by peeling and boiling. Avoiding potatoes with green skins or a tinge of green when the skin is scraped is probably helpful.

Pfuhl (1899) reported a poisoning episode in 56 German soldiers following the consumption of potatoes. All 56 soldiers recovered. In 1918, 60 adults were poisoned, and one 5-year-old child died from potato toxicity (Harris and Cockburn, 1918). Eating potato leaves as a fresh vegetable has been reported to cause similar toxicity to that of the potato flesh, including one death among about 50 poisoned individuals in Cyprus in 1932 (Willimott, 1933). Willimott detailed the symptoms including fever, gastrointestinal pain, nausea or vomiting, diarrhea, weakness, depression, and in

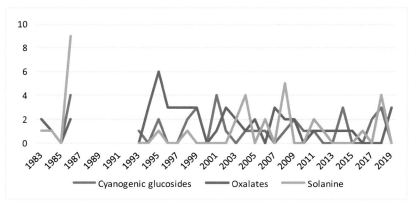

Fig. 1 AAPCC annual report data on major adverse effects of foodborne plant toxins, 1983–2019.

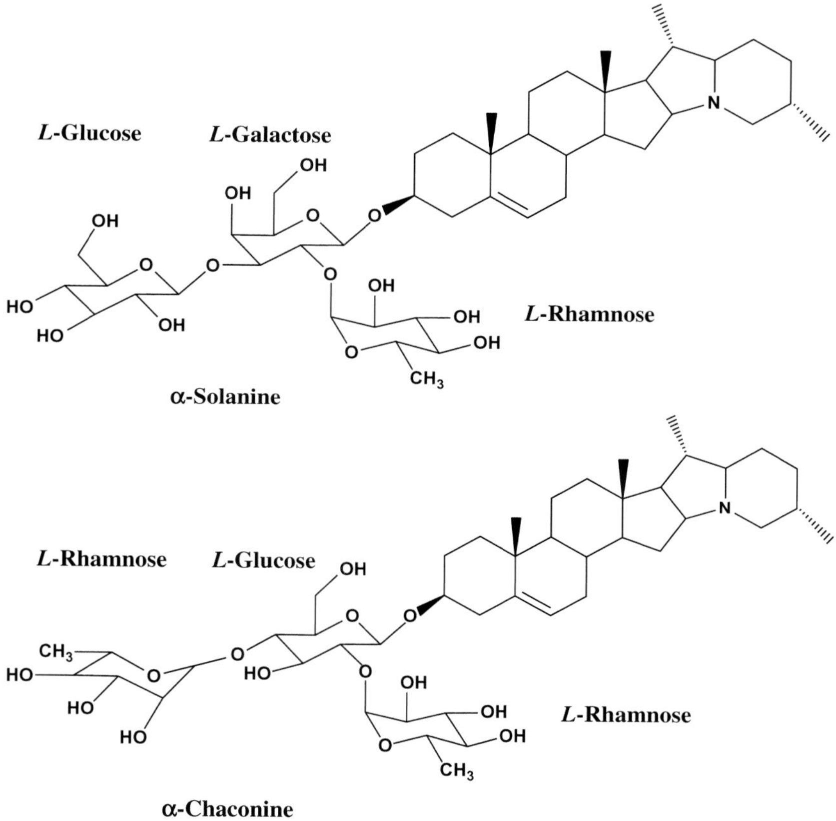

Fig. 2 Potato glycoalkaloids.

the one child, convulsions. The death, within 2 days, of a vigorous 52-year-old man, the eldest victim, was attributed to neurocardiogenic syncope. All the other victims recovered within a few days. In another report, four family members were poisoned by eating potatoes with the skins, one family member was spared because this person ate only the potato flesh (Wilson, 1959).

In 1970 the Lenape potato, cultivar B4151-6, introduced by Akeley et al. (1968), touted to be good for making potato chips due to its high solids content, was shown to have two- to fivefold more GAs than other potato cultivars (Zitnak and Johnston, 1970). This cultivar was then withdrawn from the market before many people could be poisoned, apparently due to the action of an anonymous Ontario potato breeder who tried eating this cultivar and became nauseous and then contacted Dr. Zitnak. The Lenape potato is exemplary of the need for caution in performing genetic modification of food species, either by traditional breeding or genetic engineering.

Another historical example of GA poisoning occurred a few years later. Seventy-eight schoolboys were poisoned by eating potatoes left over from the previous school year. Three of the boys lapsed into comas but all recovered from an estimated dose of 1.4–1.6 mg total potato glycoalkaloids/kg body weight (McMillan and Thompson, 1979). Based on the US Poison Control Center database since 1983 and the lack of scientific journal reports of similar outbreaks since 1979, GA toxicity seems to be limited in scope and severity (Fig. 1) over the past 40 years. A probabilistic model published in 2009 showed that the mean chronic intake of potato GAs in the Czech Republic, Sweden, and the Netherlands was 0.25, 0.29, and 0.59 mg/kg/day, respectively, well below the 1–3 mg/kg seen as a critical effect dose for these compounds. This assessment indicated that human poisoning from potato GAs is likely to be rare (Ruprich et al., 2009).

A few acute human dosing trials have been done. Harvey et al. (1985) reported that no acute adverse effects were discerned in three adults eating ~1 mg GAs/kg for 7 days. Hellenäs et al. (1992b) showed that 6 of 7 adults ingesting ~1 mg GAs/kg from one dose of potatoes noticed a bitter taste and had nausea; one of the six had diarrhea. One ascending dose human trial of potato GAs offers limited confirmation of the critical effect dose, in that one of the 2–3 participants ingesting the greatest GA dose, 1.25 mg/kg, vomited ~4 h postdosing. None of the other six single doses given to 203 participants at 0.3, 0.5, 0.7, 0.95, or 1.10 mg/kg showed toxic effects (Mensinga et al., 2005).

Glycoalkaloids cause acute toxic effects significant enough to receive regulatory attention. Potato GAs have been determined to have a lowest observed adverse effect level (LOAEL) in humans of 1 mg total GA/kg body weight per day for acute gastrointestinal effects (EFSA Panel on Contaminants in the Food Chain (CONTAM) et al., 2020). Using a Margin of Exposure (MOE) approach, if the estimated exposure was 10-fold less than the LOAEL, giving a MOE of 10, the risk was considered negligible. Human health risk for potato GAs was estimated by the EFSA panel to be nonnegligible for infants, toddlers, children, and adolescents at the probable maximum estimated mean exposure, but only at the maximum estimated 95th percentile of exposure for adults, elders, and the very elderly.

The EFSA panel investigated GA contents of potatoes, across cultivar and environmental conditions, and in potato products, such as flakes and mashed potato mixes. Because these GAs are cholinesterase inhibitors, and therefore insecticidal (Spochacz et al., 2018), they constitute a natural defense tactic for the potato plant. Potato genotype seemed to be the most significant factor in the glycoalkaloid content, but extremes of climate, variations in soil, and other factors can influence the amount of GAs in potatoes. Some countries, such as the Netherlands, have registries of potato cultivars, and cultivars for market in the Netherlands are not allowed to exceed a standard cultivar, Innovator, in GA content of 152 mg/kg.

Probing the mechanism of GA toxicity has posed many challenges. Solanine and chaconine are among a plethora of saponins in edible plants. Saponins with their soap-like character may disrupt membranes (Price et al., 1987). This may partly explain the effect of potato GAs to cause gastrointestinal (GI) distress. Modeling some aspects of human GI distress is challenging because the traditional test species, rodents, do not vomit, probably due to their lack of this aspect of brainstem function (Horn et al., 2013). Nausea (as indicated by food aversion) and diarrhea from potato GAs might be studied in rodents, but almost no such studies seem to have been done. Azim et al. (1983) showed diarrhea and weight loss in rabbits fed green potatoes (~50 mg GA/kg body weight) for 20 days or less; rabbits fed potatoes containing only ~20 mg GAs/kg showed no apparent adverse effects. Friedman et al. (1996) reported that solanine and chaconine suppressed body weight in female adult Swiss-Webster mice fed both compounds simultaneously for 7 days at ~0.2% by weight of the diet, without suppressing feed intake, suggesting a lack of feed aversion. Perhaps because GI distress is such a common response to so many foodborne illnesses, it seemed unnecessary to study the mechanisms of these GA-induced symptoms, but rather to focus on how to avoid ingesting toxic doses of GAs. The more significant toxic effects of GAs on human health, neurotoxicity, teratogenicity, and carcinogenic have been explored.

Neurotoxicity from potato GAs was noted in human poisonings, including convulsions, depression, and coma. Plants often produce insecticidal compounds, especially under stress. Compounds identified as cholinesterase inhibitors (Dubois et al., 1949) have been known for insecticidal activity since the mid-1850s (Pope et al., 2005). Acute cholinesterase-inhibiting insecticide poisoning is associated with gastrointestinal distress, like that produced by potato GAs (e.g., O'Malley and McCurdy, 1990). This information led to the investigation of GAs for this property. Solanine inhibited human serum cholinesterase ~90% at concentrations of ~3 μM, with less inhibition (~65%) in the serum of individuals previously identified as having an "intermediate" genotype for this enzyme (Harris and Whittaker, 1962).

The intermediate phenotype is present in 3%–4% of the population. The serum in a far rarer genotype, "atypical" showed only 20% inhibition of cholinesterase. Harris and Whittaker (1962) noted that Pokrovskii had first reported a similar finding (in Russian) in 1956, suggesting that serum cholinesterase inhibition could be a method for detecting potato GAs. Nigg et al. (1996) also reported serum GA concentrations like those reported by Hellenäs et al. (1992b) in their study. Human butyrylcholinesterase was inhibited between 10% and 86% after a potato meal (~9 nM solanine, ~16 nM chaconine). These studies suggested that cholinesterase inhibition may underlie the signs and symptoms of acute human poisoning by potato GAs. By extrapolation from the long-term effects of organophosphate insecticides and cholinesterase inhibitors (Eyer, 1995; Clegg and van Gemert, 1999; Costa, 2005), these authors concluded that asymptomatic exposure to potato GAs was unlikely to be of concern for neurotoxicity.

The teratogenicity of potato GAs has also been studied. Renwick (1972) advanced a hypothesis that potato GAs might underlie the increased incidence of neural tube defects in regions with greater potato consumption. Renwick et al. (1984) showed that neural tube defects could be produced in Syrian golden hamsters by potato GAs. Friedman et al. (1991) used the FETAX frog embryo assay to show that chaconine was teratogenic and both chaconine and solanine were embryotoxic. However, Hellenäs et al. (1992a) infused chaconine in rats from day 6 to 13 of gestation, producing serum concentrations 20-fold greater than that seen in humans dosed with GAs at the apparent lowest observed adverse effect level (Hellenäs et al., 1992b): no terata were observed in 143 rat fetuses from this study. A prospective study compared the incidence of neural tube defects (NTDs) in offspring of 27 women who scrupulously avoided potatoes throughout their pregnancy versus 61 women who did not avoid potatoes; NTDs did not differ statistically between the two groups (Nevin and Merrett, 1975). Another prospective study showed that serum GA content was greater in women who bore offspring without NTDs than in those whose offspring had NTDs (Harvey et al., 1986). Given the difficulties of extrapolating teratogenic effects from animal models to humans where animals have a very different time course and environment of gestational development than do humans, more weight should be given to human studies of developmental effects of potato GAs. The very limited human data suggest little concern for developmental toxicity from eating potatoes. But women planning pregnancy would be well advised to err on the side of safety and avoid green potatoes, before and during gestation. Countries should maintain standards for GA content of potatoes for human food to assure safety, such as those adopted for potato cultivars in the Netherlands.

Carcinogenicity most often begins with mutagenicity. Potato GAs were not mutagenic in the Ames Assay or micronucleus tests conducted in mice (Friedman and Henika, 1992), confirming an earlier negative Ames Assay conducted with solanine (Ness et al., 1984). No studies have been reported that examined the effects of GAs during tumor promotion. Numerous studies in vitro have shown the efficacy of GAs, generally in micromolar concentrations against a variety of neoplastic cells (Friedman, 2015). Solanine inhibited the invasive ability of melanoma cell line A2058 at doses of $\sim$9–23 μM (Lu et al., 2010). Pancreatic tumor cell invasion was inhibited by 3-mM solanine in vitro and pancreatic tumor xenograft invasion was inhibited in vivo in mice by 6-mg solanine/kg body weight (Lv et al., 2014). Given the greater order of magnitude needed for the anticancer effects compared with the concentrations of GAs reported in humans after dosing with minimally toxic amounts of GAs (Hellenäs et al., 1992a, 1992b), GAs appears to have limited anticancer potential without the accompanying toxic side effects.

Although potato GAs are a minor concern for acute toxicity, implications for developmental toxicity following an acute GA exposure during gestation remain to be resolved. Humans would be well advised to avoid green potatoes or a bitter taste from these typically mild and hunger-satisfying foods. Overall, these plant toxins seem to be of minor concern, but rare serious illnesses or fatalities from plant substances warrant the continued vigilant coordination of efforts of toxicologists, food scientists, plant breeders, and regulatory entities (Hopkins, 1995; Slanina, 1990). Countries would be well advised to follow the lead of the Netherlands to have GA standards for potato cultivars that protect humans from these toxins.

Mycotoxins

Fungal toxins pose a range of acute and long-term health concerns and include both poisonings by mushrooms and mycotoxins. Mycotoxins are produced by fungi that colonize food crops whereas mushrooms are consumed directly as food. Both the mycotoxins and the toxins from mushrooms are secondary metabolites produced by these organisms. Although this chapter focuses on mycotoxins, mushroom poisoning will be considered briefly. The symptoms and signs of mushroom poisoning vary from slight gastrointestinal discomfort to death. Most poisonous mushrooms contain gastrointestinal irritants but usually cause no long-term damage. However, there are several toxins with specific, and sometimes deadly, effects. Examples of such toxins include cyclopeptides (amatoxin), gyromitrins (monomethylhydrazine), orellanine, muscarine, and psilocybin. Wild mushroom hunters would be well advised to consult expert mycologists to avoid such potentially toxic and/or lethal problems. Many regions have local mycological organizations that may be helpful (https://namyco.org/clubs.php).

Mycotoxins are secondary metabolites produced as a result of mold infection of crops such as cereals, dried fruits, nuts, and spices both before and after harvest. The most agriculturally important mycotoxins are the aflatoxins, which can cause acute toxicoses and hepatocellular carcinomas and growth impairment; fumonisins, associated with esophageal cancer and neural tube defects; deoxynivalenol and other trichothecenes, which are immunotoxic and a cause of gastroenteritis; and ochratoxin A (OTA), which has been associated with renal diseases.

A recent review of mycotoxicoses (Pitt and Miller, 2017) provides a basis for elaboration on several examples of mycotoxins of concern to long-term human health. The most important and well studied of the mycotoxins is aflatoxin B1 (AFB1), named for the fungal species of its origin, *Aspergillus flavus*. AFB1 is a known human liver carcinogen, through its transformation by cytochromes P-450 to a relatively stable epoxide (Kensler et al., 2011). The milestones of progress on understanding the metabolism and the ensuing carcinogenicity of AFB1 were reviewed by Kensler et al. (2011) and Rushing and Selim (2019). A stronger correlation has been shown to exist between induction of liver cancer and aflatoxin B1 and hepatitis B virus than aflatoxin B1 alone (Wu et al., 2009). Ochratoxin A produced by several *Aspergillus* and *Penicillium* species is a renal toxin and carcinogen. Another mycotoxin is the immune and gastrointestinal toxin, DON, formerly known as vomitoxin (Malir et al., 2016). These toxins will not be further discussed in this chapter.

Fumonisin B1 (FB1), named for *Fusarium moniliforme* (now *F. verticillioides*), has been associated with human esophageal cancer in South Africa and China (Marasas, 1995). Several animal studies supporting the epidemiological-based fumonisin carcinogenicity have been reviewed by Gelderblom et al. (1992). Gelineau-van Waes et al. (2009) have suggested that FB1 is also a risk factor for neural tube defects. FB1 is structurally similar to sphingosine and seems to exert its untoward effects by disrupting sphingolipid metabolism and inhibiting ceramide synthetase (Merrill Jr et al., 1997). Fumonisins are found almost exclusively in maize, which makes their biocontrol less complex than for those mycotoxins found in more diverse food sources. But due to poor absorption, biomarkers for fumonisins remain a significant challenge (Turner and Snyder, 2021).

Eluting biosynthetic pathways, identification of nontoxigenic fungal species and variants, and mechanisms of plant host resistance to toxigenic fungi have yielded useful results that have been applied to mitigation efforts. The mitigation of fungal toxins continues to be mainly the work of plant and fungal scientists. At the present, biocontrol is the most promising avenue for fumonisin mitigation and the control of mycotoxin contamination in general (Deepa et al., 2021). Postharvest mitigation by careful attention to storage conditions, optical sorting to remove mycotoxin-contaminated seeds, and government regulation, such as limiting total aflatoxins to 20 ppb or less in foods in the United States, are adding to the ever-expanding mitigation toolbox. The mitigation efforts for the aflatoxins have been recently reviewed (Pickova et al., 2021; Ayofemi Olalekan Adeyeye, 2020) as have the mitigation efforts for mycotoxins in general (Agriopoulou et al., 2020). These efforts pose significant challenges as does the development of exposure biomarkers for mycotoxins of public health concern (Turner and Snyder, 2021). The development of Afla-Guard, a nontoxigenic competitor for aflatoxin-producing fungi in peanuts, is one such example (Pickova et al., 2021) of a mitigation approach.

Deoxynivalenol (DON, Fig. 3) was first isolated, and its structure determined by Vesonder et al. (1973), as the emetic factor from *Fusarium*-infected corn. DON is the most common and highly concentrated of the trichothecene toxins, often found in wheat or corn in mg/kg amounts. DON is mainly a product of *Fusarium graminearum*, the most widely distributed toxigenic *Fusarium* species (IARC, 1993). This fungus causes a serious disease, head blight, in wheat and barley.

As reviewed by Bamburg (1983), vomiting after ingesting moldy grain has been reported occasionally in humans since 1926. Although suspected, it was not proven that DON was responsible for these incidents. The trichothecenes, including DON, are protein synthesis inhibitors

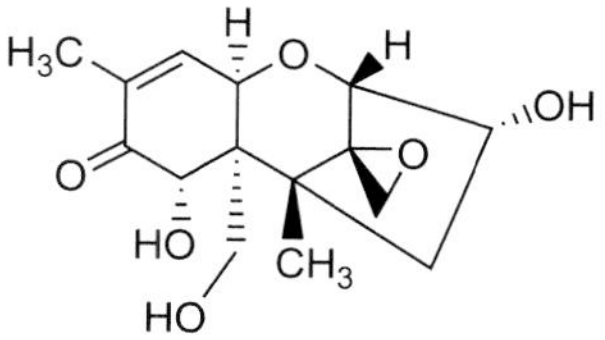

Fig. 3 Deoxynivalenol.

(Ueno and Fukushima, 1968). Early in the investigation of its toxicity, DON was identified as immunosuppressive to human mitogen-induced lymphocyte proliferation in small doses (0.3 μM) (Atkinson and Miller, 1984). Forsell and Pestka (1985) showed that DON was somewhat less potent than were nivalenol or fusarenone X. As reviewed by Rotter et al. (1996), DON was first reported to cause immunosuppression in vivo by Pestka et al. (1987) who showed decreased time to death in mice challenged with *Listeria monocytogenes.* Pestka's laboratory also showed that DON fed to mice at 25 mg/kg induced IgA and its accumulation in the glomeruli, a condition analogous to human IgA nephropathy, the most common glomerulonephritis worldwide (Pestka et al., 1989). While DON does not cause this disease in humans, it may be a helpful model to use in understanding the pathophysiology of human IgA nephropathy.

Insulin-like Growth Factor Acid-Labile Subunit (IGFALS) expression and circulating IGF-1 were suppressed in mice fed 20-mg DON/kg for 4 weeks (Amuzie and Pestka, 2010), which could underlie the growth suppression by this toxin independent of feed refusal. Prelusky and Trenholm (1993) have shown that some serotonin receptor antagonists and anticholinergic compounds, but not antihistaminic or antidopaminergic agents, effectively blocked emesis in swine orally dosed with DON. Using mink as a model for emesis, Wu et al. (2013) showed increased levels of the plasma peptide YY3-36 (PYY3-36) and 5-hydroxytryptamine (5-HT) after treatment with DON. Antagonists for the receptors for these two peptides at least partly blocked the emesis. The 5-HT3 receptor antagonist granisetron was completely effective against DON emesis in mink. These researchers also reported that the calcium-sensing receptor (CaSR) and transient receptor ankyrin-1 (TRPA1) stimulated the satiety hormone and feed refusal increased in DON-exposed mice. These same receptors seemed to be crucial for emesis in DON-exposed mink, as demonstrated by the ability of CaSR and TRPA-1 antagonists to block the emetic response while also suppressing PYY3-36 and 5-HT in mink (Wu et al., 2017). These studies supported the possibility that DON can cause vomiting in humans but does not prove that DON was the causative agent in the earlier reported human cases.

However, no epidemiological studies linking DON with growth suppression have been undertaken. Nonetheless, it is possible that DON exposure could be related to human growth suppression, given the prevalence of the occurrence of this toxin and its suggested mode of action (Lombard, 2014). Dozens of DON biomonitoring studies have been conducted over the past 40 years. Srey and colleagues (Srey et al., 2014) have reported

DON exposures above the provisional tolerable daily intake levels (PTDI) of 1 µg/kg body weight in ∼10%–30% of 166 Tanzanian children ages 6–14 months, using urinary DON as the biomarker. While several other studies have reported DON exposures below PTDI levels (Yau et al., 2016, Ali et al., 2016, Wells et al., 2016 (in pregnant women)), other studies, all in the UK, have reported that up to 32% of the vegetarians surveyed exceeded PTDI for DON (Wells et al., 2017) as did 10% of an elderly cohort (Papageorgiou et al., 2018a), and 33%–63% of children and 5%–46% of adolescents (Papageorgiou et al., 2018b).

Martins et al. (2021) compared urinary DON biomarkers with food intake in Portugal and showed that 3.2% of children and 6.0% of adolescents were likely to exceed DON's PTDI, whereas only 0.1% of the general population exceeded the PTDI. A recent report from Zhuhai, Guangdong, China, of a DON toxicity outbreak from breakfast noodles causing vomiting in 87 school children, grades 1–3, with confirmed DON exposures of 1.3–2.1 µg/kg body weight, further supports a PTDI of 1.0 µg/kg (Ruan et al., 2020). Further study, however, is needed to determine the potential human health risks of DON exposure. Vomiting caused by acute DON toxicity may be largely preventive of serious long-term effects of this toxin. Growth suppression may have significant long-term health consequences, such as impaired cognition (Beckmann et al., 2021). But connecting DON intake with such consequences, given how many factors influence cognition, will be immensely challenging.

DON may be mitigated by deep oxidation as its epoxide is key to its toxicity (Ueno et al., 1973). This physiological capacity in ruminants seems crucial for their resistance to DON toxicity (Karlovsky, 2011). Other types of biotransformation of DON in plants, such as glycosylation or acetylation, may be reversed in the mammalian digestive tract. None of these activities seem feasible for the engineering of *Fusarium* and DON-resistant grains (Karlovsky, 2011). Some humans can deepoxidate DON, as noted for the first time by Turner et al. (2010), in approximately one-third of a population of 76 male French farmers. This ability was much rarer in another population (1 of 34 adults from the UK from whom urinary DON metabolites were measured) (Turner et al., 2011). This activity is due to anaerobic gut microbes and would be of little protective value against DON, except as DON or its metabolites (such as DON-3-glucoside, DON glucuronides) could be detoxified to some extent in the lower gut, which is not thought to be a main site of action for DON toxicity. Once ingested and absorbed, DON may be at least partly detoxified by its glucuronidation, first shown by

Wu et al. (2007). Because UDP glucuronosyltransferase activity may be increased by a greater total intake of vegetables (Navarro et al., 2011), humans might be able to mitigate DON toxicity by generous intake of vegetables.

The history of DON shows a growing understanding of its toxic mechanisms and our ability to detect human exposures and assess risks. Given the shortcomings of other approaches, it seems that DON mitigation depends on developing more effective control strategies for *Fusarium* head blight (FHB) to protect the world's food supply. However, wheat varieties do not yet exist with full FHB resistance (Mesterhazy, 2020) and fungicides must be carefully applied. Plant scientists are hard at work on FHB resistance, well–illustrating the interdependent nature of mycotoxin research.

Seafood toxins

Seafood toxins have been included in the AAPCC annual reports since 2006. There were on average nine major adverse health cases resulting from seafood toxins annually over the years 2006–2019 reported in the United States, with the total number of annual cases ranging from 5 to 17. The AAPCC report includes ciguatera, saxitoxin, tetrodotoxins, and scombroid toxicosis as specifically tracked seafood toxins. Ciguatera accounted for nearly half of the cases with approximately 50,000 cases of ciguatera poisoning reported annually globally (Friedman et al., 2017). Since ciguatoxins are the predominant cause of seafood intoxications a more detailed history of ciguatera poisonings follows.

The US FDA's *Bad Bug Book* (Food and Drug Administration, 2012) in its chapter on toxins includes useful information on ciguatera, which induces gastrointestinal distress through its effects on the nervous system. A number of other shellfish toxins are described in the *Bad Bug Book* including saxitoxin (paralytic shellfish poisoning), okadaic acid (diarrhetic shellfish poisoning), brevetoxins (neurotoxic shellfish poisoning), domoic acid (amnesiac shellfish poisoning), and azaspiracid shellfish poisoning. Scombrotoxin and tetrodotoxin (pufferfish or fugu poisoning) are also described. Major historical outbreaks in the United States are noted, as well as seafood sources, and regulatory action levels that have been determined for each of the shellfish toxins. All these toxins cause to some degree gastrointestinal distress (nausea, vomiting, cramps, and diarrhea). Saxitoxin and tetrodotoxin cause rapid respiratory arrest, due to their ability to block sodium channels in the nervous system and can be fatal. Narahashi et al. (1964) were the first to report the mode of action for tetrodotoxin to be blockage of the sodium channels, and shortly thereafter confirmed a similar mechanism for saxitoxin (Narahashi et al., 1967).

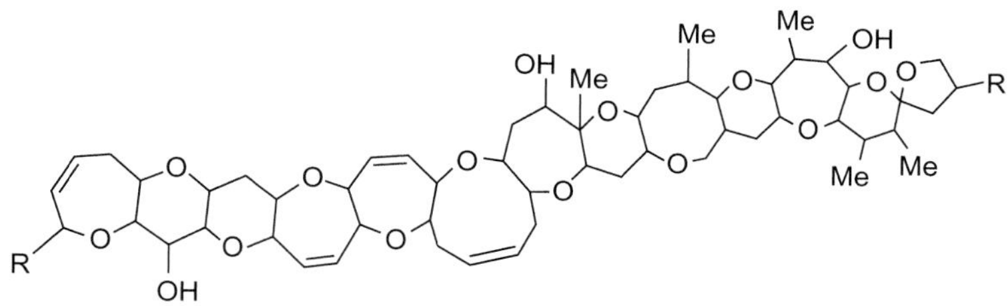

Fig. 4 An example ciguatoxin structure.

Ciguatera-related toxins (Fig. 4) cause gastrointestinal distress, including pain, vomiting, and diarrhea, and neurological effects including numbness, allodynia (touching something cold causes burning and touching something hot causes the feeling of extreme cold), muscular pain and weakness, convulsions, and respiratory depression, which may persist for weeks or become chronic even after an acute intoxication. Although rare, ciguatera may be fatal due to respiratory failure (Bagnis et al., 1970).

Mullins (2021) reviewed the accounts of fish-related poisonings from the 1500s to 1700s, finding the most credible story of ciguatera intoxication symptoms from a Spanish colony of Cuba in the late 1700s. Ciguatera (CTXs) was reported in Mexico as long ago as 1862 (Núñez-Vázquez et al., 2018). Many fish species, most commonly in tropical regions, may harbor ciguatera toxins. The toxin is the product of marine algae (dinoflagellates) of the *Gambierdiscus* species. Yasumoto et al. (1977) first identified *Gambierdiscus toxicus* as a key ciguatoxin-producing algal species. Currently, three species of *Gambierdiscus* (*G. toxicus, G. australes,* and *G. polynesiensis*) and one *Fukuyoa* species (*F. paulensis*) are known to produce CTXs (Loeffler et al., 2021). These algae require light and warmth, so tropical reefs are the main regions of concern for harvesting fish potentially containing these odorless, tasteless toxins. Fish of interest include jacks, snappers, mackerel, groupers, and barracuda in the tropical Atlantic and Pacific oceans (Food and Drug Administration, 2012; Friedman et al., 2017). Factors responsible for hazardous algal blooms remain to be fully explained. The toxins are transferred up the food chain from algae to herbivorous fish to carnivorous fish (Lewis, 2001; Mello et al., 2018) and finally to humans upon consumption of contaminated fish.

More than 30 CTX analogs have been identified, varying in their potency. A recent expert FAO/WHO panel recommended classifying CTX toxins into four groups based on structural relations (CTX4A, CTX3C, C-CTX, and I-CTX for the Caribbean and Indian CTXs, respectively).

Only CTX3C and CTX1B are commercially available (Loeffler et al., 2021). Analytical methods for CTXs continue to evolve; much work remains to standardize the extraction and testing methods. The US FDA has set guidance levels for C-CTX1 and CTX1B at 0.1 ppb and 0.01 ppb toxic equivalents, respectively, in fish, and established CTX fish-testing procedures (Loeffler et al., 2021).

Banner and colleagues began research on ciguatera in the 1950s and isolated a ciguatoxin (Banner et al., 1963). Li (1965) showed the ability of a ciguatoxin (CTX) extract from red snapper to inhibit bovine erythrocyte acetylcholinesterase and for atropine to partly reverse the toxicity of the CTX extract. However, atropine was not able to prevent the death of rats by respiratory failure from CTX extracts, showing that CTX probably exerts other mechanisms of toxicity than purely as an anticholinesterase (Rayner et al., 1968). Bidard et al. (1984) showed that purified CTX stimulated sodium entry into cultured neuroblastoma cells through voltage-dependent sodium channels. Blocking potassium or calcium channels in these cells did not alter the effects of CTX, further supporting this mechanism. CTX and brevetoxins apparently share a specific binding site on subunit 5 of sodium channels because CTX completely and competitively inhibits brevetoxin binding to rat brain membranes. CTX had a 20- to 50-fold greater affinity for these channels. This binding leaves the channel open, overstimulating the nerve cell with a constant influx of sodium (Lombet et al., 1987). Rare chronic neurological problems from permanent sodium channel opening by CTX may present as a type of chronic fatigue syndrome (Pearn, 2001). This condition was recognized as a type of chronic inflammatory response syndrome, possibly related to human leukocyte antigen (HLA) haplotypes (Ryan et al., 2015) but sorting out which specific HLA characteristics might predispose someone to this chronic condition will be quite challenging. Le Garrec et al. (2016) developed a keratinocyte-neuron coculture model to determine how CTX might cause allodynia; they identified substance P and calcitonin gene-related peptide as two downstream factors stimulated by CTX, which might facilitate improved treatment for some CTX symptoms. Protease-activated receptor-2 (PAR-2), involved with itching and pain, was shown to mediate the CTX response because PAR-2 antagonists blocked CTX-induced release of substance P in cocultured keratinocytes and neurons (L'Herondelle et al., 2021).

Even less information is available regarding the potential mechanism of CTX-induced gastrointestinal effects. Using an Ussing chamber model with rabbit distal ileum, Fasano et al. (1991) showed that CTX stimulated intestinal fluid secretion without accompanying tissue damage and suggested that calcium is the "second messenger" mediating the process.

Mannitol is hyperosmotic and the recommended treatment for CTX poisoning. Palafox et al. (1988) showed improvement in neurological symptoms in CTX-intoxicated patients within minutes of mannitol treatment; the gastrointestinal effects of CTX were, however, slower to resolve. Mannitol appears to decrease the neuronal edema to alleviate acute symptoms. Mullins and Hoffman (2017) have summarized the use of mannitol and other CTX treatments. Several case reports and case series and one prospective trial are available to support the efficacy of mannitol whereas one small randomized controlled trial showed no difference in the efficacy between mannitol and normal saline. Six other drug treatments were assessed in a few case reports or case series, but all of these treatments required much longer periods than did mannitol. Thus, although limited, the evidence supports mannitol as the preferred treatment for acute CTX intoxication.

The history of ciguatoxins shows remarkable progress in identifying these substances, their origins, and their mechanisms of action (Chinain et al., 2019, 2021; Lewis and Holmes, 1993; Pasinszki et al., 2020; Scheuer et al., 1967). The nature of the toxins makes their mitigation extremely challenging. Advances in education at all levels of the global fish supply chain, harvesting, processing, selling, and consuming are needed. Advances in technologies for the detection and regulation of these toxins are very likely to continue.

Conclusions

Inherent toxins from plants, fungi, and seafood have posed profound challenges for toxicologists and public health officials. Advances in biology and chemistry have permitted elucidation of major mechanisms of acute action for potato glycoalkaloids, deoxynivalenol, and ciguatoxins, the toxins highlighted in this chapter. Collaborative efforts over decades have led to broad agreement on regulatory guidance for these substances. Because toxins, including the three example toxins, are inherent in foods commonly consumed in many parts of the world, avoiding potatoes (GAs), wheat (DON), or several fish species (CTX) is not a practical solution to prevent these intoxications. Designing a potato without GAs does not appear to be a practicable approach (as noted before), whereas designing systems for growing wheat resistant to DON, probably by introducing nontoxigenic fungi that outcompete toxigenic *Fusarium graminearum,* might be feasible. Whereas all three toxins are environmental problems, in that certain environmental stresses favor the production of GAs, DON, and CTXs, environmental conditions favoring these toxins, especially CTX, remain elusive. Yet all three toxins can be mitigated by human interventions if the available technologies are applied.

These toxins represent, in another sense, a fundamental dilemma for toxicologists. The history of each toxin has been described with a focus on the simplest case of acute exposure. However, exposure to them and their effects on public health may be much more complex than these histories suggest because we are never exposed to only a single toxicant and only acutely, but to complex mixtures of substances (our foods or even a single food) that may be persistent and interacting in yet to be known ways to exacerbate or mitigate toxicity. All three toxins interact with our nervous systems, a complex array of neurotransmitters and receptors that might well be attenuated or inhibited by other factors in our foods, and that is just one system that these toxins interfere with. In addition, interindividual variation in human toxic responses seems certain but is largely uncharacterized. The reductionist approach, toxin by toxin, has yielded incredibly useful information, but we can only see what responses we can measure. The limits of measurement keep expanding. In any case, these toxins give us the chance to experience the wonderment and awe of our natural world, and the wonder as well as limitations of human efforts to improve our ability to survive in it while enjoying a vast array of foods.

References

Agriopoulou, S., Stamatelopoulou, E., Varzakas, T., 2020. Advances in occurrence, importance, and mycotoxin control strategies: prevention and detoxification in foods. Foods 9, 137–185.

Akeley, R.V., Mills, W.R., Cunningham, C.E., Watts, J., 1968. Lenape: a new potato variety high in solids and chipping quality. Am. Potato J. 45, 142–145.

Ali, N., Blaszkewicz, M., Degen, G.H., 2016. Assessment of deoxynivalenol exposure among Bangladeshi and German adults by a biomarker-based approach. Toxicol. Lett. 6 (258), 20–28.

Amuzie, C.J., Pestka, J.J., 2010. Suppression of insulin-like growth factor acid-labile subunit expression—a novel mechanism for deoxynivalenol-induced growth retardation. Toxicol. Sci. 113, 412–421.

Assin, A.S., 2012. Ricin poisoning causing death after ingestion of herbal medicine. Ann. Saudi Med. 32, 315–317. https://doi.org/10.5144/0256-4947.2012.315.

Atkinson, H.A., Miller, K., 1984. Inhibitory effect of deoxynivalenol, 3-acetyldeoxynivalenol and zearalenone on induction of rat and human lymphocyte proliferation. Toxicol. Lett. 23, 215–221.

Audi, J., Belson, M., Patel, M., Schier, J., Osterloh, J., 2005. Ricin poisoning: a comprehensive review. JAMA 294, 2342–2351.

Avilés-Gaxiola, S., Chuck-Hernández, C., Serna Saldívar, S.O., 2018. Inactivation methods of trypsin inhibitor in legumes: a review. J. Food Sci. 83, 17–29.

Ayofemi Olalekan Adeyeye, S., 2020. Aflatoxigenic fungi and mycotoxins in food: a review. Crit. Rev. Food Sci. Nutr. 60, 709–721.

Azim, A., Shaikh, H.A., Ahmad, R., 1983. Toxic effects of high glycoalkaloid feeding on the protein digestibility and growth of rabbits. J. Pharm. Univ. Karachi 2, 15–24.

Bagnis, R., Berglund, F., Elias, P.S., van Esch, G.J., Halstead, B.W., Kojima, K., 1970. Problems of toxicants in marine food products. 1. Marine biotoxins. Bull. World Health Organ. 42, 69–88.

Bamburg, J.R., 1983. Biological and biochemical actions of the trichothecene mycotoxins. Prog. Mol. Subcell. Biol. 8, 41–110.

Banner, A.H., Helfrich, P., Scheuer, P.J., Yoshida, T., 1963. Research on ciguatera in the tropical Pacific. Proc. Gulf Caribbean Fish. Inst. 6, 84–98.

Beckmann, J., Lang, C., du Randt, R., Gresse, A., Long, K.Z., Ludyga, S., Müller, I., Nqweniso, S., Pühse, U., Utzinger, J., Walter, C., Gerber, M., 2021. Prevalence of stunting and relationship between stunting and associated risk factors with academic achievement and cognitive function: a cross-sectional study with South African primary school children. Int. J. Environ. Res. Public Health 18, 4218–4235.

Bidard, J.N., Vijverberg, H.P., Frelin, C., Chungue, E., Legrand, A.M., Bagnis, R., Lazdunski, M., 1984. Ciguatoxin is a novel type of Na+ channel toxin. J. Biol. Chem. 259, 8353–8357.

Bray, G.A., Heisel, W.E., Afshin, A., et al., 2018. The science of obesity management: an endocrine society scientific statement. Endocr. Rev. 39, 79–132.

Bronstein, A.C., Spyker, D.A., Cantilena Jr., L.R., Green, J.L., Rumack, B.H., Giffin, S.L., 2009. Annual Report of the American Association of Poison Control Centers' National Poison Data System (NPDS): 27th Annual Report. Clin. Toxicol. (Phila) 48, 979–1178. Erratum in: Clin Toxicol (Phila). 2014, 52:1284.

Chinain, M., Gatti, C.M., Roué, M., Darius, H.T., 2019. Ciguatera poisoning in French Polynesia: insights into the novel trends of an ancient disease. New Microbes New Infect. 31, 100565.

Chinain, M., Gatti, C.M.I., Darius, H.T., Quod, J.P., Tester, P.A., 2021. Ciguatera poisonings: a global review of occurrences and trends. Harmful Algae 102, 101873.

Clegg, D.J., van Gemert, M., 1999. Expert panel report of human studies on chlorpyrifos and/or other organophosphate exposures. J. Toxicol. Environ. Health B Crit. Rev. 2, 257–279.

Costa, L.G., 2005. Current issues in organophosphate toxicology. Clin. Chim. Acta 366, 1–13.

Deepa, N., Achar, P.N., Sreenivasa, M.Y., 2021. Current perspectives of biocontrol agents for management of Fusarium verticillioides and its fumonisin in cereals—a review. J. Fungi (Basel) 7, 776–796.

Desfosses, M., 1820. Extrait d'une lettre à M. Robiquet. J. Pharm. 6, 374–376.

Dubois, K.P., Doull, J., Salerno, P.R., Coon, J.M., 1949. Studies on the toxicity and mechanisms of action of p-nitrophenyl diethylthionophosphate (parathion). J. Pharmacol. Exp. Ther. 95, 79–91.

EFSA Panel on Contaminants in the Food Chain (CONTAM), Schrenk, D., Bignami, M., Bodin, L., Chipman, J.K., Del Mazo, J., Hogstrand, C., Hoogenboom, L.R., Leblanc, J.C., Nebbia, C.S., Nielsen, E., Ntzani, E., Petersen, A., Sand, S., Schwerdtle, T., Vleminckx, C., Wallace, H., Brimer, L., Cottrill, B., Dusemund, B., Mulder, P., Vollmer, G., Binaglia, M., Ramos Bordajandi, L., Riolo, F., Roldán-Torres, R., Grasl-Kraupp, B., 2020. Risk assessment of glycoalkaloids in feed and food, in particular in potatoes and potato-derived products. EFSA J. 18, e06222.

Essers, A.J., Alink, G.M., Speijers, G.J., Alexander, J., Bouwmeister, P.J., van den Brandt, P.A., Ciere, S., Gry, J., Herrman, J., Kuiper, H.A., Mortby, E., Renwick, A.G., Shrimpton, D.H., Vainio, H., Vittozzi, L., Koeman, J.H., 1998. Food plant toxicants and safety risk assessment and regulation of inherent toxicants in plant foods. Environ. Toxicol. Pharmacol. 5, 155–172.

Eyer, P., 1995. Neuropsychopathological changes by organophosphorus compounds—a review. Hum. Exp. Toxicol. 14, 857–864.

Fasano, A., Hokama, Y., Russell, R., Morris Jr., J.G., 1991. Diarrhea in ciguatera fish poisoning: preliminary evaluation of pathophysiological mechanisms. Gastroenterology 100, 471–476.

Food and Drug Administration, 2012. Bad Bug Book, Foodborne Pathogenic Microorganisms and Natural Toxins, second ed., pp. 193–217.

Forsell, J.H., Pestka, J.J., 1985. Relation of 8-ketotrichothecene and zearalenone analog structure to inhibition of mitogen-induced human lymphocyte blastogenesis. Appl. Environ. Microbiol. 50, 1304–1307.

Friedman, M., 2006. Potato glycoalkaloids and metabolites: roles in the plant and in the diet. J. Agric. Food Chem. 54, 8655–8681.

Friedman, M., 2015. Chemistry and anticarcinogenic mechanisms of glycoalkaloids produced by eggplants, potatoes, and tomatoes. J. Agric. Food Chem. 63, 3323–3337.

Friedman, M.A., Fernandez, M., Backer, L.C., Dickey, R.W., Bernstein, J., Schrank, K., Kibler, S., Stephan, W., Gribble, M.O., Bienfang, P., Bowen, R.E., Degrasse, S., Flores Quintana, H.A., Loeffler, C.R., Weisman, R., Blythe, D., Berdalet, E., Ayyar, R., Clarkson-Townsend, D., Swajian, K., Benner, R., Brewer, T., Fleming, L.E., 2017. An updated review of Ciguatera Fish poisoning: clinical, epidemiological, environmental, and public health management. Mar. Drugs 15, 72–113.

Friedman, M., Henika, P.R., 1992. Absence of genotoxicity of potato alkaloids alpha-chaconine, alpha-solanine and solanidine in the Ames Salmonella and adult and foetal erythrocyte micronucleus assays. Food Chem. Toxicol. 30, 689–694.

Friedman, M., Henika, P.R., Mackey, B.E., 1996. Feeding of potato, tomato and eggplant alkaloids affects food consumption and body and liver weights in mice. J. Nutr. 126, 989–999.

Friedman, M., Rayburn, J.R., Bantle, J.A., 1991. Developmental toxicology of potato alkaloids in the frog embryo teratogenesis assay—Xenopus (FETAX). Food Chem. Toxicol. 29, 537–547.

Gelderblom, W.C., Marasas, W.F., Vleggaar, R., Thiel, P.G., Cawood, M.E., 1992. Fumonisins: isolation, chemical characterization and biological effects. Mycopathologia 117, 11–16.

Gelineau-van Waes, J., Voss, K.A., Stevens, V.L., Speer, M.C., Riley, R.T., 2009. Maternal fumonisin exposure as a risk factor for neural tube defects. Adv. Food Nutr. Res. 56, 145–181.

Hajslova, J., Schulzova, V., Botek, P., Lojza, J., 2004. Natural toxins in food crops and their changes during processing. Czech J. Food Sci., 29–34.

Harris, F.W., Cockburn, T., 1918. Alleged poisoning by potatoes. Am. J. Pharm. 90, 722–726.

Harris, H., Whittaker, M., 1962. Differential inhibition of the serum cholinesterase phenotypes by solanine and solanidine. Ann. Hum. Genet. 26, 71–76.

Harvey, M.H., Morris, B.A., McMillan, M., Marks, V., 1986. Potato steroidal alkaloids and neural tube defects: serum concentrations fail to demonstrate a causal relation. Hum. Toxicol. 5, 249–253.

Harvey, M.H., Morris, B.A., McMilllan, M., Marks, V., 1985. Measurement of potato steroidal alkaloids in human serum and saliva by radioimmunoassay. Hum. Toxicol. 4, 503–512.

Hellenäs, K.E., Cekan, E., Slanina, P., Bergman, K., 1992a. Studies of embryotoxicity and the incidence of external malformations after continuous intravenous infusion of alpha-chaconine in pregnant rats. Pharmacol. Toxicol. 70, 381–383.

Hellenäs, K.E., Nyman, A., Slanina, P., Lööf, L., Gabrielsson, J., 1992b. Determination of potato glycoalkaloids and their aglycone in blood serum by high-performance liquid chromatography. Application to pharmacokinetic studies in humans. J. Chromatogr. 573, 69–78.

Hopkins, J., 1995. The glycoalkaloids: naturally of interest (but a hot potato?). Food Chem. Toxicol. 33, 323–328.

Horn, C.C., Kimball, B.A., Wang, H., Kaus, J., Dienel, S., Nagy, A., Gathright, G.R., Yates, B.J., Andrews, P.L., 2013. Why can't rodents vomit? A comparative behavioral, anatomical, and physiological study. PLoS One 8, e60537.

IARC, 1993. Toxins derived from Fusarium graminearum, F. culmorum and F. crookwellense: zearalenone, deoxynivalenol, nivalenol and fusarenone X. IARC Monogr. Eval. Carcinog. Risks Hum. 56, 397–444.

Karlovsky, P., 2011. Biological detoxification of the mycotoxin deoxynivalenol and its use in genetically engineered crops and feed additives. Appl. Microbiol. Biotechnol. 91, 491–504.

Kensler, T.W., Roebuck, B.D., Wogan, G.N., Groopman, J.D., 2011. Aflatoxin: a 50-year odyssey of mechanistic and translational toxicology. Toxicol. Sci. 120 (Suppl 1), S28–S48.

Le Garrec, R., L'Herondelle, K., Le Gall-Ianotto, C., Lebonvallet, N., Leschiera, R., Buhe, V., Talagas, M., Vetter, I., Lewis, R.J., Misery, L., 2016. Release of neuropeptides from a neuro-cutaneous co-culture model: a novel in vitro model for studying sensory effects of ciguatoxins. Toxicon 116, 4–10.

Lewis, R.J., 2001. The changing face of ciguatera. Toxicon 39, 97–106.

Lewis, R.J., Holmes, M.J., 1993. Origin and transfer of toxins involved in ciguatera. Comp. Biochem. Physiol. C Comp. Pharmacol. Toxicol. 106, 615–628.

L'Herondelle, K., Pierre, O., Fouyet, S., Leschiera, R., Le Gall-Ianotto, C., Philippe, R., Buscaglia, P., Mignen, O., Talagas, M., Lewis, R.J., Michel, L., Misery, L., Le Garrec, R., 2021. PAR2, keratinocytes, and Cathepsin S mediate the sensory effects of ciguatoxins responsible for ciguatera poisoning. J. Invest. Dermatol. 141, 648–658.

Li, K.M., 1965. Ciguatera fish poison a cholinesterase inhibitor. Science 147, 1580–1581.

Loeffler, C.R., Tartaglione, L., Friedemann, M., Spielmeyer, A., Kappenstein, O., Bodi, D., 2021. Ciguatera mini review: 21st century environmental challenges and the interdisciplinary research efforts rising to meet them. Int. J. Environ. Res. Public Health 18, 3027–3054.

Lombard, M.J., 2014. Mycotoxin exposure and infant and young child growth in Africa: what do we know? Ann. Nutr. Metab. 64 (Suppl 2), 42–52.

Lombet, A., Bidard, J.N., Lazdunski, M., 1987. Ciguatoxin and brevetoxins share a common receptor site on the neuronal voltage-dependent Na+ channel. FEBS Lett. 219, 355–359.

Lu, M.K., Shih, Y.W., Chang Chien, T.T., Fang, L.H., Huang, H.C., Chen, P.S., 2010. α-Solanine inhibits human melanoma cell migration and invasion by reducing matrix metalloproteinase-2/9 activities. Biol. Pharm. Bull. 33, 1685–1691.

Lv, C., Kong, H., Dong, G., Liu, L., Tong, K., Sun, H., Chen, B., Zhang, C., Zhou, M., 2014. Antitumor efficacy of α-solanine against pancreatic cancer in vitro and in vivo. PLoS One 9, e87868.

Malir, F., Ostry, V., Pfohl-Leszkowicz, A., Malir, J., Toman, J., 2016. Ochratoxin A: 50 years of research. Toxins (Basel) 8, 191–240.

Marasas, W.F., 1995. Fumonisins: their implications for human and animal health. Nat. Toxins 3, 193–198.

Martins, C., Torres, D., Lopes, C., Correia, D., Goios, A., Assunção, R., Alvito, P., Vidal, A., De Boevre, M., De Saeger, S., Nunes, C., 2021. Deoxynivalenol exposure assessment through a modelling approach of food intake and biomonitoring data—a contribution to the risk assessment of an enteropathogenic mycotoxin. Food Res. Int. 140, 109863.

Mattson, S.N., Bernes, G.A., Doyle, L.R., 2019. Fetal alcohol spectrum disorders: a review of the neurobehavioral deficits associated with prenatal alcohol exposure. Alcohol. Clin. Exp. Res. 43, 1046–1062.

McMillan, M., Thompson, J.C., 1979. An outbreak of suspected solanine poisoning in schoolboys: examination of criteria of solanine poisoning. Q. J. Med. 48, 227–243.

Mello, F.D., Braidy, N., Marçal, H., Guillemin, G., Nabavi, S.M., Neilan, B.A., 2018. Mechanisms and effects posed by neurotoxic products of cyanobacteria/microbial eukaryotes/dinoflagellates in algae blooms: a review. Neurotox. Res. 33, 153–167.

Mensinga, T.T., Sips, A.J., Rompelberg, C.J., van Twillert, K., Meulenbelt, J., van den Top, H.J., van Egmond, H.P., 2005. Potato glycoalkaloids and adverse effects in humans: an ascending dose study. Regul. Toxicol. Pharmacol. 41, 66–72.

Merrill Jr., A.H., Schmelz, E.M., Wang, E., Dillehay, D.L., Rice, L.G., Meredith, F., Riley, R.T., 1997. Importance of sphingolipids and inhibitors of sphingolipid metabolism as components of animal diets. J. Nutr. 127, 830S–833S.

Mesterhazy, A., 2020. Updating the breeding philosophy of wheat to Fusarium Head Blight (FHB): resistance components, QTL identification, and phenotyping—a review. Plants (Basel) 9, 1702–1735.

Mullins, M.E., 2021. Ciguatera fish poisoning in the age of discovery and the age of enlightenment. Clin. Toxicol. 10, 1–5.

Mullins, M.E., Hoffman, R.S., 2017. Is mannitol the treatment of choice for patients with ciguatera fish poisoning? Clin. Toxicol. (Phila) 55, 947–955.

Narahashi, T., Haas, H.G., Therrien, E.F., 1967. Saxitoxin and tetrodotoxin: comparison of nerve blocking mechanism. Science 157, 1441–1442.

Narahashi, T., Moore, J.W., Scott, W.R., 1964. Tetrodotoxin bloackage of sodium conductance increase in giant lobster axons. J. Gen. Physiol. 47, 965–974.

Navarro, S.L., Saracino, M.R., Makar, K.W., Thomas, S.S., Li, L., Zheng, Y., Levy, L., Schwarz, Y., Bigler, J., Potter, J.D., Lampe, J.W., 2011. Determinants of aspirin metabolism in healthy men and women: effects of dietary inducers of UDP-glucuronosyltransferases. J. Nutrigenet. Nutrigenom. 4, 110–118.

Ness, E., Joner, P.E., Dahle, H.K., 1984. Alpha-solanine tested for mutagenicity with the Ames test. Acta Vet. Scand. 25, 145–147.

Nevin, N.C., Merrett, J.D., 1975. Potato avoidance during pregnancy in women with a previous infant with either anencephaly and/or spina bifida. Br. J. Prev. Soc. Med. 29, 111–115.

Nigg, H.N., Ramos, L.E., Graham, E.M., Sterling, J., Brown, S., Cornell, J.A., 1996. Inhibition of human plasma and serum butyrylcholinesterase (EC 3.1.1.8) by alpha-chaconine and alpha-solanine. Fundam. Appl. Toxicol. 33, 272–281.

Núñez-Vázquez, E.J., Almazán-Becerril, A., López-Cortés, D.J., Heredia-Tapia, A., Hernández-Sandoval, F.E., Band-Schmidt, C.J., Bustillos-Guzmán, J.J., Gárate-Lizárraga, I., García-Mendoza, E., Salinas-Zavala, C.A., Cordero-Tapia, A., 2018. Ciguatera in Mexico (1984⁻2013). Mar. Drugs 17, 13–41.

O'Malley, M.A., McCurdy, S.A., 1990. Subacute poisoning with phosalone, an organophosphate insecticide. West J. Med. 153, 619–624.

Padmaja, G., 1995. Cyanide detoxification in cassava for food and feed uses. Crit. Rev. Food Sci. Nutr. 35, 299–339.

Palafox, N.A., Jain, L.G., Pinano, A.Z., Gulick, T.M., Williams, R.K., Schatz, I.J., 1988. Successful treatment of ciguatera fish poisoning with intravenous mannitol. JAMA 259, 2740–2742.

Papageorgiou, M., Wells, L., Williams, C., White, K.L.M., De Santis, B., Liu, Y., Debegnach, F., Miano, B., Moretti, G., Greetham, S., Brera, C., Atkin, S.L., Hardie, L.J., Sathyapalan, T., 2018a. Occurrence of deoxynivalenol in an elderly cohort in the UK: a biomonitoring approach. Food Addit. Contam. Part A Chem. Anal. Control Expo. Risk Assess. 35, 2032–2044.

Papageorgiou, M., Wells, L., Williams, C., White, K., De Santis, B., Liu, Y., Debegnach, F., Miano, B., Moretti, G., Greetham, S., Brera, C., Atkin, S.L., Hardie, L.J., Sathyapalan, T.,

2018b. Assessment of urinary deoxynivalenol biomarkers in UK children and adolescents. Toxins (Basel) 10, 50–63.

Pasinszki, T., Lako, J., Dennis, T.E., 2020. Advances in detecting ciguatoxins in fish. Toxins (Basel) 12, 494–521.

Pearn, J., 2001. Neurology of ciguatera. J. Neurol. Neurosurg. Psychiatry 70, 4–8.

Pestka, J.J., Moorman, M.A., Warner, R.L., 1989. Dysregulation of IgA production and IgA nephropathy induced by the trichothecene vomitoxin. Food Chem. Toxicol. 27, 361–368.

Pestka, J.J., Tai, J.H., Witt, M.F., Dixon, D.E., Forsell, J.H., 1987. Suppression of immune response in the B6C3F1 mouse after dietary exposure to the Fusarium toxins deoxynivalenol (vomitoxin) and zearalenone. Food Chem. Toxicol. 25, 297–304.

Pfuhl, E., 1899. [Regarding an outbreak of illness due to poisoning by solanine in potatoes] Über eine Massenerkrankung durch Vergiftung mit stark solaninhaltigen Kartoffeln. Deutsch. Med. Wochenschr. 25, 753–754.

Pickova, D., Ostry, V., Toman, J., Malir, F., 2021. Aflatoxins: history, significant milestones, recent data on their toxicity and ways to mitigation. Toxins (Basel) 13, 399–422.

Pitt, J.I., Miller, J.D., 2017. A concise history of mycotoxin research. J. Agric. Food Chem. 65, 7021–7033.

Pope, C., Karanth, S., Liu, J., 2005. Pharmacology and toxicology of cholinesterase inhibitors: uses and misuses of a common mechanism of action. Environ. Toxicol. Pharmacol. 19, 433–446.

Prelusky, D.B., Trenholm, H.L., 1993. The efficacy of various classes of anti-emetics in preventing deoxynivalenol-induced vomiting in swine. Nat. Toxins 1, 296–302.

Price, K.R., Johnson, I.T., Fenwick, G.R., 1987. The chemistry and biological significance of saponins in foods and feeding stuffs. Crit. Rev. Food Sci. Nutr. 26, 27–135.

Rayner, M.D., Kosaki, T.I., Fellmeth, E.L., 1968. Ciguatoxin: more than an anticholinesterase. Science 160, 70–71.

Renwick, J.H., 1972. Hypothesis: anencephaly and spina bifida are usually preventable by avoidance of a specific but unidentified substance present in certain potato tubers. Br. J. Prev. Soc. Med. 26, 67–88.

Renwick, J.H., Claringbold, W.D., Earthy, M.E., Few, J.D., McLean, A.C., 1984. Neural-tube defects produced in Syrian hamsters by potato glycoalkaloids. Teratology 30, 371–381.

Rietjens, I.M., Martena, M.J., Boersma, M.G., Spiegelenberg, W., Alink, G.M., 2005. Molecular mechanisms of toxicity of important food-borne phytotoxins. Mol. Nutr. Food Res. 49, 131–158.

Roerecke, M., Vafaei, A., Hasan, O.S.M., et al., 2019. Alcohol consumption and risk of liver cirrhosis: a systematic review and meta-analysis. Am. J. Gastroenterol. 114, 1574–1586.

Rotter, B.A., Prelusky, D.B., Pestka, J.J., 1996. Toxicology of deoxynivalenol (vomitoxin). J. Toxicol. Environ. Health 48, 1–34.

Ruan, F., Chen, J.G., Chen, L., Lin, X.T., Zhou, Y., Zhu, K.J., Guo, Y.T., Tan, A.J., 2020. Food poisoning caused by deoxynivalenol at a school in Zhuhai, Guangdong, China, in 2019. Foodborne Pathog. Dis. 17, 429–433.

Ruprich, J., Rehurkova, I., Boon, P.E., Svensson, K., Moussavian, S., Van der Voet, H., Bosgra, S., Van Klaveren, J.D., Busk, L., 2009. Probabilistic modelling of exposure doses and implications for health risk characterization: glycoalkaloids from potatoes. Food Chem. Toxicol. 47, 2899–2905.

Rushing, B.R., Selim, M.I., 2019. Aflatoxin B1: a review on metabolism, toxicity, occurrence in food, occupational exposure, and detoxification methods. FD Chem. Toxicol. 124, 81–100. https://doi.org/10.1016/j.fct.2018.11.047.

Ryan, J.C., Wu, Q., Shoemaker, R.C., 2015. Transcriptomic signatures in whole blood of patients who acquire a chronic inflammatory response syndrome (CIRS) following an exposure to the marine toxin ciguatoxin. BMC Med. Genet. 8, 15–27.

Samtiya, M., Aluko, R.E., Dhewa, T., 2020. Plant food anti-nutritional factors and their reduction strategies: an overview. Food Prod. Process. Nutr. 2. Article 6.

Scheuer, P.J., Takahashi, W., Tsutsumi, J., Yoshida, T., 1967. Ciguatoxin: isolation and chemical nature. Science 155, 1267–1268.

Slanina, P., 1990. Solanine (glycoalkaloids) in potatoes: toxicological evaluation. Food Chem. Toxicol. 28, 759–761.

Spochacz, M., Chowański, S., Walkowiak-Nowicka, K., Szymczak, M., Adamski, Z., 2018. Plant-derived substances used against beetles-pests of stored crops and food-and their mode of action: a review. Compr. Rev. Food Sci. Food Saf. 17, 1339–1366.

Srey, C., Kimanya, M.E., Routledge, M.N., Shirima, C.P., Gong, Y.Y., 2014. Deoxynivalenol exposure assessment in young children in Tanzania. Mol. Nutr. Food Res. 58 (7), 1574–1580.

Turner, P.C., Hopton, R.P., Lecluse, Y., White, K.L., Fisher, J., Lebailly, P., 2010. Determinants of urinary deoxynivalenol and de-epoxy deoxynivalenol in male farmers from Normandy, France. J. Agric. Food Chem. 58, 5206–5212.

Turner, P.C., Hopton, R.P., White, K.L., Fisher, J., Cade, J.E., Wild, C.P., 2011. Assessment of deoxynivalenol metabolite profiles in UK adults. Food Chem. Toxicol. 49, 132–135.

Turner, P.C., Snyder, J.A., 2021. Development and limitations of exposure biomarkers to dietary contaminants mycotoxins. Toxins (Basel) 13, 314–337.

Ueno, Y., Fukushima, K., 1968. Inhibition of protein and DNA synthesis in Ehrlich ascites tumor by nivalenol, a toxic principle of Fusarium-nivale-growing rice. Experientia 24, 1032–1033.

Ueno, Y., Nakajima, M., Sakai, K., Ishii, K., Sato, N., 1973. Comparative toxicology of trichothecene mycotoxins: inhibition of protein synthesis in animal cells. J. Biochem. 74, 285–296.

Vesonder, R.F., Ciegler, A., Jensen, A.H., 1973. Isolation of the emetic principle from Fusarium-infected corn. Appl. Microbiol. 26, 1008–1010.

Watson, W.A., Litovitz, T.L., Rodgers Jr., G.C., Klein-Schwartz, W., Reid, N., Youniss, J., Flanagan, A., Wruk, K.M., 2005. Annual report of the American Association of Poison Control Centers Toxic Exposure Surveillance System. Am. J. Emerg. Med. 23, 589–666.

Wells, L., Hardie, L., Williams, C., White, K., Liu, Y., De Santis, B., Debegnach, F., Moretti, G., Greetham, S., Brera, C., Papageorgiou, M., Thatcher, N.J., Rigby, A., Atkin, S.L., Sathyapalan, T., 2017. Deoxynivalenol biomarkers in the urine of UK vegetarians. Toxins (Basel) 9, 196–208.

Wells, L., Hardie, L., Williams, C., White, K., Liu, Y., De Santis, B., Debegnach, F., Moretti, G., Greetham, S., Brera, C., Rigby, A., Atkin, S., Sathyapalan, T., 2016. Determination of deoxynivalenol in the urine of pregnant women in the UK. Toxins (Basel) 8, 306–316.

Willimott, S.G., 1933. An investigation of solanine poisoning. Analyst 58, 431.

Wilson, G.S., 1959. A small outbreak of solanine poisoning. Monthly Bull. Ministry Health (London) 18, 207–210.

Wu, W., Bates, M.A., Bursian, S.J., Flannery, B., Zhou, H.R., Link, J.E., Zhang, H., Pestka, J.J., 2013. Peptide YY3-36 and 5-hydroxytryptamine mediate emesis induction by trichothecene deoxynivalenol (vomitoxin). Toxicol. Sci. 133, 186–195.

Wu, X., Murphy, P., Cunnick, J., Hendrich, S., 2007. Synthesis and characterization of deoxynivalenol glucuronide: its comparative immunotoxicity with deoxynivalenol. Food Chem. Toxicol. 45, 1846–1855.

Wu, H.-C., Wang, Q., Yang, H.-I., Ahsan, H., Tsai, W.-Y., Wang, L.-Y., Chen, S.-Y., Chen, C.-J., Santella, R.M., 2009. Aflatoxin B1 exposure, hepatitis B1 virus infection, and hepatocellular. Cancer Epidemiol. Biomark. Prev. 18, 846–853. https://doi.org/10.1158/1055-9965.

Wu, W., Zhou, H.R., Bursian, S.J., Link, J.E., Pestka, J.J., 2017. Calcium-sensing receptor and transient receptor ankyrin-1 mediate emesis induction by deoxynivalenol (vomitoxin). Toxicol. Sci. 155, 32–42.

Yasumoto, T., Nakajima, I., Bagnis, R., Adachi, R., 1977. Finding a dinoflagellate as a likely culprit of ciguatera. Bull. Jpn. Soc. Sci. Fish. 43, 1021–1026.

Yau, A.T., Chen, M.Y., Lam, C.H., Ho, Y.Y., Xiao, Y., Chung, S.W., 2016. Dietary exposure to mycotoxins of the Hong Kong adult population from a Total Diet Study. Food. Addit. Contam. Part A Chem. Anal. Control Expo. Risk Assess. 33 (6), 1026–1035.

Zahnley, J.C., 1984. Stability of enzyme inhibitors and lectins in foods and the influence of specific binding interactions. Adv. Exp. Med. Biol. 177, 333–365.

Zitnak, A., Johnston, G.R., 1970. Glycoalkaloid content of B5141-6 potatoes. Am. Potato J. 47, 256–260.

CHAPTER 3

Vitamins and minerals

Minerva Haugabrooks[a] and Lillian Smith[b]
[a]Health and Nutrition, Lake-Sumter State College, Leesburg, FL, United States
[b]University of South Florida, Tampa, FL, United States

Introduction

What we eat and how much we eat (dietary/nutritional intake) have been studied by numerous organizations including the US Federal government for over 100 years (Dietary Guidelines for Americans, 2020). Nutrition studies and clinical research lean toward providing a list of foods with applicable nutrition content including vitamins and minerals. The Dietary Guidelines for Americans have changed over the years from being a standard table by age to specific recommendations for each life stage from birth to older adults.

Vitamins are vital for life and consist of micronutrients that function in regulating hormones, mineral absorption, and amino acid metabolism. In 1912 Casimir Funk used the term "vitamines or vital amines" to describe bioactive substances that have properties to cure and/or prevent diseases (Teleki et al., 2013). Between 1913 and 1921 Dr. Elmer V. McCollum, a biochemist from Yale University, began using laboratory animals (albino rats) to further his nutritional studies (Day, 1974), which lead to the isolation of fat- and water-soluble vitamins. During the early part of his career, Dr. McCollum pioneered the nomenclature to describe fat- and water-soluble vitamins (Simoni et al., 2002).

The two classes of vitamins are related to their solubility in water and lipids (Ravisankar et al., 2015). Vitamins soluble in water include ascorbic acid and the B vitamins (thiamin, riboflavin, niacin, vitamin B6, folate, biotin, pantothenic acid, vitamin B12). Lipid-soluble vitamins include vitamins A, D, E, and K. Vitamins are found bound within the matrices of plants; in arid bacteria, fungi, and algae; and in the muscle tissue of animals (Pennock, 1967).

Although the human body cannot produce all of the vitamins, it can synthesize specific vitamins such as vitamin D and niacin (Drouin et al., 2011).

History of Food and Nutrition Toxicology
https://doi.org/10.1016/B978-0-12-821261-5.00009-X
59

When adhering to the recommended daily allowance (RDA) for vitamin intake, the body will synthesize the water-soluble vitamins into more bioavailable forms and expel excess amounts in the urine. There are instances when this is not possible due to nutrition and metabolism disorders. Toxicants are found in everyday life in the form of environmental pollutants and lifestyle choices such as smoking. The human body has a natural defense system to detoxify and neutralize harmful toxicants and this process takes place primarily in the liver and involves intricate biochemical pathways (Grant, 1991; Liska, 1998). Vitamins that have antioxidant properties can also play a role in neutralizing harmful toxicants (Rice-Evans et al., 1997).

This chapter will not concentrate on the specifics for each life stage, but rather on an overview of the history, food sources, deficiency, and toxicity levels of vitamins and minerals, focusing on the group between 19 and 50 years of age.

The intake of vitamins and minerals will be reviewed according to their recommended daily allowance and how overconsumption can lead to toxicity. Both vitamins and minerals serve important functions in the anatomy and physiology of the body and are indispensable for good health.

We will begin our journey by discussing fat-soluble vitamins.

Fat-soluble vitamins

Vitamin A

First discovered in 1906, vitamin A is soluble in fat; it is suggested when taking vitamin A as a supplement to take it with a meal or while eating lipids. Vitamin A is found in animals and plants in two forms: preformed vitamin A and provitamin A (National Institutes of Health, 2021a,b,c,d). Preformed vitamin A is found in two forms: retinol and retinyl esters. Provitamin A carotenoids are derived from plant sources (Table 1). Some food sources of provitamin A include dark green cruciferous vegetables and citrus fruits. Dairy products, liver, and fish are excellent sources of preformed vitamin A (National Institutes of Health, 2021a,b,c,d). The amount of provitamin A and preformed vitamin A contained in food sources depends on the food matrices and the processing effects (Tang, 2014). Supplemental sources of vitamin A can include multivitamins, liquid drops, or can be consumed in pill form. Fortification of cereals and grains in food products helps prevent vitamin A deficiency in children and pregnant women (Rice et al., 2004) (Fig. 1).

Table 1 Sources of Vitamin A.

Natural sources	Supplemental sources
Pistachio nuts	Retinyl acetate
Mangos	Retinyl palmitate—preformed vitamin A
Beef liver	Beta-carotene—provitamin A
Dairy (cheese, milk)	Vitamin A combination (proformed+preformed)

From National Institutes of Health, 2021a. Strengthening Knowledge and Understanding of Dietary Supplements (Fact Sheet for Health Professionals). Retrieved from: https://ods.od.nih.gov/factsheets/VitaminA-HealthProfessional/, National Institutes of Health, 2021b. Strengthening Knowledge and Understanding of Dietary Supplements (Fact Sheet for Health Professionals). Retrieved from https://ods.od.nih.gov/factsheets/VitaminD-HealthProfessional/, National Institutes of Health, 2021c. Strengthening Knowledge and Understanding of Dietary Supplements (Fact Sheet for Health Professionals). Retrieved from: https://ods.od.nih.gov/factsheets/VitaminK-Consumer/, National Institutes of Health, 2021d. Strengthening Knowledge and Understanding of Dietary Supplements (Fact Sheet for Health Professionals). Retrieved from: https://ods.od.nih.gov/factsheets/VitaminC-HealthProfessional/.

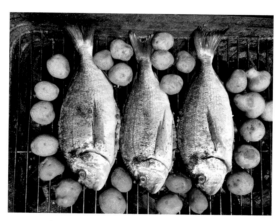

Fig. 1 Fish oils are a good source of fat-soluble vitamins.

Vitamin D

Discovered in the mid-1900s, it is found in two forms vitamin D2 and D3. Both forms of vitamin D are obtained from external sources. Vitamin D2 (ergocalciferol) is obtained from plants through irradiation of ergosterol, a plant sterol. Vitamin D3 is produced through exposure to sunlight, which converts cholesterol to cholecalciferol D3 (DeLuca, 2014). Vitamin D functions by absorption in the intestines, reabsorption in the kidneys and bones, and regulates calcium (Ca) homeostasis by increasing serum calcium (Christakos et al., 2011). It also functions by increasing cellular differentiation (Samuel and Sitrin, 2008), insulin secretion (Szymczak-Pajor et al., 2020), and possibly blood pressure regulation (Min, 2013; Wu et al., 2010). The deficiency of vitamin D can cause osteomalacia, osteoporosis, and rickets (Amrein et al., 2020). Health complications can increase the risk of vitamin D deficiency, such as inflammatory bowel disease (IBD), fat malabsorption syndrome, and aging (Sizar et al., 2021). The toxicity of vitamin D is caused by the body's unregulated metabolism of vitamin D. Vitamin D metabolites that regulate hormones are 1a 25 (OH)2D3 and 24, 25(OH)2D3 (Makris et al., 2020). High levels of these metabolites can cause increased calcium internal absorption and calcium reabsorption leading to complications such as kidney stones (Tang and Chonchol, 2013). These elevated vitamin D levels can lead to hypervitaminosis D (Marcinowska-Suchowierska et al., 2018), hyperparathyroidism (Stein et al., 2011), and tuberculosis (Talat et al., 2010) (Table 2).

Vitamin E

Evans and Bishop described vitamin E in the mid-1900s. The active form of vitamin E is a-tocopherol and comes from the Greek word tokos (offspring), pherein (to bare), and the ol (alcohol) (Merriam-Webster, 2022). Vitamin E functions as an antioxidant by stabilizing cell membranes and neutralizing reactive oxygen species (Chow, 1991; Smith et al., 2016). The interaction between vitamin E and ascorbic acid allows for the regeneration of vitamin E (Dror and Allen, 2011). Sources of vitamin E include plants and animals, with higher tocopherol content in fortified foods (Table 3). Absorption of vitamin E occurs via transportation by high-density lipoproteins and

Table 2 Sources of Vitamin D.

Natural sources	Supplemental sources
Salmon	Ergocalciferol D2
Sun exposure	Cholecalciferol D3
Fortified cereal	
Fortified orange juice	
Fortified dairy products	

From Chen, T. C., Chimeh, F., Lu, Z., Mathieu, J., Person, K. S., Zhang, A., Holick, M. F., 2007. Factors that influence the cutaneous synthesis and dietary sources of vitamin D. Arch. Biochem. Biophys., 460(2), 213-217. Vitamin D Sources Table 1; National Institutes of Health, 2021a. Strengthening Knowledge and Understanding of Dietary Supplements (Fact Sheet for Health Professionals). Retrieved from: https://ods.od.nih.gov/factsheets/VitaminA-HealthProfessional/, National Institutes of Health, 2021b. Strengthening Knowledge and Understanding of Dietary Supplements (Fact Sheet for Health Professionals). Retrieved from https://ods.od.nih.gov/factsheets/VitaminD-HealthProfessional/, National Institutes of Health, 2021c. Strengthening Knowledge and Understanding of Dietary Supplements (Fact Sheet for Health Professionals). Retrieved from: https://ods.od.nih.gov/factsheets/VitaminK-Consumer/, National Institutes of Health, 2021d. Strengthening Knowledge and Understanding of Dietary Supplements (Fact Sheet for Health Professionals). Retrieved from: https://ods.od.nih.gov/factsheets/VitaminC-HealthProfessional/ .

Table 3 Sources of Vitamin E.

Natural sources	Supplemental sources
Apples Wheat germ Hazelnut Sunflower oil	α-Tocopherol

From Reboul, E., Richelle, M., Perrot, E., Desmoulins-Malezet, C., Pirisi, V., Borel, P., 2006. Bioaccessibility of carotenoids and vitamin E from their main dietary sources. J. Agric. Food Chem. 54(23), 8749-8755.Vitamin E; Lee, G.Y., Han, S.N., 2018. The role of vitamin E in immunity. Nutrients 10(11), 1614.Vitamin E Sources.

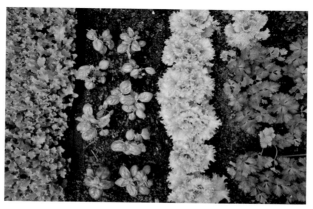

Fig. 2 Leafy vegetables are a good source of vitamin K.

deficiency is rare due to food fortification in cereals and dairy products which contain more than the recommended daily allowance (Table 6). Vitamin E deficiency can lead to problems in the brain and spinal cord due to fat malabsorption caused by genetic disorders such as ataxia with vitamin E deficiency (AVED) (Kohlschütter et al., 2020) (Fig. 2).

Vitamin K

Vitamin K was discovered in 1929 by Henrik Dam during an experiment on chicks that had a disease resembling scurvy and based on its antihemorrhagic factors it was proposed to represent the fat-soluble vitamin with the letter K representing the word Koagulation in German (Dam, 1935). Vitamin K functions by activating proteins necessary for bone growth and cell signaling (Booth, 2009). Sources of vitamin K include plants, animals, and synthetic forms (Tables 4 and 5).Vitamin K is stored in the liver, plasma, kidney, and bone marrow and is transported via intestinal absorption and

Table 4 Major sources and forms of Vitamin K.

Sources	Forms of Vitamin K
Plants—vegetable oils, green leafy vegetables	Phylloquinone (K1)
Animal—liver and fermented foods	Menaquinone (K2)
Animal feed	Menadione (K3)

From National Institutes of Health, 2021a. Strengthening Knowledge and Understanding of Dietary Supplements (Fact Sheet for Health Professionals). Retrieved from: https://ods.od.nih.gov/factsheets/VitaminA-HealthProfessional/, National Institutes of Health, 2021b. Strengthening Knowledge and Understanding of Dietary Supplements (Fact Sheet for Health Professionals). Retrieved from https://ods.od.nih.gov/factsheets/VitaminD-HealthProfessional/, National Institutes of Health, 2021c. Strengthening Knowledge and Understanding of Dietary Supplements (Fact Sheet for Health Professionals). Retrieved from: https://ods.od.nih.gov/factsheets/VitaminK-Consumer/, National Institutes of Health, 2021d. Strengthening Knowledge and Understanding of Dietary Supplements (Fact Sheet for Health Professionals). Retrieved from: https://ods.od.nih.gov/factsheets/VitaminC-HealthProfessional/.

Table 5 Plant and supplemental sources of Vitamin K.

Natural sources	Supplemental sources
Cabbage	Multivitamin
Spinach	Vitamin K
Carrot	Vitamin K with Ca, Mg or vitamin D
Whole bread	Phylloquinone and phytonadione
Soybean oil	Menaquinone-4 and menaquinone-7

From Booth, S.L., Suttie, J.W., 1998. Dietary intake and adequacy of vitamin K. J. Nutr. 128(5), 785-788. Vitmain K Sources: http://npic.orst.edu/factsheets/sulfurgen.html#symptoms; National Institutes of Health, 2021a. Strengthening Knowledge and Understanding of Dietary Supplements (Fact Sheet for Health Professionals). Retrieved from: https://ods.od.nih.gov/factsheets/VitaminA-HealthProfessional/, National Institutes of Health, 2021b. Strengthening Knowledge and Understanding of Dietary Supplements (Fact Sheet for Health Professionals). Retrieved from https://ods.od.nih.gov/factsheets/VitaminD-HealthProfessional/, National Institutes of Health, 2021c. Strengthening Knowledge and Understanding of Dietary Supplements (Fact Sheet for Health Professionals). Retrieved from: https://ods.od.nih.gov/factsheets/VitaminK-Consumer/, National Institutes of Health, 2021d. Strengthening Knowledge and Understanding of Dietary Supplements (Fact Sheet for Health Professionals). Retrieved from: https://ods.od.nih.gov/factsheets/VitaminC-HealthProfessional/.

excreted in the urine and bile. Vitamin K deficiency is caused by fat malabsorption, poor dietary intake, and drug interactions (Antagonist-warfarin). Drugs like Coumadin (warfarin) function as blood thinners by inhibiting clotting factors that are vitamin K dependent (Wells et al., 1994). Deficiency can cause calcium deposits to form in the arterial vessels and malformation in bone development, but these abnormalities are rare due to the food sources of K1 (Table 4) and natural source of K2 which allow for the body to obtain more than the adequate intake of vitamin K (Table 6).

Table 6 The RDA for fat-soluble vitamins.

Vitamin	Life Stage	Age	Males	Females	UL (μg/day)
Vitamin A (μg/day)	Adults	19 years and older	900	900	3000
Vitamin D (μg/day)	Adults	19 years and older	15	15	100
Vitamin E (mg/day)	Adults	19 years and older	15	15	1000
Vitamin K (μg/day)	Adults	19 years and older	120	90 AI[a]	Not determined[a]

RDA, recommended dietary allowance.

[a]AI—Adequate Intake is used for vitamin K due to insufficient scientific evidence to calculate an Estimated Average Requirement (EAR). UL—Tolerable Upper Intake Level.

From Institute of Medicine (US) Standing Committee on the Scientific Evaluation of Dietary Reference Intakes, 1998. Vitamin B6. In Dietary Reference Intakes for Thiamin, Riboflavin, Niacin, Vitamin B6, Folate, Vitamin B12, Pantothenic Acid, Biotin, and Choline. National Academies Press (US) and Institute of Medicine (US), 2011. Dietary Reference Intakes for Calcium and Vitamin D. National Academies Press.

Water-soluble vitamins

Vitamin C

Vitamin C was discovered in 1907 by Holst and Frohlich (Harris, 1962). Vitamin C is exclusively obtained from the diet or supplements (Table 7) its oxidized form as L-ascorbic acid because humans do not have the enzyme L-gulonolactone oxidase (Linster and Van Schaftingen, 2007). Vitamin C functions as a cofactor for enzymes and can reduce metals through enzymatic reactions such as collagen synthesis, carnitine formation (Jacob and Sotoudeh, 2002), and the production of norepinephrine (Kuhn et al., 2018). Absorption of vitamin C occurs via active transport

Table 7 Sources of ascorbic acid.

Natural sources	Supplemental sources
Oranges	Sodium ascorbate
Blueberries	Ascorbate
Potatoes	Mineral ascorbates
Broccoli	Vitamin C with bioflavonoids

From Krinsky, N. I., Beecher, G. R., Burk, R. F., Chan, A. C., Erdman, J. J., Jacob, R. A., Traber, M. G., 2000. Dietary Reference Intakes for Vitamin C, Vitamin E, Selenium, and Carotenoids. Institute of Medicine and Fediuk, K., Hidiroglou, N., Madère, R., Kuhnlein, H.V., 2002. Vitamin C in Inuit traditional food and women's diets. J. Food Compos. Anal. 15(3), 221-235.

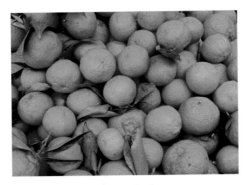

Fig. 3 Citrus fruits are a good source of vitamin C.

across the plasma membrane and excess vitamin C is filtered by the kidneys and excreted in the urine. Vitamin C deficiency is partly due to inadequate intake and poor adoption and, in rare cases, can cause scurvy (Maxfield and Crane, 2018). There is a low risk of toxicity due to vitamin C consumption because excess amounts are excreted in the urine; however, in patients with renal complications excess vitamin C can lead to the formation of oxalate stones (Grosso et al., 2013). The formation of oxalates in patients with rental complication is higher due to the metabolism of vitamin C (ascorbate) to oxalate (Chalmers et al., 1986; Baxmann et al., 2003) (Fig. 3).

Thiamin (vitamin B1)

Thiamin (vitamin B1) was discovered in the early 1900s and functions as a coenzyme during mitochondrial reactions, such as converting pyruvate to acetyl coenzyme A (Goyer, 2010). This conversion allows for acetyl CoA to enter the Krebs cycle which is important in aerobic respiration (Alabduladhem and Bordoni, 2021). It is found in the body as thiamin monophosphate, thiamine pyrophosphate, and thiamine triphosphate through phosphorylation thiamin (free form) (Pourcel et al., 2013). Once phosphorylated, it is stored in the heart, liver, kidneys, and brain and activates membrane channels critical in nerve conduction and voluntary muscle action (Martel et al., 2022). Lifestyle choices (alcoholism) greatly affect thiamin absorption and deficiency can occur in individuals with disease such as cancer (Mulholland, 2006; Gomes et al., 2021). However, the concentration of thiamine in the body will affect absorption, for example, passive absorption can occur when there are higher amounts of thiamine and active absorption occurs when there are lower amounts of thiamin present

(Collie et al., 2017). Due to the water-soluble nature of vitamin B1 there is little evidence of its toxic effects.

Riboflavin (vitamin B2)

Riboflavin (vitamin B2) contains three forms that are found in nature which are free riboflavin, flavin mononucleotide (FMN), and flavin adenine dinucleotide (FAD). Phosphorylation of riboflavin yields the other two forms (Northrop-Clewes and Thurnham, 2012). Sources of riboflavin include both animal and plant; however, fortification is also a process that increases riboflavin in the diet (Powers, 2003). Riboflavin functions as a precursor for coenzymes (flavoenzymes) involved in metabolic reactions that give rise to vitamin B6, niacin, and folic acid (Buehler, 2011). Deficiency due to riboflavin in the diet is rare but can be caused by lifestyle choices (alcoholism), anorexia, and dietary restrictions (lactose intolerance); however, when inadequate amounts of the vitamin are not ingested, it can lead to metabolic complications such as increased oxidative stress and poor intestinal absorption (Ashoori and Saedisomeolia, 2014). The excess is absorbed into the gastrointestinal tract via active transport, filtered by the kidneys, and then excreted in the urine (Powers, 2003). Although there are no immediate toxic effects of increased riboflavin intake due to limited absorption it is important to adhere to the RDA for riboflavin (Fig. 4).

Pyridoxine (vitamin B6)

Vitamin B6 was discovered in the early 1930s and by 1938 it was isolated by Samuel Lepkovsky (Rosenberg, 2012). Vitamin B6 is a cofactor in amino acid metabolisms, such as hemoglobin neurotransmitter synthesis

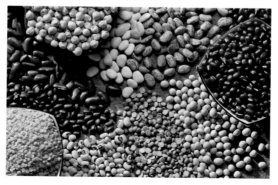

Fig. 4 Legumes are an excellent source of B vitamins.

and enzymatic reactions (Mooney et al., 2009). It also functions in lipid metabolism, immune function, and the nervous system (Ueland et al., 2017). It is phosphorylated into three forms: pyridoxal (PLP), pyridoxamine (PMP), and pyridoxine (PNP) (Coburn, 1996). The pyridoxal and pyridoxamine forms of vitamin B6 are found in animal tissues and the pyridoxine form is present in plants (Malouf and Evans, 2003). Absorption of the phosphorylated forms of vitamin B6 occurs in the small intestine by passive diffusion (Institute of Medicine US Standing Committee on the Scientific Evaluation of Dietary Reference Intakes, 1998). Deficiency of vitamin B6 is rare due to food fortification of cereal grains, plant, and animal sources; however, individuals with chronic disease (diabetes, heart disease) have lower levels of plasma vitamin B6 (Lotto et al., 2011). There are no known toxic effects of vitamin B6 but drug interactions can limit the bioavailability of the vitamin which can lead to a deficiency (Hemminger and Wills, 2020).

Folate (vitamin B9)

Folate is essential to amino acid and nucleic acid metabolism and functions as a cofactor and cosubstrate during nucleic acid synthesis. It is metabolically active when converted to tetrahydrofolate from folic acid (Smith et al., 2008). It is present in animal sources or can be obtained from nutritional supplements as folic acid. Like most B vitamins (Tables 8 and 9), deficiency is rare and is often due to malabsorption or lifestyle choices that decrease bioavailability. Folate is fortified in foods to prevent folate deficiency caused by poor absorption due to poor nutrition, health complications, age, and lifestyle habits (Alcoholism). Toxicity of B vitamins is also rare due to the water solubility of the vitamins (LiverTox, 2012).

Minerals

Minerals are solid inorganic substances found in abundance in nature. We eat these minerals in our foods. For example, sodium is widely used as table

Table 8 B Vitamins.

Vitamin	Common name	Source	Function
Vitamin B3	Niacin	Nuts, legumes	Cofactor or coenzyme
Vitamin B5	Pantothenic acid	Fortified cereals, meat	Cofactor or coenzyme
Vitamin B7	Biotin	Microbial, animal	Cofactor or coenzyme
Vitamin B12	Cobalamin	Dairy, meat	Cofactor or coenzyme

Table 9 The recommended daily allowances for water-soluble vitamins.

Vitamin	Life stage	Age	Males	Females	UL (mg/day)
Vitamin C (mg/day)	Adults	19 years and older	90	75	2000
Vitamin B1 (mg/day)	Adults	19 years and older	1.2	1.1	ND
Vitamin B2 (mg/day)	Adults	19 years and older	1.3	1.1	ND
Vitamin B3 (mg/day)	Adults	19 years and older	16	14	35
Vitamin B5 (mg/day)	Adults	19 years and older	5[a]	5[a]	ND
Vitamin B6 (mg/day)	Adults	19 years and older	1.3	1.3	100
Vitamin B7 (mg/day)	Adults	19 years and older	30[b]	30[b]	ND
Vitamin B9 (mg/day)	Adults	19 years and older	400	400	1000[b]
Vitamin B12 (mg/day)	Adults	19 years and older	2.4[b]	2.4[b]	ND

RDA, recommended dietary allowance.
[a]AI—Adequate Intake is used for vitamin B5 due to in sufficient scientific evidence to calculate an Estimated Average Requirement (EAR). UL—Tolerable Upper Intake Level.
[b]μg RAE/day used for vitamin B7, vitamin B9, and vitamin B12. ND—Not Determined due to the lack of suitable data.
From Institute of Medicine (US) Standing Committee on the Scientific Evaluation of Dietary Reference Intakes, 1998. Vitamin B6. In Dietary Reference Intakes for Thiamin, Riboflavin, Niacin, Vitamin B6, Folate, Vitamin B12, Pantothenic Acid, Biotin, and Choline. National Academies Press (US) and Institute of Medicine (US), 2011. Dietary Reference Intakes for Calcium and Vitamin D. National Academies Press.

salt and abundant in rock salts and salt water. Calcium is another mineral that exists as a mineral in our bones and teeth. Without calcium our bodies would be limp and without structure and form.

Both vitamins and minerals serve important functions in the anatomy and physiology of the body and are indispensable for good health.

The discovery of minerals

Minerals are inorganic elements with positive or negative electrical charge. In the human diet minerals are separated into three categories: major, trace, and ultra-trace. Based on nutritional need, the daily requirements differ for each group. Major minerals are needed in quantities greater than 100ppm, while trace minerals are required in quantities less than 100 ppm

(McDowell, 2017). For the purpose of this discussion, the seven common major minerals and some of trace minerals will be reviewed for historical findings, food sources, deficiency, and toxicity using the US dietary guidelines for daily intake.

When considering daily intake, the essentiality of minerals needs context relative to growth and development of the human species. Mineral is one of the nutrients and as such some are essential or must be eaten in the diet regularly. For example, 19th century depictions of iron deficiency denotes chlorosis as a serious health problem affecting women (Nashawaty et al., 2021). Today, iron deficiency exists but with interventions of iron-fortified foods and supplements, the ravaging effects of reduced iron intake have been reduced. Since antiquity, minerals have been used in many cultures and in foods. For example, salt or sodium is one of the major minerals and has been a seasoning and preservative in food preparation for thousands of years (Müller, 2011).

Calcium, potassium, magnesium, phosphorus, chloride, and sulfur are the other 6 major minerals that have appreciable historical context. The famous misquoted (Witkamp and van Norren, 2018) Hippocrates phrase "let food be thy medicine and medicine be thy food" seems to support this long-suspected notion that antiquity has evidence of the value of nutrients in the prevention and healing of living organisms. These nutrients in food mirror nutrients in our bodies.

Minerals in the body are present in the earth's crust. The science of nutrition incorporates biology, anatomy, and physiology, which are disciplines that reflect the functions of minerals in food history and toxicology. The quantity of food and consequently the nutrients consumed is foundational to good health, making the phrase "the dose makes the poison" (Fernandez and Paoletti, 2021) a fitting description for reviewing the history and current intake patterns of minerals in our foods. These seven major minerals that are in the diet promote good health. The trace and ultra-minerals are needed in smaller quantities in the diet. Some have no established daily value and not recommended as additives in food or supplements.

Major minerals, known as macrominerals, are essential minerals that the body needs in relatively large amounts. These minerals are required in gram quantities per day and play crucial roles in various physiological processes. Trace minerals are called microminerals, and are essential minerals needed by the body in smaller quantities, typically measured in milligrams or micrograms. Although they are required in lesser amounts, trace minerals are equally vital for proper functioning of the body. Ultra-trace minerals, sometimes referred

Table 10 List of minerals—major, trace, and ultra-trace.

Major minerals	Trace minerals	Ultra-trace minerals
Calcium	Iron	Boron
Sodium	Iodine	Nickel
Potassium	Fluoride	Vanadium
Magnesium	Zinc	Arsenic
Phosphorus	Selenium	Nickel
Chloride	Chromium	Aluminum
Sulfur	Copper	Lead
	Manganese	mercury
	Cobalt	
	Molybdenum	

to as trace elements, are minerals that are required by the body in very small quantities, typically measured in micrograms or even nanograms. These minerals are present in the body in extremely low concentrations but still play important roles in various biological processes (Mazur and Lutz, 2019). See Table 10 for the list of minerals in each category.

Adequate intake (AI) and upper limits (UL) are reference values established to guide the intake of minerals and prevent deficiency or excessive intake, respectively (Institute of Medicine, 2006). The AI value ensures that most individuals are obtaining an adequate amount of the mineral to support their physiological functions and maintain good health. The UL value serves as a guideline to prevent excessive consumption, as very high intakes of certain minerals can lead to toxicity or other negative health consequences. See Table 11.

The recommended daily intake for selected ultra-trace minerals is very low and with no over dosage information (Lenntech, 2022). See Table 12.

Calcium

As a mineral, calcium was used for thousands of years as a building material for the Egyptian pyramids. It was commonly known as limestone. Limestone is abundant globally (GlobeNewsWire, 2021). The Romans used it as plaster of Paris to set broken bones in the early years (McDowell, 2017). Today, it is still used in building materials but has the coveted function of being the strong and sure builder of bones and teeth in human growth and development.

It is essential to humans and not only functions to strengthen bones, carry signals to the nerves, but enables blood clotting, helps muscle relaxation, maintains blood pressure, and supports the immune system.

Table 11 Biological functions and recommended intake for adults 19–50 years.

Major minerals	Trace minerals	Ultra-trace minerals
Calcium Found in bones, blood, and functions to form bones and teeth AI 1300 mg[a] UL is 2500 mg[a]	*Iron* Found in proteins, enzymes, myoglobin and hemoglobin which attracts and delivers oxygen to cells AI not established but RDA is 8 mg for males and 18 mg for females[a] UL 45 mg[a]	*Boron* Not enough evidence to establish a clear function in the human diet AI not established[a] UL is 20 mg[a]
Sodium Found in extracellular fluids and helps maintain fluid balance. It is an electrolyte AI 15 g[a] UL 2.3 g[a]	*Iodine* Found in thyroid hormones and functions in the regulation of metabolic processes AI not established but RDA is 150 µg for both males and females[a] UL 1100 µg[a]	*Nickel* Not enough evidence to establish a clear function in the human diet AI not established[a] UL 1 mg[a]
Potassium Found in cells and blood and functions for proper fluid balance, nerve transmission and muscle contraction especially in heart beat and heart health AI 4.7 g[a] UL inadequate data to set a limit[a]	*Fluoride* Found in calcified bones and functions in the health of teeth and bones AI 4 mg for males and 3 mg for females[a] UL 10 mg[a]	*Vanadium* Not enough evidence to establish a clear function in the human diet AI not established[a] UL 1.8 mg based on adverse reaction in laboratory rates and is not justified as additives to food or supplements[a]

Magnesium	Zinc	Arsenic
Participates in many enzymatic and in maintenance of intracellular quantities of calcium and potassium	Found in structural components of proteins and enzymes And functions in genetic activity	No evidence to establish a clear function in the human diet
AI not established but RDA[a] UL 350 mg[a]	AI not established but RDA is 11 mg for males and 8 mg females[a] UL 40 mg[a]	UL not established and not justified as an additive to foods or supplements[a]
Phosphorus	Selenium	
Found in bones and functions to maintain pH of the body	Found primarily in animal tissue and function to defend oxidative stress as it is an antioxidant	
AI not established but RDA[a] (Institute of Medicine, 2006) UL 4000 mg (Institute of Medicine, 2006)[a]	AI not established but RDA is 55 μg[a] UL is 400 μg[a]	
Chloride	Chromium	Aluminum
Part of sodium chloride and Found in hydrochloric acid component of the stomach and functions to maintain proper fluid balance	Found in foods with trivalent chromium (Cr^{+3}) and functions to potentiate the action of insulin in the uptake of glucose from the cells	AI 1300 mg[a] UL is 2500 mg[a]
AI 2.3 g[a] UL 3.6 g[a]	AI 35 μg for males and 25 μg for females[a] UL not established[a]	

Continued

Table 11 Biological functions and recommended intake for adults 19–50 years.—cont'd

Major minerals	Trace minerals	Ultra-trace minerals
Sulfur	*Copper*	*Lead*
Sulfate is required in the body for the synthesis of 3'-phosphoadenosine 5'-phosphosulfate (PAPS) and functions to build complete protein molecules	Found in foods such as organ meats, bran and whole grains and functions as metalloenzymes which act in the reduction of oxygen	AI 1300 mg[a] UL is 2500 mg[a]
AI not established[a] UL not established[a]	AI not established but RDA is 900 µg for males and females[a] UL is 10,000 mg[a]	
	Manganese	*Mercury*
	Functions in the formation of bones and in the metabolism of amino acid, cholesterol, and carbohydrate	AI 1300 mg[a] UL is 2500 mg[a]
	AI 2.3 mg for males and 1.8 mg for females[a] UL 11 mg[a]	
	Cobalt	
	AI 1300 mg[a] UL is 2500 mg[a]	
	Molybdenum	
	Found in legumes, grains and nuts and functions as a cofactor for some enzymes	
	AI not established but RDA is 45 µg for males and females[a] UL 20,500 µg[a]	

AI, adequate intake; *UL*, upper limit.

[a]Adequate intake (AI) and upper limit (UL) taken from Institute of Medicine, 2006. Dietary Reference Intakes: The Essential Guide to Nutrient Requirements. The National Academies Press, Washington, DC. https://doi.org/10.17226/11537.

Table 12 Recommended daily intakes for three ultra-trace minerals.

Ultra-minerals	Recommended daily intake	Over dosage
Boron	<20 mg	No information found
Nickel	<1 mg	Products with nickel may cause skin rash in case of allergies
Vanadium	<1.8 mg (Lenntech, 2022)	No information found

Modified from Lenntech, 2022. Recommended daily intake of vitamins and minerals. Available at https://www.lenntech.com/recommended-daily-intake.htm.

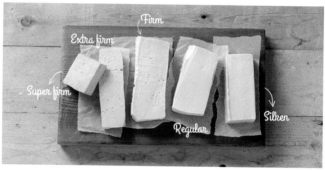

Fig. 5 Types of tofu as good sources of calcium (Tofupedia, 2015).

Foods rich in calcium are from animal sources that include milk, dairy products, and canned fish with bones (salmon, sardines). Plant-based calcium foods include fortified tofu and fortified soy beverage, greens (broccoli, mustard greens), and legumes (Fig. 5).

Deficiency of calcium is noticeable because calcium supports bone structure and prevents abnormalities. These striking deficiencies occur in both growing children and adults. In children it is called rickets (bowlegs) and in adults it is osteomalacia (soft bones) and osteoporosis (holes in the bones).

Calcium toxicity occurs when consumed in excess of 2500 mg/day and when supplements are taken.

Phosphorus

Phosphorus was first discovered in 1669 in Germany by Henning Brandt (Ashley et al., 2011). The 17th century search for the Philosopher's stone transitioned to medicinal uses, flammable matches, a limiting nutrient in crops, uses in war, to a global scarcity of phosphorus. Its place in food consumption is important to us as it is a basic component of life forms on our

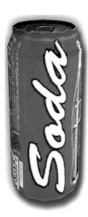

Fig. 6 An example of soft drinks that contain phosphorus.

planet. Even though it is not in free form in nature it exists in bones and teeth as calcium phosphate. It exists in plant crops and supplied in the diet from various food items.

Phosphorus is the twin to calcium as both minerals work together to strength the skeletal system. Along with calcium both are the two most abundant minerals in the body. Phosphorus is part of bones, teeth, and storage of energy in ATP and it functions in acid-base balance.

Food sources include meats, cheeses, carbonated drinks, fish, poultry, eggs, milk, and processed foods (including soda pop).

Deficiency is rare but does occur when medications cause phosphatemia.

Toxicity or upper limit (UL) is 4000 mg. Foods with high phosphorus content such as soda can cause excess intake (Wickham, 2014) (Fig. 6).

Sodium

Sodium was first isolated and discovered in 1807 by Sir Humphry Davy (Britannica, 2021), though sodium existed in nature as rock salt deposits around the world. Table salt has been a product of these rocks since antiquity.

Historically, sodium that is found in salt has been in use as far back as 6050 BC (McDowell, 2003). It has been used as a food preservative, flavor enhancer, dehydration reliever, and in deicing roads during the winter season. It has been on the generally recognized as safe (GRAS) list item and is safely regulated by the FDA (Chemicalsafetyfacts.org, 2022). Sodium is mentioned in biblical narratives many times and one of these is "ye are the salt of the earth" (Matthew 5:13) giving meaning to its essentiality to life and human existence.

Sodium is found in cells, blood, and muscles. It keeps us alive as it helps balance potassium within cells (Müller, 2011). Sodium functions to maintain fluid balance between cells, in nerve transmission, in muscle function, and fosters hydration.

Sodium food sources include table salt, soy sauce; large amounts of ingested processed foods; small amounts in milk, breads, vegetables, and unprocessed meats.

Deficiency

Hyponatremia is the condition of low sodium in the blood. However, sodium is rarely deficient in diets due to the use of processed foods.

Toxicity/UL is in consumption over 2300 mg per day. A consistently high intake of table salt (Fig. 7) will contribute to high blood pressure and increase fluid retention in chronic diseases; and increase fluids in congestive heart failure, and kidney disease.

Chloride

A compound of chloride is sodium chloride that is commonly called table salt. It is also found in potassium chloride, magnesium chloride, and calcium chloride. These chloride-containing substances are common sources of chloride which is a compound of chlorine. Chloride is essential to human life. When consumed, chloride works well with sodium and potassium which are positively charged ions. In the fluid compartments of the cell, it resides on the outside of the cell participating in fluid balance in and out of cells.

As an electrolyte, the mineral chloride functions to regulate blood pressure, blood volume, fluid balance, and is abundant in stomach's hydrochloric acid content.

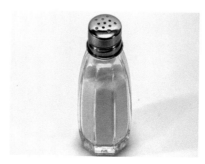

Fig. 7 Table salt is sodium chloride providing the major portion of sodium in our diets.

Food sources with chloride include table salt (sodium chloride), seaweed, lettuce, celery, olives, soy sauce; processed foods; milk, meats, breads, and vegetables.

Deficiency usually occurs during fluid loss through sweating, vomiting, and or diarrhea. Diuretics can also cause loss of chloride. Deficiency of chloride is associated with acid–base balance and salt balance (Signorelli et al., 2020).

Unless purposefully removed from the diet this mineral is not usually found to be deficient as table salt and processed foods provide more than enough chloride in our intake.

Toxicity/UL—3.6 mg is the value set by the National Academies Press.

Potassium

The potassium element was isolated in a pot by Sir Humphry Davy in 1807. Though it was connected with the flames in the lab it was later associated with food and in the production of plant fertilizers.

Food sources of potassium include meats, milk, fresh fruits and vegetables, whole grains, and legumes.

Deficiency of potassium is generally from diarrhea and not normally from poor food intake (Chemicool.com, 2012a,b). The latter contributes to hypokalemia exhibited as irregular heartbeat, fatigue, muscle cramps, and even constipation.

Toxicity/UL becomes evident in persons with poor kidney function when the excess is not removed through the urine. Impaired kidney function dictates that potassium intake from foods to be less than 4.7 g AI per day (Fig. 8).

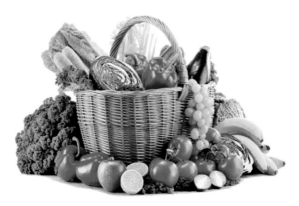

Fig. 8 Fresh fruits and vegetables are good sources of potassium. (Photo by Unknown Author is licensed under CC BY-NC.)

The UL is not set.

Magnesium

Magnesium history dates back to 1618 when a British farmer in Epsom noticed his cows' refusal to drink water from his well. That same water seemed to heal skin rashes. This began the story of Epsom salt which was later named as magnesium sulfate. However, Joseph Black recognized this element in 1755 and isolated this element through electrolysis in 1808 (WebElements, 2021).

Food sources for magnesium include nuts and seeds, legumes, leafy green vegetables; seafood; chocolate; artichokes; and "hard" drinking water.

Deficiency symptoms of magnesium are mental disorder, asthma, osteoporosis, migraines, high blood pressure, irregular heartbeat, numbness, muscle cramps, and fatigue.

Toxicity/UL

Magnesium levels do not build up in the blood except when kidney disease is present (Mazur and Litch, 2019). Intake of oral magnesium may cause diarrhea. This occurs with just the right dose of Epsom salt—magnesium sulfate. Magnesium works well with calcium, so that a toxic amount of magnesium can be abated by offering calcium (Fig. 9).

Sulfur

Sulfur is one of the minerals that was used in antiquity. It was identified in 1777 by Antoine Lavoisier (Brasted, 2021) as an element. It has been recorded in biblical history in its raw form as brimstone in Deuteronomy

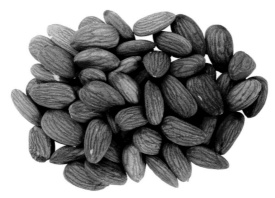

Fig. 9 Nuts are a good source of magnesium.

29:23, Job 18:15, Psalms 11:6, Isaiah 30:33, Ezekiel 38:22, Luke 17:29, and Revelation 9:17 (New International Version Bible, 2022). The dead sea collects lots of sulfur that is the primary ingredient in making a fire (Orr, 1915).

Sulfur was used by Pagan priests, and burned by the Romans as insecticides and to cleanse the air of evil spirits (Georgia Gulf Sulphur Corporation, 2021). In nature it is found in the soil, vegetation, food supply, and in the water we drink. Sulfur is part of protein molecules and is used in pesticides. It kills fungi when it is part of sulfur dusting for crops (National Pesticide Information Center, 2022).

Food sources of sulfur include foods that have protein: meats, poultry, fish, eggs, milk, legumes, and nuts.

Deficiency of dietary sulfur is unknown. Sulfur is part of protein and most people eat sufficient protein daily. Only persons with a severe protein deficiency lack this mineral.

Toxicity/UL

Sulfur is not normally toxic to humans except from overexposure in intake and breathing sulfur-laden air. Dietary required intake for sulfur has not been determined because sulfur is available from amino acids in food.

There is not sufficient research to support upper limit intake for sulfur (NAP.edu, 2006) (Fig. 10).

Selected trace minerals

Iron

The mineral iron builds hemoglobin which carries oxygen to the cells of the body. Worldwide there is an acknowledged deficiency of dietary

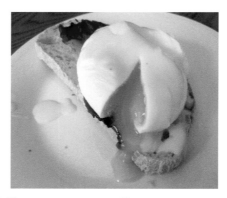

Fig. 10 Protein foods like an egg contains sulfur.

iron as evidenced by the symptoms commonly found in anemic individuals. Symptoms widely described as causing lethargy and the inability to learn.

The elemental history of iron dates back to Egypt in 3500 BC. Iron is abundant in the earth's crust, existing in various forms of iron ore from which iron II sulfate or ferrous sulfate is a common additive in foods and used to treat iron deficiency (WordPress, 2022). Iron is thought to be nontoxic and in its pure form is very reactive, rusting easily in moist air (Chemicool, 2022). Sheftel et al. (2011) noted that the history of iron is rich with stories of its ancient beginnings and is still being explored.

Food sources

Foods rich in iron include beans and legumes, tofu, dark green leafy vegetables, fortified breakfast cereals, whole grain breads, dried fruits, baked potato, and nuts.

Deficiency symptoms

The absence of good quality iron-rich foods leads to deficiency commonly called iron-deficiency anemia. In its absence hemoglobin is inadequate and is not capable of picking up enough oxygen for the cells to carry out its metabolic functions. Symptoms of iron deficiency include fatigue, weakness, headache, and reduced cognitive function in children (Fig. 11).

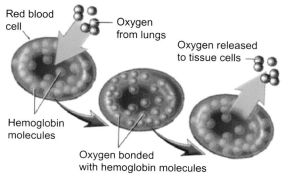

Fig. 11 Iron builds hemoglobin that picks up oxygen. (Photo by Unknown Author is licensed under CC BY-SA-NC.)

Toxicity/upper limits

Recommended amounts of iron are 18 grams for females ages 19–51 and 8 grams for males in the same age range. Considering the fact that toxicity or upper limit refers to the maximum daily intake not likely to cause harmful effects, the UL for males and females ages 14+ years is 45 grams per day (NAP.edu, 2006).

It is rare to find toxic amounts of iron as the body actively regulates iron absorption (Harvard T. H. Chan School of Public Health, 2022).

Chromium

The element chromium was discovered in Paris in 1780 by Nicolas Louis Vauquelin (Chemicool, 2022). It is an essential trace mineral and found in nature as ores. There are several forms of chromium that can cause health problems. Environmentally, chromium can affect our health when it is present in air, water, and soil (Lenntech, 2022). The hexavalent Cr^{+6} compound is toxic and carcinogenic. Trivalent chromium Cr^{+3} is not toxic and commonly found in our food sources. An individual's exposure to chromium through breathing, eating, drinking, and skin contact manifests as irritation at the point of entry. Though widely used in stainless steel devices chromium does present any hazard to humans in this form.

Food sources

Trivalent chromium is noted to help potentiate the action of insulin usage in the body (Linus Pauling Institute, 2022). Hence foods such as fruits, vegetables and whole grains, meat, and fish are good sources of chromium.

Deficiency symptoms include symptoms similar to diabetes, impaired glucose tolerance and increased insulin needs.

Toxicity/upper limits

Chromium is toxic in its hexavalent form—chromium VI. The trivalent molecule, chromium III, is found in food and is nontoxic. Chromium reacts with both saltwater and freshwater sources. For individuals, the AI recommended amount is 35 μg for males and 25 μg for females. UL has not been established (NAP.edu, 2006).

Selected ultra-trace minerals

The ultra-trace minerals are needed in small quantities and some like arsenic, lead, and mercury should not be added as additives in food or supplements.

References

Alabduladhem, T.O., Bordoni, B., 2021. Physiology, Krebs cycle. In: StatPearls. StatPearls Publishing.

Amrein, K., Scherkl, M., Hoffmann, M., Neuwersch-Sommeregger, S., Köstenberger, M., Berisha, A.T., Malle, O., 2020. Vitamin D deficiency 2.0: an update on the current status worldwide. Eur. J. Clin. Nutr. 74 (11), 1498–1513.

Ashley, K., Cordell, D., Mavinic, D., 2011. A brief history of phosphorus: from the philosopher's stone to nutrient recovery and reuse. Chemosphere 84, 737–746.

Ashoori, M., Saedisomeolia, A., 2014. Riboflavin (vitamin B2) and oxidative stress: a review. Br. J. Nutr. 111 (11), 1985–1991.

Baxmann, A.C., Mendonca, D.O.G., C., & Heilberg, I. P., 2003. Effect of vitamin C supplements on urinary oxalate and pH in calcium stone-forming patients. Kidney Int. 63 (3), 1066–1071.

Booth, S.L., 2009. Roles for vitamin K beyond coagulation. Annu. Rev. Nutr. 29, 89–110.

Brasted, R.C., 2021. Sulfur. Encyclopaedia Britannica. https://www.britannica.com/science/sulfur.

Britannica, T., 2021. Sodium. Encyclopaedia Britannica. https://www.britannica.com/science/sodium.

Buehler, B.A., 2011. Vitamin B2: riboflavin. J. Evid.-Based Complement. Alter. Med. 16 (2), 88–90.

Chalmers, A.H., Cowley, D.M., Brown, J.M., 1986. A possible etiological role for ascorbate in calculi formation. Clin. Chem. 32 (2), 333–336.

Chemicalsafetyfacts.org, 2022. Sodium Chloride. https://www.chemicalsafetyfacts.org/sodium-chloride/.

Chemicool, 2022. Iron element facts. In: "Iron." Chemicool Periodic Table. Chemicool.com. 06 Oct. 2012. Web. 3/28/2022 https://www.chemicool.com/elements/iron.html.

Chemicool.com, 2012a. Chromium. Chemicool Periodic Table. Web. 3/29/2022 https://www.chemicool.com/elements/chromium.html.

Chemicool.com, 2012b. Potassium. Chemicool Periodic Table. Web. 1/28/2022 https://www.chemicool.com/elements/potassium.html.

Chow, C.K., 1991. Vitamin E and oxidative stress. Free Radic. Biol. Med. 11 (2), 215–232.

Christakos, S., Dhawan, P., Porta, A., Mady, L.J., Seth, T., 2011. Vitamin D and intestinal calcium absorption. Mol. Cell. Endocrinol. 347 (1-2), 25–29.

Coburn, S.P., 1996. Modeling vitamin B6 metabolism. Adv. Food Nutr. Res. 40, 107–132.

Collie, J.T., Greaves, R.F., Jones, O.A., Lam, Q., Eastwood, G.M., Bellomo, R., 2017. Vitamin B1 in critically ill patients: needs and challenges. Clin. Chem. Lab. Med. (CCLM) 55 (11), 1652–1668. https://doi.org/10.1515/cclm-2017-0054.

Dam, H., 1935. The antihaemorrhagic vitamin of the chick. Biochem. J. 29 (6), 1273.

Day, H.G., 1974. Elmer Verner McCollum. Biogr. Mem. Natl. Acad. Sci. 45, 263–335.

DeLuca, H.F., 2014. History of the discovery of vitamin D and its active metabolites. BoneKEy Rep. 3.

Dietary Guidelines for Americans, 2020. History of the Dietary Guidelines. https://www.dietaryguidelines.gov/about-dietary-guidelines/history-dietary-guidelines.

Dror, D.K., Allen, L.H., 2011. Vitamin E deficiency in developing countries. Food Nutr. Bull. 32 (2), 124–143.

Drouin, G., Godin, J.R., Pagé, B., 2011. The genetics of vitamin C loss in vertebrates. Curr. Genom. 12 (5), 371–378.

Fernandez, A., Paoletti, C., 2021. What is unsafe food? Change of perspective. Trends Food Sci. Technol. 109. https://doi.org/10.1016/j.tifs.2021.01.041. https://www.sciencedirect.com/science/article/pii/S0924224421000388.

Georgia Gulf Sulphur Corporation, 2021. Our History. https://www.georgiagulfsulfur.com/sulfur/history.

GlobeNewsWire, 2021. Global Limestone Market (2021 to 2026)—Growth, Trends, COVID-19 Impact, and Forecasts. https://www.globenewswire.com/news-re-lease/2021/08/17/2281758/28124/en/Global-Limestone-Market-2021-to-2026-Growth-Trends-COVID-19-Impact-and-Forecasts.html.

Gomes, F., Bergeron, G., Bourassa, M.W., Fischer, P.R., 2021. Thiamine deficiency unrelated to alcohol consumption in high-income countries: a literature review. Ann. N.Y. Acad. Sci. 1498 (1), 46–56.

Goyer, A., 2010. Thiamine in plants: aspects of its metabolism and functions. Phytochemistry 71 (14-15), 1615–1624.

Grant, D.M., 1991. Detoxification pathways in the liver. J. Inherit. Metab. Dis., 421–430.

Grosso, G., Bei, R., Mistretta, A., Marventano, S., Calabrese, G., Masuelli, L., Giganti, M.G., Modesti, A., Galvano, F., Gazzolo, D., 2013. Effects of vitamin C on health: a review of evidence. Front. Biosci. (Landmark Ed) 18 (3), 1017–1029.

Harris, L.J., 1962. Ascorbic acid. Proc. R. Soc. Lond. Ser. B Biol. Sci. 156 (964), 295–299. Vitamin C.

Harvard T. H. Chan School of Public Health, 2022. The Nutrition Source: Iron. https://www.hsph.harvard.edu/nutritionsource/iron/.

Hemminger, A., Wills, B.K., 2020. Vitamin B6 Toxicity.

Institute of Medicine, 2006. Dietary Reference Intakes: The Essential Guide to Nutrient Requirements. The National Academies Press, Washington, DC. https://doi.org/10.17226/11537.

Institute of Medicine (US) Standing Committee on the Scientific Evaluation of Dietary Reference Intakes, 1998. Introduction to dietary reference intakes. In: Dietary Reference Intakes for Thiamin, Riboflavin, Niacin, Vitamin B6, Folate, Vitamin B12, Pantothenic Acid, Biotin, and Choline. National Academies Press, US.

Jacob, R.A., Sotoudeh, G., 2002. Vitamin C function and status in chronic disease. Nutr. Clin. Care 5 (2), 66–74.

Kohlschütter, A., Finckh, B., Nickel, M., Bley, A., Hübner, C., 2020. First recognized patient with genetic vitamin E deficiency stable after 36 years of controlled supplement therapy. J. Neurodegener. Dis. 20 (1), 35–38.

Kuhn, S.O., Meissner, K., Mayes, L.M., Bartels, K., 2018. Vitamin C in sepsis. Curr. Opin. Anaesthesiol. 31 (1), 55.

Lenntech, 2022. Recommended daily intake of vitamins and minerals. Available at https://www.lenntech.com/recommended-daily-intake.htm.

Linster, C.L., Van Schaftingen, E., 2007. Vitamin C: biosynthesis, recycling and degradation in mammals. FEBS J. 274 (1), 1–22.

Linus Pauling Institute, 2022. University of Michigan Linus Pauling Micronutrient Information Center. https://lpi.oregonstate.edu/mic/minerals/chromium#. This link leads to a website provided by the Linus Pauling Institute at Oregon State University. [Minerva Haugabrooks] is not affiliated or endorsed by the Linus Pauling Institute or Oregon State University.

Liska, D.J., 1998. The detoxification enzyme systems. Altern. Med. Rev. 3 (3), 187–198.

LiverTox, 2012. Clinical and Research Information on Drug-Induced Liver Injury [Internet]. National Institute of Diabetes and Digestive and Kidney Diseases, Bethesda (MD). Vitamin B. [Updated 2021 May 27]. Available from: https://www.ncbi.nlm.nih.gov/books/NBK548710/.

Lotto, V., Choi, S.W., Friso, S., 2011. Vitamin B6: a challenging link between nutrition and inflammation in CVD. Br. J. Nutr. 106 (2), 183–195.

Makris, K., Sempos, C., Cavalier, E., 2020. The measurement of vitamin D metabolites: part I—metabolism of vitamin D and the measurement of 25-hydroxyvitamin D. Hormones 19 (2), 81–96.

Malouf, R., Evans, J.G., 2003. Vitamin B6 for cognition. Cochrane Database Syst. Rev. 4.

Marcinowska-Suchowierska, E., Kupisz-Urbańska, M., Łukaszkiewicz, J., Płudowski, P., Jones, G., 2018. Vitamin D toxicity—a clinical perspective. Front. Endocrinol. 9, 550.

Martel, J.L., Kerndt, C.C., Doshi, H., et al., 2022. Vitamin B1 (Thiamine). In: StatPearls [Internet]. StatPearls Publishing, Treasure Island (FL). [Updated 2021 Oct 16] Available from: https://www.ncbi.nlm.nih.gov/books/NBK482360/.

Maxfield, L., Crane, J.S., 2018. Vitamin C Deficiency.

Mazur, E., Litch, N., 2019. Lutz's Nutrition and Diet Therapy.

McDowell, L., 2003. Minerals in Animal and Human Nutrition History, second ed. Elsevier, https://doi.org/10.1016/B978-0-444-51367-0.X5001-6 (Chapter 3).

McDowell, L., 2017. Mineral History: The Early Years, first ed. Design Publishing, Inc, Sarasota. https://books.google.co.uk/books?id=Z4otDwAAQBAJ&printsec=frontcover&redir_esc=y#v=onepage&q&f=false.

Merriam-Webster, 2022. Tocopherol. In: Merriam-Webster.com Dictionary. Retrieved February 3, 2022, from: https://www.merriam-webster.com/dictionary/tocopherol.

Min, B., 2013. Effects of vitamin D on blood pressure and endothelial function. Korean J. Physiol. Pharmacol. 17 (5), 385–392.

Mooney, S., Leuendorf, J.E., Hendrickson, C., Hellmann, H., 2009. Vitamin B6: a long known compound of surprising complexity. Molecules 14 (1), 329–351.

Mulholland, P.J., 2006. Susceptibility of the cerebellum to thiamine deficiency. Cerebellum 5 (1), 55–63.

Müller, M.A., 2011. Pinch of sodium. Nat. Chem. 3, 974. https://www.nature.com/articles/nchem.1205. https://doi.org/10.1038/nchem.1205.

NAP.edu, 2006. Dietary reference intake: the essential guide to nutrient intake. In: Sulfate, pp. 397–401. https://www.nap.edu/read/11537/chapter/45#400.

Nashawaty, M., Mahmoud, A., Hassan, S., Taha Osman Mohammed, T.O., Hoenig, L.J., 2021. Nutrition and Art 19th Century Images of Scurvy, Chlorosis and Pellagra. https://www.sciencedirect.com/science/article/pii/B9780128195871000057.

National Institutes of Health, 2021a. Strengthening Knowledge and Understanding of Dietary Supplements (Fact Sheet for Health Professionals). Retrieved from: https://ods.od.nih.gov/factsheets/VitaminA-HealthProfessional/.

National Institutes of Health, 2021b. Strengthening Knowledge and Understanding of Dietary Supplements (Fact Sheet for Health Professionals). Retrieved from https://ods.od.nih.gov/factsheets/VitaminD-HealthProfessional/.

National Institutes of Health, 2021c. Strengthening Knowledge and Understanding of Dietary Supplements (Fact Sheet for Health Professionals). Retrieved from: https://ods.od.nih.gov/factsheets/VitaminK-Consumer/.

National Institutes of Health, 2021d. Strengthening Knowledge and Understanding of Dietary Supplements (Fact Sheet for Health Professionals). Retrieved from: https://ods.od.nih.gov/factsheets/VitaminC-HealthProfessional/.

National Pesticide Information Center, 2022. Sulphur. http://npic.orst.edu/factsheets/sulfurgen.html.

New International Version Bible, 2022. Deuteronomy 29:23; Job 18:15; Psalms 11:6; Isaiah 30:33; Ezekiel 38:22; Luke 17:29; Revelation 9:17. https://www.biblestudytools.com/niv/.

Northrop-Clewes, C.A., Thurnham, D.I., 2012. The discovery and characterization of riboflavin. Ann. Nutr. Metab. 61 (3), 224–230.

Orr, J., 1915. Entry for 'BRIMSTONE'. In: International Standard Bible Encyclopedia. https://www.biblestudytools.com/encyclopedias/isbe/brimstone.html.

Pennock, J.F., 1967. Occurrence of vitamins K and related quinones. Vitam. Horm. 24, 307–329.

Pourcel, L., Moulin, M., Fitzpatrick, T.B., 2013. Examining strategies to facilitate vitamin B1 biofortification of plants by genetic engineering. Front. Plant Sci. 4, 160.

Powers, H.J., 2003. Riboflavin (vitamin B-2) and health. Am. J. Clin. Nutr. 77 (6), 1352–1360. https://doi.org/10.1093/ajcn/77.6.1352.

Ravisankar, P., Reddy, A.A., Nagalakshmi, B., Koushik, O.S., Kumar, B.V., Anvith, P.S., 2015. The comprehensive review on fat soluble vitamins. IOSR J. Pharm. 5 (11), 12–28.

Rice, A.L., West Jr., K.P., Black, R.E., 2004. Vitamin A deficiency. In: Comparative Quantification of Health Risks: Global and Regional Burden of Disease Attributable to Selected Major Risk Factors. vol. 1, pp. 0211–0256. Chapter 4 page 211-257.

Rice-Evans, C., Miller, N., Paganga, G., 1997. Antioxidant properties of phenolic compounds. Trends Plant Sci. 2 (4), 152–159.

Rosenberg, I.H., 2012. A history of the isolation and identification of vitamin B6. Ann. Nutr. Metab. 61 (3), 236–238.

Samuel, S., Sitrin, M.D., 2008. Vitamin D's role in cell proliferation and differentiation. Nutr. Rev. 66 (Suppl_2), S116–S124.

Sheftel, A.D., Mason, A.B., Ponka, P., 2011. The long history of iron in the Universe and in health and disease. Biochim. Biophys. Acta 1820 (3), 161–187. https://doi.org/10.1016/j.bbagen.2011.08.002. Epub 2011 Aug 9. PMID: 21856378; PMCID: PMC3258305.

Signorelli, G.C., Bianchetti, M.G., Jermini, L.M.M., Agostoni, C., Milani, G.P., Simonetti, G.D., Lava, S.A.G., 2020. Dietary chloride deficiency syndrome: pathophysiology, history, and systematic literature review. Nutrients 12 (11), 1–10. https://doi.org/10.3390/nu12113436). https://moh-it.pure.elsevier.com/en/publications/dietary-chloride-deficiency-syndrome-pathophysiology-history-and.

Simoni, R.D., Hill, R.L., Vaughan, M., 2002. Nutritional biochemistry and the discovery of vitamins: the work of Elmer Verner McCollum. J. Biol. Chem. 277 (19), e8–e10.

Sizar, O., Khare, S., Goyal, A., Bansal, P., Givler, A., 2021. Vitamin D deficiency. In: StatPearls [Internet]. StatPearls Publishing.

Smith, A.D., Kim, Y.I., Refsum, H., 2008. Is folic acid good for everyone? Am. J. Clin. Nutr. 87 (3), 517–533.

Smith, L.F., Patterson, J., Walker, L.T., Verghese, M., 2016. Chemopreventive potential of sunflower seeds in a human colon cancer cell line. Int. J. Cancer Res. 12 (1), 40–50.

Stein, E.M., Dempster, D.W., Udesky, J., Zhou, H., Bilezikian, J.P., Shane, E., Silverberg, S.J., 2011. Vitamin D deficiency influences histomorphometric features of bone in primary hyperparathyroidism. Bone 48 (3), 557–561.

Szymczak-Pajor, I., Drzewoski, J., Śliwińska, A., 2020. The molecular mechanisms by which vitamin D prevents insulin resistance and associated disorders. Int. J. Mol. Sci. 21 (18), 6644.

Talat, N., Perry, S., Parsonnet, J., Dawood, G., Hussain, R., 2010. Vitamin D deficiency and tuberculosis progression. Emerg. Infect. Dis. 16 (5), 853.

Tang, G., 2014. Vitamin A value of plant food provitamin A—evaluated by the stable isotope technologies. Int. J. Vitam. Nutr. Res. 84 (Suppl. 1), 25–29.

Tang, J., Chonchol, M.B., 2013. Vitamin D and kidney stone disease. Curr. Opin. Nephrol. Hypertens. 22 (4), 383–389.

Teleki, A., Hitzfeld, A., Eggersdorfer, M., 2013. 100 years of vitamins: the science of formulation is the key to functionality. Kona Powder Part. J. 30, 144–163.

Tofupedia, 2015. Types of Tofu. http://www.tofupedia.com/en/tofu-bereiden/soorten-tofu/.

Ueland, P.M., McCann, A., Midttun, Ø., Ulvik, A., 2017. Inflammation, vitamin B6 and related pathways. Mol. Asp. Med. 53, 10–27.

WebElements, 2021. Magnesium: Historical Information at WebElements. https://www.webelements.com. (Accessed January 2022).

Wells, P.S., Holbrook, A.M., Crowther, N.R., Hirsh, J., 1994. Interactions of warfarin with drugs and food. Ann. Intern. Med. 121 (9), 676–683.

Wickham, E., 2014. Phosphorus content in commonly consumed beverages. J. Ren. Nutr. 24 (1). https://doi.org/10.1053/j.jrn.2013.10.002. https://www.jrnjournal.org/article/S1051-2276(13)00181-7/fulltext#relatedArticles.

Witkamp, R.F., van Norren, K., 2018. Let thy food be thy medicine…when possible. Eur. J. Pharmacol. 836, 102–114. https://doi.org/10.1016/j.ejphar.2018.06.026.

WordPress, 2022. Periodic Table: Iron. Iron Element | History, Uses, Facts, Physical & Chemical Characteristics. periodic-table.com.

Wu, S.H., Ho, S.C., Zhong, L., 2010. Effects of vitamin D supplementation on blood pressure. South. Med. J. 103 (8), 729–737.

CHAPTER 4

Food additives toxicology

Roger Clemens[a], Peter Pressman[b], and A. Wallace Hayes[c]
[a]University of Southern California, School of Pharmacy, D.K. Kim International Center for Regulatory Science, Los Angeles, CA, United States
[b]Polyscience Consulting, Chatsworth, CA, United States
[c]University of South Florida, College of Public Health, Tampa, FL, United States

Introduction

A cursory overview of food regulations promulgated since 1906 reveals that all, except the Food Safety and Modernization Act of 2011, were triggered by a spectrum of adverse events. The only exception to these reactive legislative actions and regulatory promulgations was the Food Safety Modernization Act of 2011. This act was a major proactive reformation to provide additional safety of the food supply through the implementation of five key elements. Those elements are prevention, inspection, imported food, partnerships, and cooperation. A critical, but unfortunate, component of US food regulations is the Delaney Clause, which was introduced into the US food law milieu in 1958. This clause stipulated that "no additive shall be deemed to be safe if it is found to induce cancer when ingested by man or animal." Part of the contention with this clause is that virtually any substance in the food supply, including those that are innate to fruits and vegetables, even at low doses of exposure, might prove carcinogenic or otherwise toxic in some individuals at some time, and under some circumstances; hence, the intimidating challenge within the gamut of food toxicology. Jointly, these regulations were developed to impart to consumers that measures taken by regulatory agencies and food manufacturers assure the safety of the US food supply by initiating critical steps in quality assurance and effective and nonmisleading communications.

A series of food and health surveys conducted in the United States since 2010 indicate consumers have changed their attitudes and behaviors toward foods and food ingredients, beliefs about food production and food technologies, and pursuit of plant-based foods and related dietary patterns. Interestingly, the primary sources of food safety information stem from food labels and websites, whereas television, magazines, and newspapers have

History of Food and Nutrition Toxicology
https://doi.org/10.1016/B978-0-12-821261-5.00001-5
87

little impact on informing consumers about food safety in any accurate or standardized fashion. During the past decade, consumers have become more aware of dietary components that may affect their health, such as dietary fats, sugars, and sodium. There appears to be more interest than ever before on health promotion, including weight management and risk reduction for noncommunicable diseases, all of which call for foods that are safer and more nutritious. Unfortunately, much of the information accessible to the public fails to provide consumers and even scientists with the critical essence of original research on food science, medicine, nutrition, and public health topics. Many traditional systematic reviews and metaanalyses are fraught with statistical modeling errors and incomplete coverage of the topics as evidenced by the prejudiced inclusion and exclusion criteria applied to peer-reviewed publications.

Moreover, there are dramatically shifting recommendations, acrimony, and abject confusion among consumers, scientists, and healthcare professionals alike about topics such as ultra-processed foods, GMO ingredients, flavoring agents, color additives, preservatives, dietary fats and sugars, and alternative sources of protein.

Safety assessment

Safety assessment of food ingredients, either intended as a food additive or GRAS substance, entails the same key elements. Those elements include manufacturing process, specifications, dietary exposure, and safety assessments (ADME, toxicology, genotoxicity, tolerance, corroborative animal and clinical studies, allergenicity, and global regulatory approvals) which were finalized in 2016 (FDA, 2016). The essence of GRAS has been challenged by several organizations, including the Center for Food Safety, Breast Cancer Prevention Partners, the Environmental Working Group, and the Center for Science in the Public Interest (Case 1: 17-cv-03833-VSB, Filed 09/30/21). These organizations filed a complaint that contended the GRAS process lacks transparency and had inherently a conflict of interest (COI) despite the COI draft guidance in 2017 (FDA, 2017). Perhaps the most contentious point advanced by the plaintiffs was that the GRAS process did not require the sponsor to notify the FDA of its self-affirmation of the reviewed ingredient. However, on September 30, 2021, the US District Court of the Southern District of New York upheld the GRAS self-affirmation process and dismissed the lawsuit. An analysis of this judgment noted that H.R. 3699, which was introduced in the House of Representatives (June 4,

2021), would have mandated GRAS sponsors to notify the agency of ingredients that have undergone the self-affirmation process while also reestablishing the Food Advisory Committee which was disbanded in December 2017. Congress is unlikely to rally sufficient support for the bill due to the thousands of food ingredients that may be affected (McGuffin, Personal Communication; H.R.3699, 2021).

Food additives

Background: According to the "Everything Added to Food in the United States" (EAFUS) database, now known as Substances Added to Food inventory maintained by the Center for Food Safety and Applied Nutrition (CFSAN), there are nearly 4000 direct and indirect substances added to the food supply (FDA, Substances Added to Food (formerly EAFUS), 2021b). This searchable database includes food additives and color additives that are listed in FDA regulations (21 CFR § 172, 173 and § 73, 74, respectively) and flavoring substances evaluated by the Flavor Extract Manufacturers Association (FEMA) and the Joint Expert Committee on Food Additives (JECFA). FEMA issues an updated GRAS report biennially, which is published in *Food Technology* sponsored by the Institute of Food Technologists. The CFSAN database includes prohibited substances that are listed in FDA regulations (21 CFR § 189) as prohibited from use in food, delisted color additives in FDA regulations, and some GRAS substances as reviewed by FEMA. In addition, the database represents only a partial list of food ingredients, such as those from non–FDA entities, and does not indicate an FDA approval or evaluation by the agency. Another critical component of food ingredient safety is the 1958 Delaney Clause, which prohibits the addition of any chemical to the food supply that causes cancer in humans or animals, regardless of exposure or dose (Merrill, 1997).

There are more than 30 classifications of food additives according to the Code of Federal Regulations within the United States. Those classifications include, but are not limited to, preservatives, flavors, leavening agents, humectants, emulsifiers, drying agents, nonnutritive sweeteners, antimicrobial agents, pH control agents, and dough strengtheners (see Table 1). The purpose and basic functions of these food additives are shown in the table given in https://www.accessdata.fda.gov/scripts/cdrh/cfdocs/cfcfr/CFRSearch.cfm?CFRPart=18. The substances in these classifications may be used directly or indirectly as a food component that affects the characteristics of

Table 1 Categories of direct food additives as stated in the US regulations (21 CFR 184).

1. Anticaking agents and free-flow agents
2. Antimicrobial agents
3. Antioxidants
4. Colors and color adjuncts
5. Curing and pickling agents
6. Dough strengtheners
7. Drying agents
8. Emulsifiers and emulsifier salts
9. Enzymes
10. Firming agents
11. Flavor enhancers
12. Flavor agents and adjuvants
13. Flour-treating agents
14. Food preservatives
15. Formulation aids
16. Fumigants
17. Humectants
18. Leavening agents
19. Lubricants and release agents
20. Nonnutritive sweeteners
21. Nutrient supplements
22. Nutritive sweeteners
23. Oxidizing and reducing agents
24. pH control agents
25. Processing aids
26. Propellants, aerating agents, and gases
27. Sequestrants
28. Solvents and vehicles
29. Stabilizers and thickeners
30. Surface-active agents
31. Surface-finishing agents
32. Synergists
33. Texturizers

any food, such as nutritional value, stability, and sensory qualities. Many food additives are ingredients that received *prior sanction* GRAS status from the FDA (21 CFR § 182) since they had a long history of use without adverse events. Examples of these food additives include anticaking agents; preservatives that function as antimicrobials, such as ascorbic acid, potassium sorbate, and potassium bisulfite; sequestrants (e.g., disodium phosphate, dipotassium phosphate); stabilizers (e.g., Chondrus extract); and nutrients, including ascorbic acid (vitamin C) and tocopherols (vitamin E).

There is also a list of indirect food additives (21 CFR 186) that are considered GRAS and have a long history of use by the food industry. Some of these indirect food ingredients may be used in food contact surfaces, such as packaging materials. These include sodium salts of several fatty acids produced by plants and animals, pulp from natural plant sources, dextrans from microbial fermentation, iron oxides which may function as a red-brown pigment in food packaging materials, and even nature-derived clay or kaolin that is used in antidiarrheal medications, as well as a coating and filling for paper.

Food additives do not include pesticides, food colors per se, or substances that have been reviewed at Generally Recognized As Safe (GRAS). It is important to note that as of September 1, 2021, more than 1000 new food ingredients have been reviewed or are pending review by the FDA via the GRAS petition process since 1998. Hundreds more food ingredients have likely been examined by experts through the GRAS affirmation process that was initiated in 1972. The standards for GRAS documentation were finalized in 2016 and excluded the Delaney Clause.

Food colorants, both exempt and certified, are reviewed by experts under the provisions presented in the 1960 Color Additives amendment (21 U.S.C. 301). As of 2015, there are nine certified and 27 color additives exempt from batch certification for food applications as stated in the Federal regulations, such as 21 CFR 74 and 21 CFR 73, respectively (https://www.fda.gov/industry/color-additive-inventories/summary-color-additives-use-united-states-foods-drugs-cosmetics-and-medical-devices#table1A; Accessed September 1, 2021).

Food colors

Within the United States, food colors are regulated by the FDA through the Color Additives Amendment of 1960. This amendment outlines the general provisions to assess the safety and usage of pigments in the food supply. Basically, there are two classifications of food colors: those that are water soluble, known as dyes, and those that are fat soluble, known as lakes. From a statutory perspective, the United States does not have natural colors, even though many colors in the food supply originate from natural sources. There are certified colors (each batch of color is certified through extensive analytical analyses prior to use) and exempt colors. Consumers consider exempt (exempt from certification) colors as natural, since they are derived from natural sources.

The initial food color and health controversy emerged in the 1970s. The Feingold hypothesis suggested that artificial food additives and colors were linked to hyperkinesis and learning disabilities among children (Feingold, 1975). A controversy ensued among consumers and the medical community, which culminated in a regulation based on public pressure, not scientific evidence. That regulation stipulates those foods and pharmaceutical agents with the yellow color tartrazine must be labeled with a warning statement. That statement notes the "product contains FD&C Yellow No. 5 (tartrazine) which may cause allergic-type reactions (including bronchial asthma) in certain susceptible persons. Although the overall incidence of FD&C Yellow No. 5 (tartrazine) sensitivity in the general population is low, it is frequently seen in patients who also have aspirin hypersensitivity" (FDA, 2020).

As the public's reaction to the tartrazine issue prompted concerns within the medical community, the subsequent clinical evidence suggested that those children who presented with allergy-related atopic dermatitis tended to be more sensitive to the consumption of foods with this colorant (Feketea and Tsabouri, 2017). This condition, a common inflammatory skin disorder, affects about 13% of all children (NEA, 2021).

Consumer negative reactions to food colors were heightened following the 2007 publication of the South Hampton study. This study suggested that the consumption of artificial food color additives (5-mg sunset yellow, 2.5-mg carmoisine, 7.5-mg tartrazine, and 5-mg ponceau 4R) by children altered their behavior patterns and contributed to their hyperactivity (McCann et al., 2007). Despite this study being rejected by the European Food Safety Authority due to some inconsistencies in the data and conclusions (EFSA, 2008, Scientific Opinion of the Panel on Food Additives, Flavorings, Processing Aids and Food Contact Materials (AFC) on a request from the commission on the results of the study by McCann et al. (2007) on the effect of some colors and sodium benzoate on children), several organizations and parents called for the banning of artificial colors (Potera, 2010).

More recently, titanium dioxide, a color additive, has been the focus of potential safety issues. Current regulations in the United States state that TiO_2 may be safely used for coloring foods generally, as long as the level does not exceed 1% by weight of the food (21 CFR 73.575). This age-old, food-grade pigment confers a white color or opacity due to its unique light-reflecting properties. It is common in food products, such as creamers and confections, and nonfood products, including toothpaste, paint, sunscreen, cosmetics, and even packaging materials. Its small particle size, 200–300 nm in diameter, and the absence of classic risk assessment have raised safety concerns (Winkler et al., 2018). While the United States continues to support the safety of TiO_2 since consumer exposure is below a level that may be considered harmful, including cancer, the European Union recently classified E171 as a suspected carcinogen upon inhalation (particles $\leq 10\,\mu m$) and has banned its use in foods effective in 2022.

Flavoring agents

The safety of flavoring agents is reported biennially by the Flavor Extract Manufacturers Association (FEMA) (https://www.femaflavor.org/). Their reports are published in *Food Technology* sponsored by the Institute of Food Technologists based in Chicago, Illinois, and published by the Joint FAO/WHO Expert Committee on Food Additives (JECFA), an independent international scientific advisory body managed through the United Nations. FEMA's important safety assessments are conducted independent of the FDA, yet are performed under a 1959 memorandum with the FDA. The organization's charge, like any other expert GRAS panel, is to protect public health through the effective safety evaluation of flavor ingredients using the best available scientific procedures and information.

Flavoring agents impart a characteristic flavor profile. For example, vanillin, a phenolic aldehyde, in vanilla ice cream and a variety of confectionery products, or chocolate or essential oils, such as almond and lemon. Another common spectrum of flavoring agencies is ginger extract composed of an array of terpenes and phenolic compounds that is commonly found in non-alcoholic and alcoholic beverages.

The most recent listing of flavoring agents (GRAS 29) was published in March 2020 (Cohen et al., 2020). This publication includes the results of an expert review of 64 new flavorings under their conditions of intended use, and for 76 flavorings with new use levels and/or usage in new food categories. One substance, methyl eugenol was removed from the FEMA GRAS status.

Interestingly in 2018, the FDA stated that benzophenone (a plant metabolite, previously found in sunscreen products), ethyl acrylate (naturally occurs in fruit pulp), eugenyl methyl ether (naturally occurs in fruit, such as apples), myrcene (an essential oil component from bay leaves and hops), pulegone (naturally occurs in the mint plant leaves and flowering tops), pyridine (found in the leaves and roots of *Atropa belladonna* (belladonna), and *Althaea officinalis* (marshmallow) are no longer permitted for use in foods even though these substances are innate to plants. Styrene, which occurs naturally in strawberries, cinnamon, coffee, and beef, is also a synthetic flavoring and adjuvant used to make food service packaging. Styrene and its adjuvants are no longer permitted for use in food (FDA, 2018). The withdrawal of these plant-derived, yet synthetic flavorings or flavor enhancers was based on new evidence that indicated these substances induce cancer in laboratory animals even though the approved usage levels of these substances did not pose a public health risk. This action follows stipulations under the Delaney Clause (Merrill, 1997).

The safety review action by FEMA includes classic toxicological studies, including ADME and genotoxicity evaluation of flavoring agents for their intended use (Smith et al., 2018; Gooderham et al., 2020). Meanwhile, FEMA continues to update the safety assessment criteria for flavoring agents, as evidenced by the organization's 2018 publication (Cohen et al., 2018). In addition to the classic multigenerational toxicity studies, the updated criteria emphasized the importance of genotoxicity assessments, the protocols of which typically follow ICH S2 (R1) criteria, even though these criteria were originally designed for and applied to pharmaceutical agents (ICH, 2013).

An example of FEMA efforts on behalf of public safety of food flavoring agents is their assessment of citrus-derived components (Cohen et al., 2019). In this case, 54 natural flavor complexes derived from botanicals of the Citrus genus were affirmed as GRAS under their conditions of intended use as flavoring ingredients. The assessment included history of use; an array of sources, such as citrus peel oils, essential oils with and without terpenes, and extracts; the total chemical composition of the sources, plus current usage levels; assessment of per capita intake or estimated daily intake (EDI); manufacturing methods; application of the threshold of toxicological concern (TTC) concept in addition to data on the ADME; toxicology and genotoxicity of members of the generic chemical groups; and the standard FEMA evaluation maze for natural flavoring complexes. Overall, the FEMA criteria for their GRAS affirmation are the same safety assessment standards applied to other food ingredients as evaluated by other specialists based on their training and expertise.

Preservatives

A 2021 survey among 1000 adult consumers in the United States indicated that 64% seek foods that have "clean" labeling (IFIC, 2021). Despite the absence of "clean" labeling standards, consumers contend that foods that do not contain ingredients that are artificial, or synthetic, are preferred. A 2018 survey among grocery shoppers revealed that the use of food preservatives, such as benzoates, nitrites, and sulfites, is not consistent with the naturalness of food ingredients (Lusk, 2019). This preference is not associated with ingredient safety or toxicological concern, but rather one of perception of what is natural.

These three compounds (benzoates, nitrites, and sulfites) represent many FDA-approved substances that function as antimicrobials and antioxidants in foods (21 CFR 172). For example, benzoic acid is an established and safe antimicrobial preservative, which occurs naturally in a variety of foods and spices, such as strawberries, cranberries, cayenne pepper, mustard, cloves, thyme, nutmeg, and cinnamon, but is shunned by consumers (Del Olmo et al., 2017). Similarly, nitrites, which are intrinsic to select foods, such as ham and bacon, and naturally found in some vegetables are broadly demonized (Sweazea et al., 2018). Interestingly, many dietary recommendations include an increase in vegetable consumption, which, at least from an historical perspective, represent about 80% of the total nitrite/nitrate intake (Sweazea et al., 2018). Sulfites also occur in standardized foods as well as naturally in foods, including salmon, lettuce, cabbage, tomatoes, soy, grapes, sweet peppers, onions, garlic, chives, leeks, Brussel sprouts, and asparagus, as well as beer and wine (21 CFR 130.9; Carlos and de Jager, 2007).

The current regulations within the United States state that preservatives may be used as indicated in food products that are compliant with good manufacturing practices. With respect to benzoic acid, it is a generally recognized as safe (GRAS) direct food ingredient that can be used in various meat and poultry products up to 0.1% (21 CFR 184.1021). Nitrites/nitrates usage is approved for selected foods and is not permitted to exceed 500 ppm as specified by the regulation (21 CFR 172.175). Sulfites, in the form of sulfur dioxide (SO_2), sodium bisulfite ($NaHSO_3$), potassium metabisulfite ($KHSO_3$), sodium metabisulfite ($Na_2S_2O_5$), potassium metabisulfite ($K_2S_2O_5$), and sodium sulfite (Na_2SO_3), are considered GRAS. The presence of sulfites must be declared on food labels when used as an ingredient in the food and also when used as a processing aid or when present in an ingredient used in the food (e.g., dried fruit pieces) when the concentration in the food is ≥ 10 ppm total SO_2 (Timbo et al., 2004).

Stabilizers and thickeners

Substances that function to improve the texture and mouthfeel are typically called stabilizers or thickeners. These naturally derived substances are represented by an array of proteins and complex carbohydrates, including gelatin (primarily from animal collagen, a protein in connective tissues), pectin (fundamentally from citrus fruits), guar gum (a unique complex carbohydrate from a leguminous plant, *Cyamopsis tetragonolobus*), carrageenan (a sulfated carbohydrate extracted from various marine algae), xanthan gum (derived from plant and animal sources), and whey (a major protein found in milk).

Carrageenan (CGN) is one additive around which there has been intense scrutiny, much debate, and particularly persistent and strident claims, both for its safety and possible health risks. Regarding the safety and health risks with any compound, the route of administration is a fundamental variable. Importantly, unlike many compounds in the stabilizer and thickener category, the digestibility of CGN in the human gut appears to be dependent on the degree of sulfation (20%–40%) and molecular weight (<50 kDa), but is inert to digestion enzymes and limited evidence suggests it may be partially fermented by the microflora in the distal bowel (David et al., 2018). While CGN is considered safe by the US FDA (FDA, 2022b) and JECFA (FAO/WHO, 2014), even for use in infant formula, several in vitro studies with cell lines and upon injection into the footpad of rodents suggest that CGN per se may trigger inflammatory responses (Tobacman, 2001; Harmuth-Hoene and Schwerdtfeger, 1979). Threats to CGN safety were asserted that this polysaccharide was degraded to poligeenan and that this compound is responsible for the inflammatory response. However, subsequent research indicated that CGN does not degrade to poligeenan under typical thermal food processing conditions and that poligeenan does not exhibit toxicological properties following long-term bioassay environments (McKim et al., 2019). Nonetheless, unfortunately, carrageenan has been removed from many products.

Sweeteners

The dynamics of sweeteners as food additives were recently reviewed (Carocho et al., 2017). The authors point out numerous inconsistencies among international regulatory agencies regarding the safety assessment and ultimate marketing of sweeteners in current and future markets.

Several nutritive sweeteners, also considered caloric sweeteners, are deemed GRAS. These include an array of sugars, such as glucose, galactose, and fructose, which are monosaccharides, and sucrose, lactose, and maltose that are disaccharides. Of these saccharides, sucrose and fructose have received the greatest attention from consumers and regulatory agencies since high levels of consumption have been associated with noncommunicable diseases that include obesity, diabetes, cardiovascular disease, and cancer. These two sugars are innate to plants, such as sugar cane, sugar beets, sweet peas, bananas, and peaches, plus tree and vine fruits including bananas, plums, pears, peaches, tomatoes, berries, and grapes, as well as most root vegetables like yams, sweet potatoes, parsnip, radishes, and carrots. While many dietary recommendations advise consumers not to consume more than 10% of their energy intake in the form of sucrose, the debate on the impact of dietary sucrose and health continues (Rippe and Angelopoulos, 2013). More recently, some have proposed this level should be reduced to 5% of total energy intake (Mooradian et al., 2017).

The US FDA has approved nonnutritive sweeteners, including xylitol (1963), saccharin (1970), aspartame (1981, 1983, 1996), acesulfame-K (1988, 2003), sucralose (1998), erythritol (2001), neotame (2002), stevia (2008), and advantame (2014). Each of these has been extensively reviewed for its safety, including toxicology, under conditions of use.

In 1970 cyclamate was banned by the FDA since there was evidence that a mixture of saccharin and cyclamate triggered urinary bladder cancer in laboratory animals when fed 2600 mg of the mixture for 105 weeks (Price et al., 1970). A follow-up 2-year study, also in laboratory animals, by the same investigators indicated that a cyclamate metabolite, cyclohexylamine, dosed at 15-mg/kg bw, contributed to the development of a urinary bladder tumor in 1 of 8 animals. However, a 13-week study among humans, who were screened for cyclamate/cyclohexylamine conversion and subsequently consumed calcium cyclamate tablets (equivalent to 250-mg cyclamic acid), suggested an acceptable daily intake (ADI) of 0–11 mg/kg bw/d (Renwick et al., 2004). Interestingly, only 14 individuals were considered metabolizers out of the 261 screened study volunteers, suggesting that perhaps only 5% of the general population may be at risk. Regardless, cyclamate was banned in the United States in 1969, yet remains approved and available in Canada under the Twin brand name, as well as in Europe, South America, Australia, and New Zealand.

Nutrients

In general, nutrients, as defined by the National Academies/Food and Nutrition Board, are compounds known to be essential for life and health

(Institute of Medicine, Dietary Reference Intakes: The Essential Guide to Nutrient Requirements, 2006). This report updated the Recommended Dietary Allowance (RDA) that reflects the average daily dietary intake level that is sufficient to meet the nutrient requirement of nearly all (97%–98%) healthy individuals in a group.

The upper limits of compounds, which include vitamins and minerals that consumers typically read on product labels, were recommended. These nutrients have been approved by the US FDA as recommended either via the history of use (prior to 1958) or as a food additive or GRAS substance. A 1998 report established the Tolerable Upper Intake Level (UL) of nutrients (Institute of Medicine, 1998). This is the highest level of daily nutrient intake that is likely to pose no risk of adverse health effects to almost all individuals in the general population. For *example, the RDA for vitamin A is 900-μg* **Retinol Activity Equivalents** *(RAE) for adult males* (equivalent to 3000 IU), whereas the UL for this nutrient is 3000-μg RAE (equivalent to 10,000 IU) of preformed vitamin A. This does not apply to beta-carotene and the array of other carotenoids.

The safety criteria for food additives and GRAS assessment are identical. The general processes of safety assessment are indicated in Fig. 1.

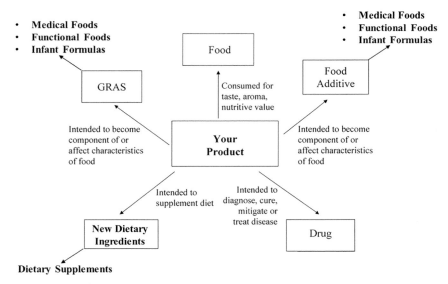

Fig. 1 GRAS vs food additive.

Processing aids

These substances, used in very small quantities, are used in the production of foods but are not required to be declared on the ingredient statement for foods destined for human consumption. Processing aids function to improve product quality, have no technical effect on the finished product, enhance nutritional value, and assist in maintaining product attributes and shelf life, and include food contact lubricants (used on food and packaging conveyor belts), antimicrobials used in equipment and wash solutions, and antifoaming agents. The enzyme, rennet, used in cheese production is considered a processing aid. To maintain chill water sanitation, ozone is frequently added to serve as an antimicrobial. Even common table salt is a processing aid as applied to some seafood. In this case, salt decreases the water activity of the product, thereby extending the shelf life of the product. Similarly, chlorine, an antimicrobial, is added to washes for fruits and vegetables, thereby extending the shelf life (Al-Mazeedi et al., 2013).

Dietary supplements

A dietary ingredient is a vitamin; a mineral; an herb or other botanical; an amino acid; a dietary substance for use by man to supplement the diet by increasing total dietary intake; or a concentrate, metabolite, constituent, extract, or combination of any of the previously mentioned dietary ingredients (FD&C Act §201(ff)(1)). A new dietary ingredient refers to a substance that was not marketed in the United States in a dietary supplement before October 15, 1994, the date of the Dietary Supplement Health Education Act (DSHEA) of 1994. These substances must be reviewed by the FDA at least 75 days prior to marketing in the United States for their safety via the New Dietary Ingredient (NDI) process as promulgated as a component of DSHEA. This review process conducted by the FDA based on the evidence submitted by the ingredient sponsor provides a "reasonable certainty of safety" (FDA, 2020). As of July 2021, more than 1200 NDI notifications had been filed with the FDA (FDA, 2022a).

Despite the NDI process, a recent report indicates that more than 50,000 dietary supplements are currently marketed as listed in the Office of Dietary Supplement's "Dietary Supplement Label Database" (Brown, 2017). The author addresses several serious adverse events associated with dietary supplement usage, including liver toxicity, kidney toxicity, heart toxicity, and cancer. These issues were discussed by the same investigator in the same issue *of Food and Chemical Toxicology*. Despite the follow-up papers that focus on these adverse events, it remains uncertain as to the direct or indirect link of dietary supplements (active or inactive ingredients) and an individual's health status. However, the author called for Phase IV postmarketing surveillance and the establishment of a dietary supplement toxicity database.

Conclusion

Undoubtedly, the global research community within the academy and the food industry has conducted an enormous amount of work over the last 200 years to advance the value and safety of food additives. The variety, abundance, and above all the safety of the US food supply have never been better. Of course, the dynamic nature of science and the accumulation of ever enlarging and improved databases on food additive toxicology lead to the need for revision of certain conclusions, better illumination of key questions, and to the development of new and clinically important questions and hypotheses. The inherent fluidity and evolution of what we know appear to have simultaneously fueled confusion, fear, and overreaction across various consumer publics, scientists and regulators themselves, and the primary care medical community. The odd disequilibrium that exists between toxicological sophistication, public fear, and outright anger, and a confused regulatory response calls for novel action and better communication among all stakeholders. Public trust and public health can only be achieved by more comprehensive, critically interpreted, and accessible communication about the science and the recommendations which it drives.

References

Al-Mazeedi, H., Regenstein, J., Riaz, M., 2013. The issue of undeclared ingredients in halal and kosher food production: a focus on processing aids. Compr. Rev. Food Sci. Food Saf. 12, 228–233. https://doi.org/10.1111/1541-4337.12002.

Brown, A., 2017. An overview of herb and dietary supplement efficacy, safety and government regulations in the United States with suggested improvements. Part 1 of 5 series. Food Chem. Toxicol. 107, 449–471. https://doi.org/10.1016/j.fct.2016.11.001.

Carlos, K.S., de Jager, L.S., 2007. Determination of sulfite in food by liquid chromatography tandem mass spectrometry: collaborative study. J. AOAC Int. 100 (6), 1785–1794. https://doi.org/10.5740/jaoacint.17-0033.

Carocho, M., Morales, P., Ferreira, I., 2017. Sweeteners as food additives in the XXI century: a review of what is known, and what is to come. Food Chem. Toxicol. 107, 302–317. https://doi.org/10.1016/j.fct.2017.06.046.

Cohen, S., Eisenbrand, G., Fukushima, S., Gooderham, N., Guengerish, F., Hecht, S., et al., 2018. Updated procedure for the safety evaluation of natural flavor complexes used as ingredients in food. Food Chem. Toxicol. 113, 171–178. https://doi.org/10.1016/j.fct.2018.01.021.

Cohen, S., Eisenbrand, G., Fukushima, S., Dooderham, N., Guengerich, F., Hecht, S.R., et al., 2019. FEMA GRAS assessment of natural flavor complexes: citrus-derived flavoring ingredients. Food Chem. Toxicol. 124, 192–218. https://doi.org/10.1016/j.fct.2018.11.052.

Cohen, S.M., Eisenbrand, G., Fukushima, S., Gooderham, N.J., Guengerich, F.P., Hecht, S.S., Rietjens, I.M.C.M., Rosol, T.J., Harman, C., Taylor, S.V., 2020. GRAS flavoring substances 29. Food Technol. (March).

David, S., Levi, C., Fahoum, L., Ungar, Y., Mayron-Holtz, E., Shpigelman, A., Lesmes, U., 2018. Revisiting the carrageenan controversy: do we really understand the digestive fate and safety of carrageenan in our foods? Food Funct. 9 (3), 1344–1352. https://doi.org/10.1039/c7fo01721a.

Del Olmo, A., Calzada, J., Nuñez, M., 2017. Benzoic acid and its derivatives as naturally occurring compounds in foods and as additives: uses, exposure, and controversy. Crit. Rev. Food Sci. Nutr. 57 (14), 3084–3103. https://doi.org/10.1080/10408398.2015.1087964.

EFSA, 2008. Scientific opinion of the panel on food additives, flavourings, processing aids and food contact materials (AFC) on a request from the commission on the results of the study by McCann et al. (2007) on the effect of some colours and sodium benzoate on chil. EFSA J. 660, 1–54. https://doi.org/10.2903/j.efsa.2008.660.

FAO/WHO, 2014. Compendium of Food Additive Specifications: FAO JECFA Monographs 16. Joint FAO/WHO Expert Committee on Food Additives.

FDA, 2016. Substances Generally Recognized as Safe. Federal Register/Vol. 81, No. 159. August 17, pp. 54961–55055.

FDA, 2017. Best Practices for Convening a GRAS Panel: Guidance for Industry, November.

FDA, 2018, October. FDA Removes 7 Synthetic Flavoring Substances from Food Additives List. Retrieved from CFSAN Constituent Updates www.fda.gov.

FDA, 2020. 21 CFR 74.1705: FD&C Yellow No. 5. In FDA, Code of Federal Regulations.

FDA, 2021, May. Substances Added to Food (Formerly EAFUS). Retrieved from. https://www.cfsanappsexternal.fda.gov/scripts/fdcc/?set=FoodSubstances.

FDA, 2022a. Submitted 75-Day Premarket Notifications for New Dietary Ingredients.

FDA, 2022b. 21 CFR § 172.620—Carrageenan. Code of Federal Regulations.

Feingold, B., 1975. Hyperkinesis and learning disabilities linked to artificial food flavors and colors. Am. J. Nurs. 75, 797–803.

Feketea, G., Tsabouri, S., 2017. Common food colorants and allergic reactions in children: myth or reality? Food Chem. 230, 578–588. https://doi.org/10.1016/j.foodchem.2017.03.043.

Gooderham, N., Cohen, S., Eisenbrand, G., Fukushima, S., Guengerish, F., Hecht, S., et al., 2020. The safety evaluation of food flavoring substances: the role of genotoxicity studies. Crit. Rev. Toxicol. 50, 1–27. https://doi.org/10.1080/10408444.2020.1712589.

H.R.3699, 2021. 117th Congress (2021–2022): Toxic Free Food Act of 2021. www.congress.gov/bill/117th-congress/house-bill/3699/text.

Harmuth-Hoene, A., Schwerdtfeger, E., 1979. Effect of indigestible polysaccharides on protein digestibility and nitrogen retention in growing rats. Nutr. Metab. 23 (5), 399–407. https://doi.org/10.1159/000176285.

ICH, 2013. www.ich.org/page/safety-guidelines.

IFIC, 2021. https://ific.org/media-information/press-releases/2021-food-health-survey/.

Institute of Medicine, 1998. Dietary Reference Intakes: A Risk Assessment Model for Establishing Upper Intake Levels for Nutrients. National Academies Press, Washington, DC.

Institute of Medicine, 2006. Dietary Reference Intakes: The Essential Guide to Nutrient Requirements. The National Academies Press, Washington DC, https://doi.org/10.17226/11537.

Lusk J.L., 2019. Consumer perceptions of 'natural' foods. Food Technology Magazine. July 1.

McCann, D., Barrett, A., Cooper, A., Crumpler, D., Dalen, L., Grimshaw, K., et al., 2007. Food additives and hyperactive behaviour in 3-year-old and 8/9-year old children in the community: a randomised, double-blinded, placebo-controlled trial. Lancet 370, 1560–1567. https://doi.org/10.1016/S0140-6736(07)61306-3.

McKim, J., Willoughby Sr., J., Blakemore, W., Weiner, M., 2019. Clarifying the confusion between poligeenan, degraded carrageenan, and carrageenan: a review of the chemistry, nomenclature, and in vivo toxicology by the oral route. Crit. Rev. Food Sci. Nutr. 59 (9), 3054–3073. https://doi.org/10.1080/10408398.2018.1481822.

Merrill, R., 1997. Food safety regulation: reforming the Delaney Clause. Annu. Rev. Public Health 18, 313–340.

Mooradian, A., Smith, M., Tokuda, M., 2017. The role of artificial and natural sweeteners in reducing the consumption of table sugar: a narrative review. Clin. Nutr. ESPEN 18, 1–8. https://doi.org/10.1016/j.clnesp.2017.01.004.

NEA, 2021. Atopic Dermatitis in Children. Retrieved from National Eczema Association: https://nationaleczema.org/eczema/children/atopic-dermatitis.

Potera, C., 2010. The artificial food day blues. Environ. Health Perspect. 118, A428. https://doi.org/10.1289/ehp.118-a428.

Price, J., Biava, C., Oser, B., Vogin, E., Steinfeld, J., Ley, H., 1970. Bladder tumors in rads fed cyclohexylamine or high doses of a mixture of cyclamate and saccharin. Science 167 (3921), 1131–1132. https://doi.org/10.1126/science.167.3921.1131.

Renwick, A., Thompson, J., O'Shaughnessy, M., Walter, E., 2004. The metabolism of cyclamate to cyclohexylamine in humans during long-term administration. Toxicol. Appl. Pharmacol. 196 (3), 367–380. https://doi.org/10.1016/j.taap.2004.01.013.

Rippe, J., Angelopoulos, T., 2013. Sucrose, high-fructose corn syrup, and fructose, their metabolism and potential health effects: what do we really know? Adv. Nutr. 4 (2), 236–245. https://doi.org/10.3945/an.112.002824.

Smith, R., Cohen, S., Fukushima, S., Gooderham, N., Hecht, S., Guengerish, F., et al., 2018. The safety evaluation of food flavouring substances: the role of metabolic studies. Toxicol. Res. (Camb.) 7, 618–646. https://doi.org/10.1039/c7tx00254h.

Sweazea, K.L., Johnson, C.S., Miller, B., Gumpricht, E., 2018. Nitrate-rich fruit and vegetable supplement reduces blood pressure in normotensive healthy young males without significantly altering flow-mediated vasodilation: a randomized, double-blinded, controlled trial. J. Nutr. Metabol. https://doi.org/10.1155/2018/1729653.

Timbo, B., Moehler, K., Wolyniak, C., Klontz, K., 2004. Sulfites—a food and drug administration review of recalls and reported adverse events. J. Food Prot. 67 (8), 1806–1811. https://doi.org/10.4315/0362-028x-67.8.1806.

Tobacman, J., 2001. Review of harmful gastrointestinal effects of carrageenan in animal experiments. Environ. Health Perspect. 109 (10), 983–994. https://doi.org/10.1289/ehp.01109983.

Winkler, H., Notter, T., Meyer, U., Naegeli, H., 2018. Critical review of the safety assessment of titanium dioxide additives in food. J. Nanobiotechnol. 16 (1), 51. https://doi.org/10.1186/s12951-018-0376-8.

CHAPTER 5

Chemical contaminants in food

Brinda Mahadevan[a], Brittany Baisch[b], Susan C. Tilton[c], and A. Wallace Hayes[d]
[a]Brincor Associates, LLC, New Albany, OH, United States
[b]Enko Chem, Inc., Regulatory Toxicology, Mystic, CT, United States
[c]Environmental and Molecular Toxicology Department, Oregon State University, Corvallis, OR, United States
[d]University of South Florida, College of Public Health, Tampa, FL, United States

Introduction

Food contamination can be the result of either natural or human activity sources and is of major importance as it poses risks to the general population's health and well-being. Harmful chemicals and microorganisms in food as well as poor sanitation practices can cause adverse effects and illness in humans. This chapter focuses on chemical contaminants in foods, as opposed to microbiological contamination. The phrase 'chemical contamination' is used to indicate situations where chemicals are either present where they should not be or are at higher concentrations than the amount that is attributed as safe (Rather et al., 2017). The impact of chemical contaminants on consumer health and well-being is often apparent only after many years of exposure and a good example would be prolonged exposure to low levels (e.g., correlations to cancer) of a toxicant such as cadmium. The dietary exposure of 37 contaminants in the US food supply revealed that 20 of the contaminants in the food products analyzed had available cancer benchmark concentrations above the recommended level. These benchmark concentrations indicated that the daily exposure of the contaminants had a probability of showing untoward effects (Dougherty et al., 2000). Another study estimated the exposure of numerous dietary contaminants on children; these results found that the cancer benchmark of the contaminants was exceeded in all the children for dieldrin, arsenic, 1,1-dichloro-2,2-bis(p-chlorophenyl) ethylene (DDE), and dioxins (Vogt et al., 2012).

Chemical contaminants can occur at any time or place from the field to the plate, and typically include environmental contaminants, food processing contaminants, adulterants, and food additives as well as migrants

History of Food and Nutrition Toxicology
https://doi.org/10.1016/B978-0-12-821261-5.00007-6

from packaging materials. Chemical contaminants are both organic and inorganic molecules found in mass-produced products which include plastics, resins, pharmaceuticals, disinfectants, deodorants, detergents, petroleum products, pesticides, and biocides. Several chemical contaminants occur in food products naturally, rather than being formed or added during the manufacturing and processing of food products. Hence there is a need to focus on all potential sources of contaminants to guarantee the safety of our food supply (Hanlon et al., 2015).

The data are clearly showing that global climate change and variability can impact the degree of environmental contamination in foods. Changes in temperature and precipitation patterns increased the frequency and intensity of extreme weather events, ocean warming, and acidification and contaminants' transport pathways. For example, climate change-related acidification and changes in ocean salinity and precipitation can affect chemical contaminants in fish and shellfish (Tirado et al., 2010).

Chemical contaminants can be classified according to the source of the contamination and the mechanism by which they enter the food production supply chain. A list of chemical contaminations of different types and from different sources is found in Fig. 1.

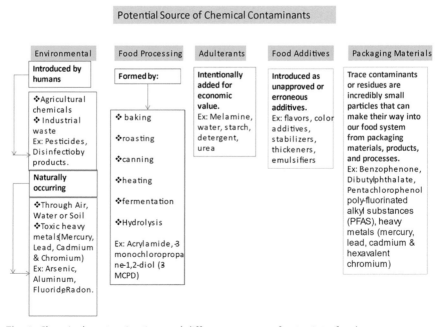

Fig. 1 Chemical contamination and different sources of entry into foods.

Historically, incidents of chemical contamination in foods and food products have not always been well documented. However, the reporting of chemical contamination in foods and food products has greatly improved in recent years. Globally, for example, the occurrence of mercury and other chemical food poisoning has been reported in several countries. Occurrences such as the poisoning that occurred in humans who ingested fish and shellfish contaminated by methyl mercury discharged in wastewater from a chemical plant into Minamata Bay, Japan (1956) or the ingestion of organomercury compounds used as seed dressings that resulted in organomercury poisoning in Iraq (1971–72) are early classical examples of chemical contamination (Fung et al., 2018). Rice contaminated with cadmium in the southern Chinese city of Guangzhou (1960), polychlorinated biphenyl (PCB) contamination in rice oil during processing in Japan (Umeda, 1972), PCBs and dibenzofurans in cooking oil in Taiwan, and PCB residue in turkeys marketed for human food in the United States (Miksch et al., 1990) are additional examples.

Food safety issues have not decreased but continue into the 21st century. Milk adulteration is a serious issue throughout the world. Some examples of adulteration of milk include the addition of water, whey, vegetable oil and protein, and milk from different species, which are economically motivated adulteration (Singh and Gandhi, 2015). In China, the 2008 contamination of infant formula with melamine affected infants and young children (El-Nezami et al., 2013). Further, the migration of packaging compounds into shelf-stable food has resulted in quality issues and acute gastrointestinal discomfort. Cross-contact from allergens continues to be a primary focal area for food toxicologists to ensure safety and quality during manufacturing and processing. Undeclared allergens are one of the leading causes of food recalls in the United States (FMI, 2020).

Toxic compounds such as nitrosamines, chloropropanols, acrylamide, furanes, or polycyclic aromatic hydrocarbons (PAHs) can be formed during food processing including cooking (Nerín et al., 2016). Although food processing has the potential to be a major contributor to chemical contamination in food, it is not considered in this chapter but is discussed elsewhere in this book.

Regulatory agencies around the world aim to protect the public from exposure to chemical contaminants that could result in adverse health effects. To standardize and minimize the risks that chemical contaminants pose to the food supply, regulatory agencies have established limits for many chemical compounds in different categories of food. Globally, there are over

40 unique chemicals that are regulated as contaminants in food, not including pesticides and veterinary and human drugs (Hanlon et al., 2015).

Substances that are added to food to maintain or improve the safety, freshness, taste, texture, or appearance of food are known as food additives. Some food additives have been in use for centuries for preservation, such as salt (meats or fish), sugar (marmalade), or sulfur dioxide (wine). Only amounts of additives shown to be safe are permitted in commercially prepared foods. The use of food additives is only justified when their use has a technological need, does not mislead consumers, and serves a well-defined technological function, such as to preserve the nutritional quality of the food or enhance the stability of the food.

The World Health Organization (WHO), in cooperation with the Food and Agriculture Organization of the United Nations (FAO), evaluates and reports on the safety of food additives, contaminants, naturally occurring toxins, and residues of veterinary drugs in food. These risk assessments are conducted by an independent, international expert scientific group—the Joint FAO/WHO Expert Committee on Food Additives (JECFA). The committee provides advice to FAO, WHO, and the member countries of both organizations, as well as to the Codex Alimentarius Commission (CAC). JECFA evaluations are based on scientific reviews of all available biochemical, toxicological, and other relevant data on a given chemical. The starting point for determining whether a food additive should be used without having harmful effects is to establish the acceptable daily intake (ADI). The ADI is an estimate of the amount of an additive in food or drinking water that can be safely consumed daily over a lifetime without adverse health effects.

In the last several decades, important developments in agricultural and food technology have greatly increased food production; however, chemical exposure from agricultural and other food production practices has resulted in major amendments to US federal food laws, including the Delaney Clause, aimed specifically at cancer-causing chemicals. Additionally, in the last 40 years, food safety research has resulted in an increased understanding of a range of untoward health effects from foodborne chemicals. The safety standard in US law is described as "reasonable certainty of no harm." The US FDA considers intakes of a chemical at or less than a chemical's Acceptable Daily Intake (ADI) to satisfy that standard (Wu and Rodricks, 2020). For food packaging, the Threshold of Regulation of 50 ppb indicates a proposed *de minimis* level for migrating packaging materials (US FDA, 2009).

This chapter is focused on chemical contaminants in food. The impact and influence of contaminants from sources such as pesticides, heavy metals, adulterants, processing and packing materials, and cross–contact allergens are included in the discussion. This chapter highlights the importance of collaboration among stakeholders within the supply chain, manufacturers, regulators, and academicians to ultimately ensure a safe food supply in the 21st century and beyond.

Environmental contaminants are introduced into food products by avenues other than during the manufacturing and production process. Therefore it is important to evaluate risk from other exposure pathways to ensure that such exposure is not contributing to contamination. Dietary risk assessments rely on multiple types of data, including food consumption data, typically obtained from the USDA's National Health and Nutrition Examination Survey (NHANES) database, combined with data from crop residues, drinking water levels, and residential exposures (https://www.cdc.gov/nchs/nhanes/index.htm; Reeves et al., 2019). These estimates provide an upper-limit value for exposures that likely overestimates risk to human health. To aid in these assessments, multiple tools have been developed through the EPA, FDA, EU, and other organizations to estimate exposure via ingestion of food or water (Table 1). Overall, there are multiple pathways for contamination of food and the risks that chemical contaminants pose in food are highly dependent on the types of ingredients and the location or conditions under which the crop is grown or sourced (Hanlon et al., 2016). In addition, the sources of contamination can vary broadly and include an intentional application (e.g., pesticide use), deposition of particulate matter onto edible produce (e.g., from atmospheric deposition), and uptake from contaminated soil and water (US Environmental Protection Agency, 2020).

Examples of chemical contaminants in food that are regulated include mycotoxins, metals, pesticides, polycyclic aromatic hydrocarbons (PAHs), polychlorinated dibenzo-para-dioxins (PCDDs), polychlorinated dibenzofurans (PCDFs), polychlorinated biphenyls (PCBs), solvents, and contaminants such as melamine and acrylamide. Some of the many tools for monitoring and estimating exposure for two common chemical contaminants, pesticide residues and heavy metals, in food and water are discussed as follows.

Pesticide residue monitoring

The US EPA defines a pesticide as any substance that is intended as a plant growth regulator, used as a nitrogen stabilizer, or used to prevent or destroy any pest. Pesticides include essentially any chemical used to mitigate pests

Table 1 Exposure assessment tools for estimating environmental chemical contamination in food and water.

Organization	Tool	Description
EPA	ExpoFIRST	A stand-alone tool that draws from data in the EPA's *Exposure Factors Handbook* for development of human exposure scenarios
EPA	Models for Pesticide Risk Assessment: Health Effects Models	Provides links to aquatic, terrestrial, and atmospheric exposure models as well as health effects models used to assess the risk of a pesticide to human health or the environment
EPA	Stochastic Human Exposure and Dose Simulation (SHEDS)	A model that can be used to simulate chemical exposures for a population over time
EPA	Human Health Water Quality Criteria and Methods for Toxics	Provides links to the Human Health Water Quality Criteria Table as well as supporting documents for the 2015 updated criteria
EPA	Food Safety; Pesticide Residues in Food	Provides information on assessing pesticide residues in food
EU	Food Contaminants Web Pages	Provide information about specific contaminants, general information about sampling and analysis of contaminants, and EU legislation governing potential food contaminants
EU	Rapid Alert System for Food and Feed (RASFF)	Tool to ensure the flow of information to enable swift reaction when risks to public health are detected in the food chain
EU	Rapid Assessment of Contaminant Exposure (RACE)	Provides estimates of different population groups' acute and chronic exposure to chemical contaminants from single foods
EU	Pesticide Residue Intake Model (PRIMo)	A model to calculate deterministic acute and chronic dietary exposure to pesticide residues
FDA	Total Diet Study (TDS)	Determines levels of various contaminants, including pesticide residues, and nutrients in foods
FDA	Pesticide Residue Monitoring Program Reports and Data	Summaries from the Food and Drug Administration of pesticide residues measured in food
FDA	FDA-iRISK	A web-based system designed to analyze data concerning microbial and chemical hazards in food and return an estimate of the resulting health burden on a population level
ILSI/JIFSAN	Heavy Metal Screening Tool	An aid for rapid risk assessments of heavy metals in food ingredients and food projects
USDA	Pesticide Data Program	A national pesticide residue monitoring program and produces the most comprehensive pesticide residue database in the United States

that cause plant diseases throughout the food production and processing chain from farm to storage and distribution to the consumer. Under the US EPA's Federal Insecticide, Fungicide, and Rodenticide Act (FIFRA), pesticides must have robust data packages to substantiate safety for human health and the environment within the scope of a specified intended use and use level. In the United States, both the USDA and FDA have testing methods to monitor pesticide residues on food (Table 1). These programs test for pesticides used around the world, including those that do not have approved tolerances in the United States. In addition, the EPA and FDA have developed tools for estimating exposure to chemical contaminants by ingestion of food and water that rely on residue screening data in addition to food consumption data and toxicological data on anticipated health effects. The FDA iRISK tool is an example of a publicly available online tool designed to analyze data for chemical and microbial hazards in food and provides an estimate of human health risk (Table 1). As analytical capabilities for detecting chemical contaminants in food improve (Medana, 2020), contaminants will be identified with more regularity at concentrations approaching parts per billion or parts per trillion range that may or may not pose an adverse effect in humans making an estimation of risk more difficult for those chemical contaminants without established regulatory limits (Kroes et al., 2000; Hanlon et al., 2016). Even as testing methods improve, recent data from the FDA and USDA monitoring of pesticides show that no samples for domestic cereals, eggs, and fish and only a small percentage of fruits (2.2%), vegetables (3.8%), and meat (0.13%) samples contained residue levels above tolerance amounts. Although most of the pesticides that exceed tolerance levels represent those pesticides that do not have established regulatory values (Reeves et al., 2019).

The Codex Alimentarius Commission (CAC) was created in 1963 by the Food and Agriculture Organization (FAO), the World Health Organization (WHO), and other bodies to develop food standards, guidelines, and codes of practice, for protecting the health of consumers, ensuring fair trade practices, and promoting coordination of work on food standards, including evaluating pesticide residue data and recommending maximum permissible limits (Wu and Rodricks, 2020).

In Europe, the European Food Safety Authority (EFSA) serves to conduct independent research and advises on potentially harmful substances in food, including pesticide residues. EFSA utilizes dietary exposure estimates from individual-level food consumption data for conducting exposure assessments and establishing allowable maximum residue levels (Lebelo et al., 2021).

To support their efforts, EFSA has established several open-access tools to estimate dietary exposure to foodborne chemicals (Ioannidou et al., 2021). In particular, RACE (Rapid Assessment of Contaminant Exposure) is a tool to provide a simplified risk assessment of chemical contaminants in food within the framework of the Rapid Alert System for Food and Feed (RASFF) (Table 1). RACE allows authorities the ability to provide a rapid evaluation of risk through estimates of acute and/or chronic dietary exposure to food contaminants from food consumption data and then decide the need for notification. Another online tool, Pesticide Residue Intake Model (PRIMo), allows for members of the agricultural/food industry to estimate acute and chronic dietary exposure to pesticide residues to support risk management decisions. Examples of how PRIMo has been successfully used to support risk assessments include the evaluation of deltamethrin residues in carob to establish a maximum residue level for consumption (Anastassiadou et al., 2020) and pyridaben residues on Egyptian strawberries and cucumber to understand health risks under different field conditions (Malhat et al., 2021).

Heavy metals and dietary metal intake

Many varieties of metals exist in the environment from both natural and anthropogenic sources and can serve as potential sources of contamination of food products. Soil and water contaminated with heavy metals, such as arsenic, cadmium, lead, mercury, and chromium, are a primary source of contaminants in the food chain. While dietary exposure to heavy metals in the United States has, for the most part, been found to fall below tolerable exposure limits (Mahaffey et al., 1975; Tran et al., 2015), there are examples of heavy metals exceeding tolerance limits in food products both globally and in the United States (Thompson and Darwish, 2019).

Since heavy metal contamination in food can lead to a variety of toxic effects and adverse health outcomes in humans, particularly neurodevelopmental effects in children, it is important to develop screening-level assessment tools for risk analysis (Wani et al., 2015). The International Life Sciences Institute (ILSI) and the Joint Institute for Food Safety and Applied Nutrition (JIFAN) have developed a web-based heavy metal screening tool that can be used as an aid for rapid risk assessments of heavy metals in foods and food products (Tran et al., 2015). The heavy metal dietary intake screening tool utilizes reference values and background exposure levels from the US EPA, the Joint FAO/WHO Expert Committee on Food Additives (JECFA), EFSA, and the Agency for Toxic Substances and Disease Registry

(ATSDR) along with food consumption data from NHANES and the Total Dietary Study (TDS, Table 1) to provide information regarding consumption and maximum allowable levels. The heavy metal dietary intake screening tool has been utilized to evaluate safety concerns for contaminated food products, including a case in which lead was detected in processed cheese and another case in which cadmium was detected in a concentrated apple juice product (Tran et al., 2015). In both cases, the metal concentrations were assessed with estimated exposure and consumption data to support risk management. Tools such as this provide an important resource for integrating food consumption, exposure, and toxicity data for risk assessment and management purposes.

Chemical contaminants in drinking water

Estimating contaminant exposure from ingestion requires data on concentration, dietary parameters, and time frames. In particular, knowledge of the chemical contaminants in drinking and groundwater is important for estimating overall exposure by ingestion and for evaluating the potential contamination of food products. In terms of pesticide contamination, drinking water exposures are calculated using models that take into account physical properties of the chemical and data regarding use rates and environmental variables (e.g., soil type and precipitation) (Reeves et al., 2019). Inorganic compounds are the largest proportion of contaminants in drinking water. Drinking water sourced from groundwater can be contaminated with heavy metals from natural or industrial sources. These exposures, which are more prevalent in low- or middle-income countries, are associated with several adverse health effects ranging from reproductive effects to cancers (Rather et al., 2017). The WHO has reported that nearly half the population in developing counties suffers from health problems due to a lack of potable water or contaminated drinking water (WHO, 1992).

Well-known examples of metal contamination in drinking water globally continue to emphasize the need to monitor drinking sources. For example, it is estimated that approximately 150 million people from more than 70 countries are at risk of arsenic contamination in their drinking water either from industrial or natural sources (Ozturk et al., 2011). Arsenic toxicity is associated with several adverse health outcomes, including cancer, reproductive, cardiovascular, renal, and skin-related diseases. Arsenic poisoning in South and Southeast Asian countries has impacted millions of individuals and further highlights concerns about the potential long-term health effects from chronic dietary exposures. The WHO has established several health-based drinking water guidelines for risk assessment, which have been adopted as standards in numerous countries (Van Leeuwen, 2000).

In the United States, the EPA sets legal limits for more than 90 contaminants in drinking water and enforces drinking water standards, in collaboration with individual states, through the Safe Drinking Water Act. In April 2014, a change in the water source in Flint, MI, resulted in lead leaching into the drinking water from the aging distribution system that contained a high percentage of lead pipes resulting in long-term health concerns associated with elevated blood lead levels in children in the Flint community (Hanna-Attisha et al., 2016). While this event highlighted concerns about metals in drinking water, historically private wells, which are not regulated as part of the Safe Drinking Water Act, are a more common source of lead contamination than most city water (Gibson et al., 2020).

Adulterants

Adulteration can be incidental when substances inadvertently contaminate food as a result of negligence or improper facility sanitation or supply chain quality controls. Adulteration can also be intentional when an ingredient is replaced with another substance or contaminated such that the quality of the food is debased (Banerjee et al., 2017; Spink, 2014; Schieber, 2018; Singh and Gandhi, 2015; Cavin et al., 2019).

Often, economic gain is a motivating factor for debasing food quality. An example would be adulterating fruit juices with sugars if crop yields are low or too expensive to manage otherwise (Kelly et al., 2021; Kelly et al., 2003; Day et al., 2001). In 2012 there was fraudulent activity in Europe to replace expensive beef with horse meat or the addition of diethylene glycol for glycerin in Australian wine. These are examples of concern over the integrity of the food supply chain, but fortunately, they did not introduce unreasonable human health risks. However, depending on the hazard profile and ingested dose of the adulterant, a detrimental public health crisis could have resulted.

Melamine

Melamine is a chemical used in cleaning and commercial products and plastics. The adulteration case with melamine is another example of an economic adulterant but this time, the public health outcome was significant.

The chemical was used to increase the nitrogen content of diluted or powdered milk, giving it the appearance of higher protein content. Of an estimated 294,000 victims, 6 babies died from kidney stones and other kidney damages, and an estimated 54,000 were hospitalized in China (Bhalla et al., 2009). Investigations revealed that batches of infant formula from various commercial brands contained melamine, and in some cases, the levels were 100- or 1000-fold higher than US FDA tolerable daily intakes. Nearly 70 countries took action with import warnings, bans, and recalls of infant formula manufactured in the affected regions of China.

Additional veterinary health effects were documented following the deaths of dogs and cats in the United States and the EU in 2004 and 2007. The animals died from kidney failure and sample analyses revealed melamine as well as cyanuric acid in the pet food.

The mode of action of melamine-induced kidney damage has been investigated (Mielech et al., 2021). Some of the pets and children suffered from acute kidney injury while others developed more chronic kidney disease. Melamine is excreted in the urine but also precipitates in the distal renal tubules, forming intratubular green radial crystals and crystalluria. The crystal deposition was more severe in pet food cases where cyanuric acid was also present as an adulterant. Cyanuric acid is white, odorless, and is a chlorine stabilizing agent used for water treatment. It forms a lattice structure with melamine at slightly acidic pH, as would be present in the proximal nephron (Bhalla et al., 2009). Lithiasis within the urinary system was the immediate health effect (Liu, 2014; Hu et al., 2013). A prospective cohort study by Gao et al. (2016) noted that the formation of kidney stones if left untreated or without being removed led to chronic glomerular and tubular kidney injuries. Aside from the immediate health crisis caused by the melamine incidents, the availability of infant formula in the affected regions of China indicated subsequent effects for several years (Tang, 2015).

Food packaging contaminants

Emerging new packaging technologies and the growing use of virgin, recycled, and reclaimed materials have impacted food packaging safety issues. Aside from the hazard profile and purity of the materials postprocess, an understanding of the contaminants in the packaging matrices and if they are in direct contact with food is important. The potential for migration into the food from packaging must be considered an industry best practice, even if extremely challenging. There is a lack of industry standards in terms of how to measure or sometimes what to measure. Through a survey of packaging required for a portfolio and by tiering the materials into buckets based on process, contact with food, and the potential for exposure are good starting places for establishing a packaging food safety program. Understanding the risk of contaminant exposure via food from packaging materials can be a daunting task and requires knowledge of the supply chain, production processes, and the composition of packaging materials. The physicochemical properties of indirect food contact materials can help predict if they can migrate through specific materials. Many food manufacturers have conducted detailed investigations to ensure the absence of migration. Product recalls over the past 20 years, however, have revealed the need for industry standards, practical methods, and agreed-upon guidance for developing packaging food safety programs.

In 2012 Advent calendars were recalled in the EU due to mineral oil in the printing ink migrating into the chocolate candies. Due to the hydrophobic properties of the mineral oils, the oils had the potential to migrate out of the printing ink and through plastic wrappers. In recent years, innovative solutions have been introduced to block the mineral oil migration.

A second recall of candy Advent calendars occurred in Denmark in 2019 resulting from customer complaints of the chocolates tasting like cardboard. Following an investigation by the Danish authorities, the calendars were deemed appropriate for food contact with a conclusion of no health risk. Although details of the investigation were not published in the public domain, this example raises the importance of not only understanding food toxicology and safety concerns, but also regulatory concerns and the role of food quality, taste, and perception. It can be difficult, at times, to discern if there is an overlap between a food safety concern and a quality issue.

Adhesives are compounds of interest in the food industry, such as those used in packaged cereals, snacks, and other shelf-stable items. A cereal recall in the United States in 2010 was prompted by consumer complaints regarding the taste and smell as well as symptoms of nausea and diarrhea. The suspected compound was methylnaphthalene and it was suspected that sensitive subpopulations of consumers may have developed symptoms. The compound, even at low ppb levels, has a strong odor that can easily be detected. Interestingly, methylnaphthalene is GRAS and this example is difficult to discern between food quality and food safety. Undoubtedly, a collaborative effort between sustainability and product stewardship experts, packaging engineers, supply chain quality, and toxicologists within the industry, academia, and regulatory agencies is essential for establishing best practices in this area.

Tools for the detection of adulterants

As economic adulteration becomes more sophisticated and widespread, analytical tools and methods for detecting food fraud are increasingly important. This field is known as food authentication. In the past 10 years, more sophisticated techniques with greater sensitivity have been developed. However, many techniques are new and expensive and require specific protocol development depending on the substances and compounds of interest. In some cases, species differentiation is the goal rather than the detection of specific chemicals. Further, the presence of substances or chemical compounds at trace levels can often be misperceived as a health risk, and therefore risk assessments and communications to internal stakeholders and the general public become increasingly important

Table 2 provides examples of methods that have been useful for detecting contaminants and adulterants in food.

Allergen cross-contact

Although other sections of this textbook will highlight the importance of allergen management for human health and food integrity, the risk of allergen cross-contact via contamination or insufficient sanitation practices

Table 2 Examples of successful methods for food authentication.

Method	Adulterants Detected
Attenuated Total Reflection—Fourier Transfer Infrared (ATR-FTIR) Spectroscopy	Hazelnut, canola, and sunflower oils in sesame oil; urea in milk (Chapman et al., 2018)
Polymerase Chain Reaction (PCR)	Meat species identification (Teen Teh and Dykes, 2014)
Matrix-Assisted Laser Desorption Ionization-Time of Flight Mass Spectrometry (MALDI-TOF-MS) or Liquid Chromatography Electron Spray Ionization Mass Spectrometry (LC-ESI-MS)	Milk speciation (Cuollo et al., 2010)
Proton Nuclear Magnetic Resonance Spectroscopy (^{1}H NMR)	Differentiation of wild or farmed fish species (Vidal et al., 2012)
Gas Chromatography triple quadrapole Mass Spectrometry (GC-MS/MS)	BPA migration from packaging (Ruiz-Matute et al., 2018)
High Performance Liquid Chromatography (HPLC)	Melamine in milk and pet food (Filazi et al., 2012)

is critical. Avoidance of allergen cross-contact is the primary goal, wherein storage, quality, and supply chain sanitation practices must be part of an over-all Allergen Control Plan (Food Allergy Research and Resource Program, 2008) (08FARP-003 Brochure (pdf version) (unl.edu).

For example, sanitation between manufacturing runs of allergen-containing and nonallergen production must be up to industry standards (Food Allergy Research and Resource Program, 2008) (08FARP-003 Brochure (pdf version) (unl.edu). Sanitation should result in no visible res-idue and involve several individual inspections of the line before startup. In cases where the certainty of no cross-contact is not guaranteed, such as when it is not physically possible to fully inspect the equipment a whereby "may contain" or other cross-contact types of product labeling may be nec-essary. At a minimum, food-allergic consumers would be aware of the risk. Importantly, precautionary allergen labeling is not beneficial unless war-ranted. It can become a burden to modify practices overtime to try to justify the removal of the language since consumers with specific food allergies would be accustomed to avoiding the product and proof to remove labeling could be met with increased scrutiny (Allen and Taylor, 2018). There are also cases where there may be no visible residue but due to the viscosity and characteristics of the food matrix potentially binding to certain equipment and forming a film, the residue is not always visible. Swabbing for certain food-allergic proteins may be necessary. These are simply examples of what may be necessary within food manufacturing sites, but allergen manage-ment experts should always be consulted to ensure that an end-to-end al-lergen control plan from the supply chain, storage, production, sanitation, and then to labeling is appropriate.

The highest risk to allergic consumers occurs in cases of unintentional allergen cross-contact, where the product does not have appropriate label-ing by FDA or USDA standards, or to ensure food safety (Sheehan et al., 2018). Food allergens present in low ppm ranges can cause very serious, life-threatening reactions. This is why undeclared food allergens are the pri-mary reason for food recalls in the United States (FMI, 2020) and are one of the leading causes of recalls worldwide (HACCP Mentor, 2021). Not only is the health risk problematic but hundreds of thousands of pounds of food must also be destroyed, and reputational risk can be economically devastating.

In 2015 an FDA Consumer Advisory was issued that suggested that those with peanut allergies avoid ground or powdered cumin (Food Safety News, 2015; Living Allergic, 2016). Dozens of allergic reactions were reported to

Table 3 Food allergen cross-contact resources.

Reference	Description and significance
Sarver et al. (2021)	Describes on-the-go portable assays that can be utilized for on-site, rapid, and sensitive detection of various allergenic proteins. Methodologies like these have future promise during audits of the supply chain when qualifying a new vendor, where unbeknownst allergenic proteins may be present
Goodman et al. (2016)	"AllergenOnline"—an allergen database to assess novel food proteins for potential cross-reactivity with known allergens. Such a database can be leveraged for understanding cross-reactivity and considerations for consumer health and product labeling within a portfolio
Gupta et al. (2017)	Provides a perspective on supply chain allergen management programs and how they are impacted by economic factors. Such considerations help with supply chain audits and maintaining collaborative partnerships with suppliers

regulatory authorities and not only were cumin spices in scope for recall, but also meat products and spice kits or products containing cumin. Upon investigation, the levels of peanut were in some cases 5-10% of the cumin as supplied. Experts speculated that at such high levels, it was likely to be intentional adulteration rather than cross-contact due to residue. Whether or not cumin was intentionally adulterated was never resolved with certainty. Such investigations often deal with a complex international supply chain, with the challenges of investigating remote geographies after elapsed time.

Table 3 provides additional resources of the current state of cross-contact allergen detection of residues.

Future directions for food safety

The past few years have witnessed an upsurge in incidences relating to food safety issues, which can be attributed to different factors as alluded to in this chapter. The rapid change in climatic conditions, presence of a mixture of nonfood residues in food as a result of industrial development, new agricultural practices, and environmental pollution are all playing a pivotal role in food safety. In such situations, ensuring the ingredients and any potential contaminants or adulterants in the products do not present a significant public health risk can be a challenge. The use of botanicals and dietary supplements derived from natural substances as an addition for improved quality of life or claimed medical benefits has become increasingly more frequent in the United States and other global geographies. Hence manufacturers and regulators may have to acclimatize to the specific food safety challenges that natural ingredients bring to the table. Rapid advances are being made in analytical methods, research approaches, and authentication tools to address the implications this holds for supply chain integrity and food safety. However, the challenge in identifying fraudulent ingredients is that the methods of adulteration vary widely. The addition of peanut protein to cumin powder or the dilution of natural curcumin with synthetic curcuminoids is just two examples of a variety of adulteration methods recently observed in the industry (Press release, 2017).

Dietary supplements, as defined by the Dietary Supplement Health and Education Act of 1994 (DSHEA) in the United States, are products intended to supplement the diet that contain vitamins, minerals, amino acids, other dietary substances, and/or herbs or other botanicals (Abdel-Rahman et al., 2011). Botanical dietary supplements (BDS) are generally available as whole plants, plant parts, powdered plant material, or plant extracts. These supplements may also be marketed in various forms, including powders, tablets, capsules, gummies, teas, tinctures, and essential oils. Extensive use of botanical dietary supplements, combined with a paucity of toxicity data, has fueled interest in developing approaches for ensuring the safety of BDS (Shipkowski et al., 2019). In the United States, the FDA functions to regulate BDS through Good Manufacturing Practices (cGMP) and postmarket surveillance along with New Dietary Ingredient (NDI) requirements. Recently, recognizing the inherent BDS challenges of complexity and variability, the National Toxicology Program (NTP) initiated discussions and held a workshop titled "Addressing Challenges in the Assessment of Botanical Dietary Supplement Safety" to identify and improve the understanding to ensure the safety of botanical dietary supplements (Rider et al., 2018).

The outcome of the workshop was directed toward comprehending the hazards associated with BDS and recommendations for continued progress that included three areas. They were the following: (1) developing and applying approaches for identifying toxicologically active constituents; (2) developing and validating methods for determining "sufficient similarity" of complex BDS; and (3) establishing recommendations for conducting evaluations of absorption, distribution, metabolism, and elimination (ADME) of BDS including the underlying kinetics of these processes (Rider et al., 2018).

Genetically modified contamination is the unwanted escape and spread of Genetically Modified Organisms (GMOs) or genetic material from GMOs to non-GM plants, animals, and foods. This dispersal can occur through pollen spread and seed escape and mixing of food and feed. GM contamination is living pollution that can self-replicate.

In conclusion, food safety and nutrition are interlinked as they can impact health and malnutrition in different age groups. In light of numerous chemical contamination incidents, food safety in the 21st century may need to expand beyond improving the nutritional profile and transparency of ingredients. For example, the botanical dietary supplement industry through collaboration with research agencies, such as the NTP, National Institute of Environmental Health and Safety (NIEHS), and National Institute of Health (NIH), may be able to conduct toxicity testing for specific botanicals rendering them safe and provide useful information to consumers for better decision making.

Acknowledgment

Thanks to Ms. Yashoda Murali, sophomore student, New Albany High School, New Albany, Ohio, for creating Fig. 1 for this chapter.

References

Abdel-Rahman, A., Anyangwe, N., Carlacci, L., Casper, S., Danam, R.P., Enongene, E., Erives, G., Fabricant, D., Gudi, R., Hilmas, C.J., Hines, F., Howard, P., Levy, D., Lin, Y., Moore, R.J., Pfeiler, E., Thurmond, T.S., Turujman, S., Walker, N.J., 2011. The safety and regulation of natural products used as foods and food ingredients. Toxicol. Sci. 123 (2), 333–348. https://doi.org/10.1093/toxsci/kfr198.

Allen, K.J., Taylor, S.L., 2018. The consequences of precautionary allergen labeling: safe haven or unjustifiable burden? J. Allergy Clin. Immunol. Pract. 6 (2). https://doi.org/10.1016/j.jaip.2017.12.025.

Anastassiadou, M., Bernasconi, G., Brancato, A., Cabrera, L.C., Ferreira, L., Greco, L., Jarrah, S., Kazocina, A., Leuschner, R., Magrans, J.O., Miron, I., Nave, S., Pedersen, R., Reich, H., Rojas, A., Sacchi, A., Santos, M., Theobald, A., Vagenende, B., Verani, A., 2020. Modification of the existing maximum residue level for deltamethrin in carobs/Saint John's breads. EFSA (European Food Safety Authority) J. 18 (10), 6271. https://doi.org/10.2903/j.efsa.2020.6271.

Banerjee, D., Chowdhary, S., Chakraborty, S., Bhattacharyya, R., 2017. Recent advances in detection of food adulteration. In: Food Safety in the 21st Century: Public Health Perspective, pp. 145–160, https://doi.org/10.1016/B978-0-12-801773-9.00011-X.

Bhalla, V., Grimm, P.C., Chertow, G.M., Pao, A.C., 2009. Melamine nephrotoxicity: an emerging epidemic in an era of globalization. Kidney Int. 75 (8), 774–779. https://doi.org/10.1038/ki.2009.16.

Cavin, C., Cottenet, G., Fuerer, C., Tran, L.A., Zbinden, P., 2019. Food fraud vulnerabilities in the supply chain: an industry perspective. In: Encyclopedia of Food Chemistry, pp. 670–678, https://doi.org/10.1016/B978-0-08-100596-5.21788-5.

Chapman, J., Power, A., Chandra, S., Roberts, J., Cozzolino, D., 2018. Countering the 'Fake News' of food: the role of chemometrics with vibrational spectroscopy techniques. Ref. Mod. Food Sci. https://doi.org/10.1016/B978-0-08-100596-5.22373-1.

Cuollo, M., Caira, S., Fierro, O., Pinto, G., Picariello, G., Addeo, F., 2010. Toward milk speciation through the monitoring of casein proteotypic peptides. Rapid Commun. Mass Spectrom. 24 (11). https://doi.org/10.1002/rcm.4564.

Day, M.P., Correia, P., Hammond, D.A., 2001. 13C-IRIS: an improved method to detect the addition of low levels of C4-derived sugars to juices. J. AOAC Int. 84 (3). https://doi.org/10.1093/jaoac/84.3.957.

Dougherty, C.P., Holtz, S.H., Reinert, J.C., Panyacosit, L., Axelrad, D.A., Woodruff, T.J., 2000. Dietary exposures to food contaminants across the United States. Environ. Res. 84 (2). https://doi.org/10.1006/enrs.2000.4027.

El-Nezami, H., Tam, P.K.H., Chan, Y., Lau, A.S.Y., Leung, F.C.C., Chen, S.F., Lan, L.C.L., Wang, M.F., 2013. Impact of melamine-tainted milk on foetal kidneys and disease development later in life. Hong Kong Med. J. 19 (6), S34–S38.

Filazi, A., Sireli, U., Ekici, H., Can, H., Karagoz, A., 2012. Determination of melamine in milk and dairy products by high performance liquid chromatography. J. Dairy Sci. 95, 602–608. https://doi.org/10.3168/jds.2011-4926.

FMI, 2020. Undeclared Allergens Continue to be the Leading Cause of U.S. Food Recalls. Accessed 26 Aug 2021.

Food Allergy Research & Resource Program, 2008. Components of an Effective Allergen Control Plan: A Framework for Food Processors.

Food Safety News, 2015. https://www.foodsafetynews.com/2015/04/china-toughens-up-food-safety-laws-with-new-amendments/.

Fung, F., Wang, H.S., Menon, S., 2018. Food safety in the 21st century. Biom. J. 41 (2), 88–95. https://doi.org/10.1016/j.bj.2018.03.003.

Gao, J., Wang, F., Kuang, X., Chen, R., Rao, J., Wang, B., Li, W., Liu, H., Shen, Q., Wang, X., Xu, H., 2016. Assessment of chronic renal injury from melamine-associated pediatric urolithiasis: an eighteen-month prospective cohort study. Ann. Saudi Med. 36 (4), 252–257.

Gibson, J.M., Fisher, M., Clonch, A., Macdonald, J.M., Cook, P.J., 2020. Children Drinking Private Well Water Have Higher Blood Lead Than Those With City Water., https://doi.org/10.1073/pnas.2002729117/-/DCSupplemental.

Goodman, R.E., Ebisawa, M., Ferreira, F., Sampson, H.A., van Ree, R., Vieths, S., Baumert, J.L., Bohle, B., Lalithambika, S., Wise, J., Taylor, S.L., 2016. AllergenOnline: a peer-reviewed, curated allergen database to assess novel food proteins for potential cross-reactivity. Mol. Nutr. Food Res. 60 (5). https://doi.org/10.1002/mnfr.201500769.

Gupta, R.S., Taylor, S.L., Baumert, J.L., Kao, L.M., Schuster, E., Smith, B.M., 2017. Economic factors impacting food allergen management: perspectives from the food industry. J. Food Prot. 80 (10). https://doi.org/10.4315/0362-028X.JFP-17-060.

Hanlon, P., Brorby, G.P., Krishan, M., 2016. A Risk-Based Strategy for Evaluating Mitigation Options for Process-Formed Compounds in Food: Workshop Proceedings., https://doi.org/10.1177/1091581816640262.

Hanlon, P.R., Hlywka, J.J., Scimeca, J.A., 2015. A risk-based strategy for controlling chemical contaminants as relevant hazards in food ingredients. Food Prot. Trends 35 (2), 89–100.

Hanna-Attisha, M., Lachance, J., Sadler, R.C., Schnepp, A.C., 2016. Elevated blood lead levels in children associated with the flint drinking water crisis: a spatial analysis of risk and public health response. Am. J. Public Health 106, 283–290. https://doi.org/10.2105/AJPH.2015.303003.

Hu, P., Wang, J., Hu, B., Lu, L., Zhang, M., 2013. Clinical observation of childhood urinary stones induced by melamine-tainted infant formula in Anhui province, China. Arch. Med. Sci. https://doi.org/10.5114/aoms.2013.33350.

Ioannidou, S., Cascio, C., Gilsenan, M.B., 2021. European Food Safety Authority open access tools to estimate dietary exposure to food chemicals. Environ. Int. 149. https://doi.org/10.1016/j.envint.2020.106357.

Kelly, S.D., Abrahim, A., Rinke, P., Cannavan, A., 2021. Detection of exogenous sugars in pineapple juice using compound-specific stable hydrogen isotope analysis. npj Sci. Food. https://doi.org/10.1038/s41538-021-00092-5.

Kelly, S.D., Rhodes, C., Lofthouse, J.H., Anderson, D., Burwood, C.E., Dennis, M.J., Brereton, P., 2003. Detection of sugar syrups in apple juice by δ2H‰ and δ13C‰ analysis of hexamethylenetetramine prepared from fructose. J. Agric. Food Chem. 51 (7). https://doi.org/10.1021/jf021044p.

Kroes, R., Galli, C., Munro, I., Schilter, B., Tran, L.-A., Walker, R., Würtzen, G., 2000. Threshold of toxicological concern for chemical substances present in the diet: a practical tool for assessing the need for toxicity testing. Food Chem. Toxicol. 38 (2–3), 255–312. https://doi.org/10.1016/S0278-6915(99)00120-9.

Lebelo, K., Malebo, N., Jonas Mochane, M., Masinde, M., Hardisson de la Torre, A., Rubio, C., Javier Carrascosa Iruzubieta, C., 2021. Chemical contamination pathways and the food safety implications along the various stages of food production: a review. Int. J. Environ. Res. Public Health. https://doi.org/10.3390/ijerph18115795.

Liu, J., 2014. Infant formula safety in China. World J. Pediatr. 10. https://doi.org/10.1007/s12519-014-0447-3.

Living Allergic, 2016. Special Report: Investigating Motive and Spice Safety in the Big Peanut-Tainted Cumin Recalls. allergicliving.com. (Accessed 26 August 2021).

Mahaffey, K.R., Corneliussen, P.E., Jelinek, C.F., Fiorino, J.A., 1975. Heavy metal exposure from foods. In: Environmental Health Perspectives. Vol. 12.

Malhat, F., Saber, E.-S., Anagnostopoulos, C., Shokr, A., 2021. Dissipation behavior and dietary risk assessment of pyridaben in open field strawberries and cucumber under Egyptian cultivation conditions. Environ. Sci. Pollut. Res. https://doi.org/10.1007/s11356-021-14752-2.

Medana, C., 2020. Analysis of chemical contaminants in food. Toxics 8, 27. https://doi.org/10.3390/toxics8020027.

HACCP Mentor, 2021. https://haccpmentor.com/food-allergen-cross-contact/.

Mielech, A., Puścion-Jakubik, A., Socha, K., 2021. Assessment of the risk of contamination of food for infants and toddlers. Nutrients 13, 2358.

Miksch, D., Means, W., Johns, J., 1990. Food Safety: Residues in Animal-Derived Foods. Issued: 8e90, University of Kentucky Agricultural Communication Services. http://www2.ca.uky.edu/agcomm/pubs/ip/ip11/ip11.htm. (Accessed 12 August 2021).

Nerín, C., Aznar, M., Carrizo, D., 2016. Food contamination during food process. Trends Food Sci. Technol. 48, 63–68. https://doi.org/10.1016/J.TIFS.2015.12.004.

Ozturk, M., Metin, M., Altay, V., Bhat, R.A., Ejaz, M., Gul, A., Unal, B.T., Hasanuzzaman, M., Nibir, L., Nahar, K., Bukhari, A., Dervash, M.A., Kawano, T., 2011. Arsenic and human health: genotoxicity, epigenomic effects, and cancer signaling. Biol. Trace Elem. Res. https://doi.org/10.1007/s12011-021-02719-w.

Rather, I.A., Koh, W.Y., Paek, W.K., Lim, J., 2017. The sources of chemical contaminants in food and their health implications. Front. Pharmacol. 8 (Nov). https://doi.org/10.3389/fphar.2017.00830.

Reeves, W.R., McGuire, M.K., Stokes, M., Vicini, J.L., 2019. Assessing the safety of pesticides in food: how current regulations protect human health. Adv. Nutr. 10 (1), 80–88. https://doi.org/10.1093/advances/nmy061.

Rider, C.V., Walker, N.J., Waidyanatha, S., 2018. Getting to the root of the matter: challenges and recommendations for assessing the safety of botanical dietary supplements. Clin. Pharmacol. Ther. 104 (3), 429–431. https://doi.org/10.1002/cpt.1088.

Ruiz-Matute, A.I., Rodríguez-Sánchez, S., Sanz, M.L., Soria, A.C., 2018. Chromatographic technique: gas chromatography (GC). In: Modern Techniques for Food Authentication, pp. 415–458, https://doi.org/10.1016/B978-0-12-814264-6.00012-8.

Sarver, R.W., Almy, D.J., Bergeron, E.R., Strong, B.F., Steiner, B.A., Donofrio, R., Lupo, A.J., Gray, R.L., Sperry, A.K., 2021. Overview of portable assays for the detection of mycotoxins, allergens, and sanitation monitoring. J. AOAC Int. 104 (1). https://doi.org/10.1093/jaoacint/qsaa113.

Schieber, A., 2018. Introduction to food authentication. In: Modern Techniques for Food Authentication, pp. 1–21, https://doi.org/10.1016/B978-0-12-814264-6.00001-3.

Sheehan, W.J., Taylor, S.L., Phipatanakul, W., Brough, H.A., 2018. Environmental food exposure: what is the risk of clinical reactivity from cross-contact and what is the risk of sensitization. J. Allergy Clin. Immunol. Pract. 6 (6). https://doi.org/10.1016/j.jaip.2018.08.001.

Shipkowski, K.A., Betz, J.M., Birnbaum, L.S., Bucher, J.R., Paul, M., Hopp, D.C., Mackay, D., Oketch-rabah, H., Walker, N.J., Rider, C.V., 2019. Naturally complex: perspectives and challenges associated with botanical dietary supplement safety assessment. Food Chem. Toxicol. 919, 963–971. https://doi.org/10.1016/j.fct.2018.04.007.

Singh, P., Gandhi, N., 2015. Milk preservatives and adulterants: processing, regulatory and safety issues. Food Rev. Int. 31 (3), 236–261. https://doi.org/10.1080/87559129.2014.994818.

Spink, J., 2014. Safety of food and beverages: risks of food adulteration. Encycl. Food Safety 3, 413–416. https://doi.org/10.1016/B978-0-12-378612-8.00300-0.

Tang, L., 2015. Infant formula crisis in China: a cohort study in Sichuan province. Health Popular Nutr. 1 (1), 117–122.

Teen Teh, A.H., Dykes, G.A., 2014. Meat species determination. In: Encyclopedia of Meat Sciences, pp. 265–269, https://doi.org/10.1016/B978-0-12-384731-7.00209-9.

Thompson, L.A., Darwish, W.S., 2019. Environmental chemical contaminants in food: review of a global problem. J. Toxicol. https://doi.org/10.1155/2019/2345283.

Tirado, M.C., Clarke, R., Jaykus, L.A., McQuatters-Gollop, A., Frank, J.M., 2010. Climate change and food safety: a review. Food Res. Int. 43 (7), 1745–1765. https://doi.org/10.1016/j.foodres.2010.07.003.

Tran, N.L., Barraj, L.M., Scrafford, C., Bi, X., Troxell, T., 2015. Partitioning of dietary metal intake—a metal dietary exposure screening tool. Risk Anal. 35 (5). https://doi.org/10.1111/risa.12322.

Umeda, G., 1972. PCB Poisoning in Japan. Ambio 1 (4).

US Environmental Protection Agency, 2020. Exposure Assessment Tools by Routes—Ingestion. [Cited August 10, 2021]. Available from: https://www.epa.gov/expobox/exposure-assessment-tools-routes-ingestion.

US FDA, 2009. http://www.fda.gov/NewsEvents/PublicHealth-Focus/ucm179005.htm. (Accessed 12 August 2021).

Van Leeuwen, F.X.R., 2000. Safe drinking water: the toxicologist's approach. Food Chem. Toxicol. 38 (Suppl.1), S51–S58. https://doi.org/10.1016/S0278-6915(99)00140-4.

Vidal, N.P., Manzanos, M.J., Goicoechea, E., Guillén, M.D., 2012. Quality of farmed and wild sea bass lipids studied by 1H NMR: usefulness of this technique for differentiation on a qualitative and a quantitative basis. Food Chem. 135 (3), 1583–1591. https://doi.org/10.1016/J.FOODCHEM.2012.06.002.

Vogt, R., Bennett, D., Cassady, D., Frost, J., Ritz, B., Hertz-Picciotto, I., 2012. Cancer and non-cancer health effects from food contaminant exposures for children and adults in California: a risk assessment. Environ. Health: A Global Access Sci. Source 11 (1). https://doi.org/10.1186/1476-069X-11-83.

Wani, A.L., Ara, A., Usmani, J.A., 2015. Lead toxicity: a review. Interdiscip. Toxicol. 8 (2), 55–64. https://doi.org/10.1515/intox-2015-0009.

WHO, 1992. Our Planet, Our Health. Report of the WHO Commission on Health and Environment. World Health Organization, Geneva.

Wu, F., Rodricks, J.V., 2020. Forty years of food safety risk assessment: a history and analysis. Risk Anal. 40. https://doi.org/10.1111/risa.13624.

CHAPTER 6

Food allergy, intolerance, and sensitivity

Kevin N. Boyd[a] and Joseph L. Baumert[b]

[a]The Hershey Company, Hershey, PA, United States
[b]Food Allergy Research and Resource Program (FARRP), Department of Food Science and Technology, University of Nebraska, Lincoln, NE, United States

Introduction

Food allergy is not a new phenomenon but has certainly garnered significant attention over the past 10–20 years as prevalence and awareness have continued to rise (Kattan, 2016; Sampson, 2016). Although estimates vary greatly as to the number of food-allergic individuals, a significant contributor to the differences in estimates can be attributed to some self-reporting vs. physician-diagnosed allergy (Gupta et al., 2018, 2019; Lyons et al., 2020). Nevertheless, food allergy continues to be a growing public health concern. While some allergies, such as those to milk and egg, are more likely to be outgrown as a child gets older; others, such as peanut and tree nut, are more likely to be lifelong (Savage and Johns, 2015; Wood, 2003). Moreover, other food allergies, such as an allergy to shellfish, are more prevalent in adults. Although the cascade of intracellular events and the immune response following exposure to an allergen are well understood (Helm and Burks, 2000; Sampson et al., 2018), the explanation as to why some individuals develop food allergies while most do not remains unknown. While many factors have been suggested to contribute to the increase in the prevalence of food allergies over the last 20–30 years, recent clinical data supports the dual-allergen exposure hypothesis. The dual-allergen exposure hypothesis suggests that allergic sensitization to foods occurs through low-dose skin (cutaneous) exposure, whereas consistent high-dose oral exposure to food allergens that are introduced early in an infant's diet contributes to tolerance (Du Toit et al., 2018). Studies such as the LEAP Study (Learning Early About Peanut allergy) and other follow-on studies have demonstrated that the occurrence of peanut allergy can be significantly reduced when peanut is introduced into an infant's diet (Du Toit et al., 2015).

History of Food and Nutrition Toxicology
https://doi.org/10.1016/B978-0-12-821261-5.00010-6

Although the majority of this chapter will focus on immunoglobulin-E-mediated reactions (i.e., IgE-mediated food allergy), there are several terms related to food hypersensitivities that will be briefly described. When discussing food hypersensitivities, one factor is parsing between food allergy, celiac disease, food intolerance, and food sensitivity as these terms have distinct meanings but might be used in an interchangeable/overlapping manner in some cases (e.g., nontechnical settings, subject/patient descriptions). Understanding the true terminology and the definitions of each of these terms is even more important with the increasing popularity of over-the-counter food sensitivity tests because sensitization to a food by itself does not automatically equate to a food allergy (i.e., if there is no clinical response).

Food allergy is defined as an immune-mediated response to the ingestion of a food. Food allergies can be IgE mediated or non–IgE mediated, with IgE-mediated food allergies involving Type I hypersensitivity reactions that result in the rapid onset of symptoms that can potentially lead to anaphylaxis. Non–IgE-mediated food allergies involve Type IV reactions, which are cell mediated and have a slower onset. The mechanisms of non–IgE-mediated immune reactions are not as well characterized, may not easily be associated with particular foods as they are delayed reactions, and do not typically result in anaphylaxis (Cianferoni, 2020). The immune-mediated responses are primarily elicited by proteins in food; however, there are examples of nonprotein-mediated food allergies. There can also be allergic reactions to raw fruits or vegetables, which is known as oral allergy syndrome or pollen food allergy syndrome. Pollen food allergy syndrome typically involves mild reactions, such as itching (pruritus) of the lips, tongue, and mouth due to a contact reaction to labile proteins found in fruits and vegetables (Webber and England, 2010; Price et al., 2015). Individuals who experience pollen food allergy syndrome are typically sensitized to pollen from sources such as birch, ragweed, mugwort, or grasses. Upon ingestion of certain fruits or vegetables, these individuals will experience mild reactions to homologous proteins found in some fruits and vegetables due to sensitization to environmental pollens (Price et al., 2015).

Unlike food allergies, which by definition involve the immune system, food intolerances involve physiological responses that are not driven by the immune system. Food intolerances typically result in gastrointestinal discomfort and are not life threatening (Tuck et al., 2019). Compared with a food allergy where patients practice strict avoidance, individuals with a food intolerance may be able to consume a small amount of food to which they are intolerant without experiencing discomfort. The most common food intolerance is lactose intolerance, which has an interesting story linked to evolution and the need for a gene in chromosome 2 to code for the lactase enzyme, beta-galactosidase (Anguita-Ruiz et al., 2020). A deficiency in the lactase enzyme leads to a decreased efficiency in the small intestine's ability to metabolize lactose into simple sugars that can be absorbed into the bloodstream. Bacteria in the gastrointestinal system then feed on the lactose and produce fatty acids and gases that can lead to bloating and gastrointestinal discomfort. Individuals with lactose intolerance may be able to consume up to 12 g of lactose during a single eating occasion so complete avoidance of lactose-containing foods may not be needed by all individuals. The severity of symptoms associated with ingestion of milk by an individual who is lactose intolerant is very different than ingestion by an individual with an IgE-immune-mediated allergy to milk protein. Favism is another food intolerance that also involves a metabolic deficiency in the enzyme (i.e., glucose-6-phosphate dehydrogenase; G6PD) needed to break down beta-glucosides (vicine and convicine), which are found in some foods such as fava beans (Luzzatto and Arese, 2018). Vicine and convicine are hydrolyzed in the gastrointestinal tract into divicine and isouramil, which are highly reactive redox compounds. Once these compounds are transferred into the blood by epithelial cells in the gastrointestinal tract, they can produce reactive oxygen species, such as hydrogen peroxide and superoxide anion, that rapidly oxidize NADPH and glutathione (Luzzatto and Arese, 2018). Red blood cells that lack sufficient production of G6PD needed to reverse glutathione depletion succumb to oxidative damage, which results in acute hemolytic anemia. This can become severe in some individuals.

Reference may also be made to food sensitivity. Although the term hypersensitivity may be used to broadly cover immune-mediated allergies, intolerances, and sensitivities, sensitivity itself is a term that does not have a precise definition. Sensitivity is commonly used to describe situations where an individual associates a variety of potential physiological responses with a food. Food intolerances may also be included in the broader designation of food sensitivities. Food sensitivities may also include idiosyncratic responses where the mechanisms and underlying factors leading to an adverse response to a food or food component are not known. In addition, the causal relationship may also be uncertain. Although the underlying causes and/or relationships from a food are unknown, the associated effects are typically mild. One of the most common current examples of a food sensitivity is nonceliac gluten sensitivity (NCGS) or nonceliac wheat sensitivity

(NCWS), which involves potential reactivity to gluten or other wheat proteins and results in gastrointestinal symptoms (e.g., abdominal pain and bloating), headaches, fatigue, and/or "foggy mind" (Leonard et al., 2017). Nonceliac gluten sensitivity/nonceliac wheat sensitivity resolves with the removal of gluten or wheat from the diet, and NCGS/NCWS is different from celiac disease as the autoantibodies produced in celiac patients are not present. In addition, damage to the villi in the small intestine is not observed during biopsy.

Celiac disease is an autoimmune disease in which gluten found in wheat, barley, rye, and hybridized strains of these grains triggers an inflammatory reaction that damages the small intestine and negatively affects the small intestine's ability to absorb nutrients from food. This can lead to a myriad of potential long-term effects if gluten is not avoided (Caio et al., 2019). While celiac disease is managed like a food allergy (i.e., avoidance of gluten in the diet) and also involves an immunological response, the mechanisms and clinical manifestations are distinct (Green et al., 2015). The primary difference is that a food allergy to wheat, for example, would elicit an immediate Type I hypersensitivity reaction in a wheat-allergic patient, whereas the response in a patient with celiac disease would typically be delayed and would not drive the same type of visual objective symptoms seen in a wheat-allergic patient experiencing an IgE-mediated reaction. In addition, while wheat is one of the priority allergens, IgE-mediated allergy to rye and barley is not common. Individuals with celiac disease, however, must avoid wheat, barley, rye, and hybridized strains of these grains as they all contain various protein fractions that share common amino acid sequences and result in observed clinical cross-reactivity in celiac patients following exposure to these grains. Although these protein fractions have specific names in each of the grains from which they are derived (i.e., gliadin in wheat, hordein in barley, and secalin in rye), specific prolamin protein fractions from these grains are collectively referred to as gluten. In the United States, wheat is a priority allergen that requires labeling of the allergen source as outlined in the Food Allergy Labeling and Consumer Protection Act (FALCPA) of 2004. In addition, the United States has enacted regulations that establish labeling requirements for products bearing voluntary gluten-free claims. Other countries, such as Canada and the European Union, include cereal grains containing gluten, which encompasses wheat, rye, barley, and hybridized strains (and perhaps even oats) into their priority allergen lists. The following section will discuss the regulations around allergens in more detail.

Food allergen regulations and management in manufacturing

As mentioned at the beginning of the chapter, food allergies are not a new phenomenon, but regulations around allergen labeling and "formal" management criteria are more recent. The Codex Alimentarius, which is a set of international food standards, guidelines, and codes of practice that are developed through a joint food safety program between the Food and Agriculture Organization (FAO) of the United Nations and the World Health Organization (WHO), included a list of foods and ingredients known to cause hypersensitivity as part of the Labeling of Prepackaged Foods standard in 1999 (Codex Alimentarius, 2018). Some countries have adopted these allergens, whereas others have developed their own lists and implemented local regulations. In the United States, the passage of FALCPA in 2004 defined eight priority allergenic food sources and required these allergenic foods to be labeled by their common name on prepackaged food items when they, or components derived from the named allergens, are intentional ingredients in a food (including natural flavors or processing aids). In 2021, the Food Allergy Safety, Treatment, Education, and Research (FASTER) Act was signed into law, which covered several elements related to food allergy, including adding sesame as the 9th major allergen in the United States.

The use of precautionary or advisory allergen labeling statements (e.g., may contain) is not addressed in FALCPA. These voluntary statements are allowed based on the discretion of the food manufacturer with the only regulatory stipulation being that (1) these statements are truthful and not misleading, and (2) that they are not used in lieu of good manufacturing practices, including established allergen controls and cleaning practices. The potential for cross contact, or the unintended presence of an allergen in a product due to the supply chain and/or manufacturing process, is not addressed in FALCPA. Management of allergens in the supply chain and within manufacturing facilities has been addressed by food manufacturers through prerequisite programs and allergen control programs for many years; however, allergen management was "formalized" in regulation with the passage of the Food Safety Modernization Act (FSMA) in 2011 in which allergens were incorporated as chemical hazards that must be controlled. Some countries around the world are just now implementing food allergen regulations, and laws continue to change as foods are assessed under the criteria of prevalence, severity, and potency as to whether changes need to be made to priority allergen lists. Although there is a core set of foods that commonly appears on priority allergen lists of countries around the world, there are also unique differences in regulated allergens that may be based, at least in part, on differences in diet and food consumption in different regions of the world.

Allergen management is addressed in various food safety regulations around the world, and the Codex Alimentarius also recently published an updated code of practice for allergen management (Codex Alimentarius, 2020). Many other organizations have produced, or are currently working on, "best practice" guidelines for effective allergen management. One of the unique elements of living with a food allergy compared with managing other common conditions or diseases is that we need to eat, typically multiple times a day; thus, there is a reliance and trust that is necessary between consumers and anyone providing food. This includes food manufacturers, restaurants, and even friends and family. Managing and living with a food allergy can have a significant impact on the quality of life for both the individual and his/her family (DunnGalvin et al., 2015). There is a lot of anxiety that comes with managing a food allergy, primarily stemming from the fear of unknowingly consuming an allergen and the uncertainties that are inherent with managing/living with a food allergy. There is uncertainty associated with the allergy itself in terms of individual sensitivity and the potential severity of a reaction, which can contribute to an allergic individual's daily anxiety (Turner et al., 2016). In addition, individuals managing one or more food allergies must also navigate the uncertainty associated with choosing safe foods as they must trust the information provided on a product label or that is verbally relayed to them by staff when eating away from home. In these scenarios, allergic individuals must also trust the management and handling practices of food manufacturers and food service workers. Food manufacturers have allergen controls in place throughout the supply chain to mitigate unintentional allergen cross contact and ultimately to properly label and package products. In many cases, food manufacturing facilities are managing a variety of allergens in the facility and producing products with different allergen profiles on the same manufacturing equipment.

Regulated allergens that are ingredients in a product must be declared by their common name; however, precautionary allergen labeling (e.g., may contain X) is voluntary, and food manufacturers must determine when such a statement is warranted. The intended purpose of these statements is to convey meaningful risks to food-allergic consumers and identify products that should be avoided if an individual is allergic to one of the foods that is mentioned. In reality, however, these statements are overused by manufacturers and are not used consistently among companies such that allergic consumers cannot easily make sense of products on store shelves and are often not able to make informed decisions. This can result in both the unnecessary avoidance of foods by some individuals as well as risky choices by others who begin to ignore precautionary allergen labeling because the use is so widespread and not believed to align with risk (DunnGalvin et al., 2015). For the food manufacturer, allergens are a chemical hazard that must be controlled, and management strategies must be in place to mitigate cross contact. While actively working to prevent unintentional allergen presence, manufacturers must also decide when to include precautionary allergen labeling to convey risks when allergen cross contact is unavoidable. This conundrum, combined with regulatory uncertainty and a target of "zero" (or below the limit of quantification of analytical tests) for residual allergen, contributes to the overuse of precautionary allergen labeling.

A regulatory limit of 20 ppm for gluten-free labeling has been established in many countries, which stems not only from past analytical capabilities of test methods but also from clinical evidence that intake at this level does not pose a significant risk for individuals with celiac disease. Similarly, with IgE-mediated food allergy, individuals have a threshold below which he/she will not react. With advances in statistical modeling and increased clinical data from allergic individuals that have undergone low-dose oral food challenges, population-based reference doses have been derived that can estimate the milligram amount of food protein from an allergenic source that is predicted to elicit a reaction in a certain percentage of an allergic population (Houben et al., 2020; Remington et al., 2020; Taylor et al., 2014). This information can be used as a tool for a variety of elements in allergen management, labeling, and analytical tests. Because food-allergic individuals practice strict avoidance to even tiny amounts of their allergen(s) based upon clinical advice from medical professionals, and many also have a lack of trust in food manufacturers, the concept of reference doses (or thresholds) does not immediately align with what they have likely been told since diagnosis. Moreover, most food-allergic individuals have little to no knowledge regarding their individual sensitivity/threshold as they have not undergone a graded low-dose challenge to establish their minimal eliciting dose. There are some exciting advances in food allergen diagnostics, however, that could provide patients and clinicians with this kind of data (Santos et al., 2022). This could not only have the possibility to unlock more food choices (e.g., an individual with a high threshold/low sensitivity may be able to safely consume most products that bear precautionary allergen labeling or feel comfortable at certain restaurants), but this knowledge could also decrease anxiety and potentially change the clinical management of food allergies from a one-size-fits-all approach to a patient-specific approach (Sicherer et al., 2022). Indeed, there is even a clinical trial occurring as this book chapter is being written that is investigating whether peanut- and/or tree nut-allergic individuals with a high eliciting dose are better served by ingesting low levels of their allergen below their eliciting dose rather than following a strict avoidance diet as strict avoidance could impact the development of oral tolerance (Trendelenburg et al., 2022). The concept of thresholds is the same as the goal of oral immunotherapy, or desensitization, in which patients want to get to a level that protects them from accidental low-dose exposure (Baumert et al., 2018; Remington et al., 2018, 2019). This type of knowledge by patients, combined with effective use of all available information to identify meaningful risks by food manufacturers, will decrease the unnecessary avoidance of foods by food-allergic consumers. The following sections will highlight how food manufacturers can effectively utilize risk assessment as part of their allergen management and labeling programs.

Food allergen risk assessment

Conducting a risk assessment for a food allergen follows the same general principles as any chemical risk assessment; however, there are several unique elements compared with typical chemical risk assessments (Crevel et al., 2014a). There is ongoing research to try to identify and predict the allergenicity of foods/novel foods, but in addition to the natural complexities of this research, there is the added challenge that foods, or the specific proteins in foods, are not inherently hazardous (or allergenic) and do not trigger abnormal immune responses in the vast majority of individuals. The mechanisms by which some individuals develop food allergy while most tolerate the same food with no issue are not clear. These aspects set food allergies and allergen risk assessments apart from most chemical risk assessments where the assessment may focus on ensuring an acceptable margin of safety for a sensitive subpopulation, but the hazard is relevant for the general population; thus, assessing the sensitive subpopulation, or most sensitive endpoint, serves as a surrogate for the less sensitive populations or endpoints.

Chemical risk assessments are primarily conducted for chemicals that are not intentionally added to products or that have limited exposure. Common food allergens are excellent sources of protein and other nutrients as part of a healthy diet and are either consumed directly or used in numerous products for functional and/or nutritional benefits. In addition, with other types of consumer products, exposure/product use may be self-limiting; however, food is intentionally eaten multiple times per day and systemic exposure is 100% so there is significantly more exposure than other types of consumer products. The presence of a priority/regulated allergen as an intentional ingredient, which is a hazard for individuals with a food allergy to that particular food, is managed through labeling (i.e., required to be listed in the ingredient statement) similar to other acute chemical hazards, such as corrosivity in consumer products. The actual hazard that is being assessed in an allergen risk assessment is the unintentional presence of an allergen(s) (NASEM Report, 2017). Although any food may elicit an allergic reaction, the focus is primarily on the priority/regulated allergens of various countries.

Hazard identification and characterization

Cosmetics and consumer products, or the ingredients in those products, are routinely tested for dermal sensitization using in vivo or in vitro methods. In addition, there are structural features of dermal sensitizers that help predict their skin protein binding potential and ability to cause a dermal reaction. In silico models have been developed that utilize these features to predict a chemical's sensitization potential. Hazard identification for food allergens is somewhat different than dermal sensitizers used in consumer products. In addition, the severity of a dermal sensitization reaction is not comparable to the potential severity of a food-allergic reaction. The primary intent with products that may contain low levels of potential dermal sensitizers is to avoid inducing skin sensitization; however, products may elicit dermal sensitization reactions in previously sensitized individuals. Although there are assays and tests to evaluate the dermal sensitization potential of compounds, foods are not quite the same. The allergenicity of food proteins can be modified by processing, and some, such as milk and egg, may be tolerated by some allergic individuals after being baked (Upton and Nowak-Wegrzyn, 2018). Some food allergies can also be outgrown over time as a child develops, whereas others may be foods an individual has consumed with no issue for decades and suddenly develops an allergy in adulthood. While allergens are hazards to food-allergic individuals, the hazard being assessed in allergen risk assessment is the unintentional presence of an allergen.

Hazard characterization involves defining the dose-response relationship and identifying a reference dose that can be used to compare against the exposure estimate (Houben et al., 2020; Remington et al., 2020; Westerhout et al., 2019). Whereas many chemical hazards are identified and characterized through in vivo animal data or in vitro data, human data exist for food allergens. Indeed, the hazard characterization for food allergens has been established from human data collected from clinical oral food challenges to inform the dose-response relationship. There are, however, a variety of additional factors that can impact this dose-response relationship both on the subject side and in the food processing side. There are data showing associations with IgE binding to specific proteins within foods and the potential severity of a reaction upon ingestion, but there is a wide range of variability within each allergen in terms of patient response. Human clinical data from oral food challenges have been modeled to derive population-based reference doses for the most prevalent food allergens. A panel of experts who participated in the Ad hoc Joint FAO/WHO Expert Consultation on Risk Assessment of Food Allergens recently concluded that the amount of protein from an allergenic source predicted to elicit an allergic reaction in 5% of individuals with a given allergy (i.e., ED_{05}) could be used to inform a risk assessment (FAO/WHO, 2021). Although a current approach developed in Australia and New Zealand to assist in risk assessment for the food industry (i.e., the Voluntary Incidental Trace Allergen Labeling or VITAL) recommended the use of the ED_{01} protein level, the FAO/WHO group's analysis of available data indicated that the use of the ED_{05} value is unlikely to result in more severe reactions than the use of the ED_{01} protein level and therefore would provide additional benefit in food choice while not significantly increasing the risk.

Exposure

One of the challenges in the exposure estimate for any chemical risk assessment is to balance conservative defaults with realistic, data-driven information. Whereas many consumer product assessments look at dermal exposure, inhalation exposure, and perhaps incidental oral exposure with factors such as dermal absorption or how much of the inhaled dose is absorbed impacting the estimated exposure, exposure assessments for food are much less complicated regarding the route of exposure and systemic uptake. Although the route of exposure in food allergen cross contact assessments is focused on oral exposure, estimating the potential unintentional presence of protein that could end up in a product is inherently challenging as the presence is actively trying to be prevented, and large-scale food manufacturing is a dynamic process with a variety of factors that could impact that estimation and/or change the accuracy of that estimate on any given day. These factors create additional uncertainty and variability that must be taken into account.

In food allergen exposure assessments, there are two primary elements: (1) the amount of unintentional allergen presence in a food, and (2) the amount of food consumed that would contain the allergenic residue of concern. One might reason that this latter aspect is rather simple; however, there are still some challenges with estimating food consumption for various products, particularly for acute exposure to a single item vs. looking at data for a typical diet. Food allergen assessments are also different from other dietary assessments of a chemical where the focus may be on a subchronic or chronic endpoint and utilize an average exposure over time. Food packages contain recommended serving sizes, but these are typically based on nutritional intake and not necessarily reflective of consumer behavior. There are food intake databases that can be used for information, and sometimes the risk assessor can estimate based on a pack type (e.g., even if an item has multiple servings as the recommendation, certain items in a nonreclosable package, for example, are likely to be consumed in a single eating occasion).

The other more challenging element is estimating the potential presence of an unintentional allergen, which could be present from agricultural commingling (e.g., soy in wheat flour from crop production, harvesting, and shared storage), unavoidable introduction at an ingredient supplier, some source within the supply chain, and/or introduced during the production process of the final marketed food product. All of these potential sources need to be taken into account. Because allergens are a chemical hazard that must be managed, this unintentional presence is almost always sporadic and hard to accurately estimate. If an assessor was able to get an accurate estimate and consistently characterize what might unintentionally be there, then there is a question as to whether something could be done to prevent the cross contact. These challenges result in conservative exposure assessments, which limit the utility of these assessments for proactive precautionary labeling, especially as manufacturers currently must work toward a target of "zero" (or below the limit of quantification of analytical tests) for the residual allergen (Crevel et al., 2014b). When performing a risk assessment for an incident, exposure estimates can be more accurate as specific data can be generated based on the facts uncovered during the investigation. Other factors that add complexity are the form of the allergen and whether the unintentional cross contact is likely to be homogenous. For example, particulate forms of an allergen (e.g., pieces of nuts) may pose a risk and would likely not be homogeneously interspersed throughout a product; thus, the exposure estimate for the small fraction that might have a particulate piece of an allergen would be high, but the majority of the product may not contain any unintentional allergen. In addition, batch production processes may be more likely to result in homogeneous dispersion and a more accurate exposure estimate than continuous processes.

Risk characterization

The current management plan for food-allergic consumers is strict avoidance. With the fear of a life-threatening reaction, this equates to a black-and-white approach where the thought of risk or risk assessment seems foreign. In addition, the general advice for food-allergic patients is that no amount of allergen is safe and no prior reaction can predict a future reaction. Again, there is a disconnect between this information and the concept of thresholds and risk assessment, even though many food-allergic consumers are interested/open to the idea of oral immunotherapy, which is essentially desensitization that allows the individual to tolerate some amount of an allergen (i.e., a threshold). These individuals would still be allergic to the food, but raising their threshold/eliciting dose improves quality of life by opening up food choices and minimizing the risk of a severe reaction due to unintentional ingestion of a small amount of allergen through cross contact. One challenge in characterizing the risk of unintentional allergen presence in food is that production is dynamic, and the risk can increase or decrease at different points in time, which is different than some chemical contaminant assessments that are not dependent on cleaning/sanitation or the sequence of production. While food allergen risk assessment clearly serves a valuable function in managing an incident, there is also utility in assessments to evaluate the potential risks of unintentional allergen presence and provide some consistency and meaning to voluntary precautionary allergen labeling on foods (e.g., may contain X).

As additional clinical data become available to continue to inform population-based thresholds and our understanding of risk, the reference doses for each allergen can continue to be refined. Because these reference doses are small amounts of protein for many allergens, exposure assessments cannot be unnecessarily conservative or everything will still appear to be a risk. With some of the complexities in exposure estimates for some types of production processes (i.e., continuous processes with allergen particulate), the unintentional allergen presence may be even more sporadic (e.g., affect 1:100 units, or 1:10,000, or 1:100,000, or 1:1,000,000). In such situations, 99%–99.9999% of the product produced may not pose a risk to a food-allergic consumer, but a small fraction of the product produced may pose a significant risk in the rare instance that a particulate is present as the exposure to the unintended allergen could be quite high. In a practical sense, if the unintended particulate allergen cross contact only occurs in a fraction of a percent of the product produced, then the chances that someone with the same allergy as the potential particulate cross contact would happen to purchase/consume an impacted consumer unit are very low; however, the food allergen risk assessment is conducted for the sensitive population (i.e., the food-allergic consumer). Nevertheless, this type of information provides context, and decisions based upon stakeholder consensus must be made on what constitutes an acceptable risk that will be operationally achievable while protecting food-allergic consumers and not further restricting food choices (Crevel et al., 2014b).

In addition to allergen controls throughout the supply chain, the consumer-facing piece of risk management is precautionary allergen labeling. As precautionary allergen labeling is intended to communicate a potential risk to the food-allergic consumer, the alignment on an approach and guidance for this type of risk management is best done in a collaborative manner with all stakeholders (i.e., food manufacturers, researchers, food safety regulators, clinicians, and patient advocacy groups). There are multiple such efforts currently ongoing that will produce guidance for food manufacturers on these topics. In addition, there are exciting advances in diagnostics that will hopefully provide more confidence in the accuracy of a food allergy diagnosis (Foong et al., 2021; Suárez-Fariñas et al., 2021) and provide patients with an indication of their sensitivity or threshold range (Hourihane et al., 2017). Oral food challenge data and dose-response modeling have demonstrated that some patients can tolerate large doses of his/her allergen of concern, whereas others react to very small amounts (Taylor et al., 2014; Remington et al., 2020). Clinicians and patients have not had this information on an individual level beyond those that participated in clinical trials; thus, most patients receive the same clinical management advice irrespective of their specific circumstances. With better diagnostic information, patients may be able to adopt more individualized management plans, and the idea that not every encounter with an allergen will produce a life-threatening reaction will assist in quality of life and trust in food products that may utilize the same reference dose data to provide more meaning and consistency to precautionary allergen labeling. In situations when a given allergen is not an intentional ingredient in a product, but the product is not marketed as "free from" the allergen, there is confusion as to what could be encompassed in this "middle area." This is the realm where risk assessment can provide for meaningful and transparent application of precautionary allergen labeling. For example, a low level of residual, sporadic, unintentional allergen cross-contact (despite following good manufacturing practices) that would result in consumption (i.e., exposure) below an identified reference dose would not be included in a precautionary allergen statement as the level would be anticipated to be tolerated (i.e., not elicit a reaction) in 95%–99% of the allergic population. In addition, for the 1%–5% who are predicted to respond, this level of exposure would not be anticipated to elicit a severe reaction. The fear for allergic individuals is severe, potentially life-threatening reactions. Because of the lack of properly conducted risk assessments and transparent communication, many foods are unnecessarily labeled with precautionary allergen statements (i.e., making them appear risky) that inadvertently restrict important food choices and can impact healthy diets. Food-allergic individuals would likely be willing to accept a small risk of minor to moderate reactions if the risk of severe reaction was mitigated and the associated benefit was significantly more food choice.

Conclusions

Chemical risk assessments are commonly performed for things like cancer risk or liver toxicity and regardless of the effect, they are endpoints that we cannot visualize and immediately associate with an effect. In addition, there is a lot of conservatism built into these assessments, and cancer assessments, for example, involve repeated exposure over a long period. Again, using cancer assessments as an example, typically the accepted risk is somewhere around 1:100,000 chance of developing cancer based on exposure to a particular chemical over a lifetime. With food allergens, the effects are immediate, potentially severe to life threatening, and commonly involve children. Although individuals can be allergic to any food, in terms of prioritization and risk management, the focus is on priority/regulated allergens, and food safety regulators, clinicians, and allergen/immunology experts continue to look at prevalence, severity, and potency as criteria to evaluate priority allergen lists around the globe. Individual differences may arise in countries due to local diets and what types of foods are commonly consumed.

Currently, alternative sources of protein and food innovations are uncovering potential new allergen concerns. For example, innovations involving insect protein may elicit reactions in individuals with shellfish allergy due to the potential clinical cross-reactivity of homologous proteins found in insects and shellfish. In addition to cross-reactivity with existing allergens, exposure to new and/or concentrated forms of protein that have previously been consumed in foods (e.g., the use of pea protein isolate) may alter the immunological response. Another more recently uncovered allergy, which is believed to be induced by bites from the lone star tick, involves an immunologic reaction to galactose-alpha-1,3-galactose (i.e., alpha-gal), which is a sugar found in nonprimate mammals and can elicit a reaction following the consumption of red meat (Commins et al., 2009; Commins, 2020). There are also innovations such as dairy proteins that are generated in culture that are virtually identical to animal-derived proteins, and thus still allergenic, but can be used in products with a vegan or sustainability claim and/or focus. This can be confusing as vegan products tend to be viewed as safe by individuals with milk or egg allergy. Moreover, sustainability research and minimizing food waste have also led to innovations in food packaging materials that may use components derived from common allergens, such as almond husks or chitosan from shellfish. As food and packaging innovation continues, there will be new elements where research and risk assessments will be critical to understanding the potential impact of these ingredients, packaging, and products. There are also many exciting therapeutics in development in the food allergy area, which had been neglected for many years, but until these pharmaceutical interventions are mainstream, or the underlying cause of food allergies is discovered and managed, allergen management practices in the food and agricultural industry will continue to be critically important for protecting food-allergic consumers.

References

Anguita-Ruiz, A., Aguilera, C.M., Gil, A., 2020. Genetics of lactose intolerance: an updated review and online interactive world maps of phenotype and genotype frequencies. Nutrients 12 (9), 2689.

Baumert, J.L., Taylor, S., Koppelman, S., 2018. Quantitative assessment of the safety benefits associated with increasing clinical peanut thresholds through immunotherapy. J. Allergy Clin. Immunol. Pract. 6, 457–465.

Caio, G., Volta, U., Sapone, A., Leffler, D.A., et al., 2019. Celiac disease: a comprehensive current review. BMC Med. 17, 142.

Cianferoni, A., 2020. Non-IgE mediated food allergy. Curr. Pediatr. Rev. 16 (2), 95–105.

Codex Alimentarius, 2018. General Standard for the Labeling of Prepackaged Foods, CXS 1-1985. In: Adopted in 1985. Amended in 1991, 1999, 2001, 2003, 2005, 2008, and 2010. Revised in 2018. https://www.fao.org/fao-who-codexalimentarius/sh-proxy/en/?lnk=1&url=https%253A%252F%252Fworkspace.fao.org%252Fsites%252Fcodex%252F-Standards%252FCXS%2B1-1985%252FCXS_001e.pdf. (Accessed 28 February 2022).

Codex Alimentarius, 2020. Code of Practice on Food Allergen Management for Food Business Operators, CXC 80–2020. In: Adopted in 2020. https://www.fao.org/fao-who-co-dexalimentarius/sh-proxy/en/?lnk=1&url=https%253A%252F%252Fworkspace.fao.org%252Fsites%252Fcodex%252FStandards%252FCXC%2B80-2020%252FCX-C_080e.pdf. (Accessed 28 February 2022).

Commins, S.P., 2020. Diagnosis and management of alpha-gal syndrome: lessons from 2,500 patients. Expert Rev. Clin. Immunol. 16 (7), 667–677.

Commins, S.P., Satinover, S.M., Hosen, J., Mozena, J., et al., 2009. Delayed anaphylaxis, angioedema, or urticaria after consumption of red meat in patients with IgE antibodies specific for galactose-alpha-1,3-galactose. J. Allergy Clin. Immunol. 123 (2), 426–433.

Crevel, R.W.R., Baumert, J.L., Baka, A., Houben, G., Knulst, A.C., Kruizinga, A., Luccioli, S., Taylor, S.L., Madsen, C., 2014a. Development and evolution of risk assessment for food allergens. Food Chem. Toxicol. 67, 262–276.

Crevel, R.W.R., Baumert, J.L., Luccioli, S., Baka, A., Hattersley, S., Hourihane, J., Ronsmans, S., Timmermans, F., Ward, R., Chung, Y.J., 2014b. Translating reference doses into allergen management practice: challenges for stakeholders. Food Chem. Toxicol. 67, 277–287.

Du Toit, G., Roberts, G., Sayre, P.H., Bahnson, H.T., Radulovic, S., Santos, A.F., Brough, H.A., Phippard, D., Basting, M., Feeney, M., Turcanu, V., Server, M.L., Lorenzo, M.G., Plaut, M., Lack, G., for the LEAP Team, 2015. Randomized trial of peanut consumption in infants at high risk for peanut allergy. N. Engl. J. Med. 372, 803–813.

Du Toit, G., Sampson, H.A., Plaut, M., Burks, A.W., Akdis, C.A., Lack, G., 2018. Food allergy: update on prevention and tolerance. J. Allergy Clin. Immunol. 141, 30–40.

DunnGalvin, A., Dubois, A.E.J., Flokstra-de Blok, B.J.M., Hourihane, J.O'.B., 2015. The effects of food allergy on quality of life. In: Ebisawa, M., Ballmer-Weber, B.K., Vieths, S., Wood, R.A. (Eds.), Food Allergy: Molecular Basis and Clinical Practice. Chemical Immunology and Allergy, vol. 101. Karger, pp. 235–252.

FAO/WHO, 2021. Ad hoc Joint FAO/WHO Expert Consultation on Risk Assessment of Food Allergens, 2021. Updated in 2022. Part 2: Review and establish threshold levels in foods of the priority allergens (Summary and Conclusions). https://www.fao.org/3/cb6388en/cb6388en.pdf (https://www.fao.org/3/cb9312en/cb9312en.pdf, 04 June 2022) and https://www.fao.org/3/cb9312en/cb9312en.pdf. (Accessed 6 April 2022).

Foong, R.-X., Dantzer, J.A., Wood, R.A., Santos, A.F., 2021. Improving diagnostic accuracy in food allergy. J. Allergy Clin. Immunol. Pract. 9 (1), 71–80.

Green, P.H.R., Lebwohl, B., Greywoode, R., 2015. Celiac disease. J. Allergy Clin. Immunol. 135 (5), 1099–1106.

Gupta, R.S., Warren, C.M., Smith, B.M., et al., 2018. The public health impact of parent-reported childhood food allergies in the United States. Pediatrics 142 (6), e20181235.

Gupta, R.S., Warren, C.M., Smith, B.M., et al., 2019. Prevalence and severity of food allergies among US adults. JAMA Netw. Open 2 (1), e185630.

Helm, R.M., Burks, W.A., 2000. Mechanisms of food allergy. Curr. Opin. Immunol. 12 (6), 647–653.

Houben, G.F., Baumert, J.L., Blom, W.M., et al., 2020. Full range of population eliciting dose values for 14 priority allergenic foods and recommendations for use in risk characterization. Food Chem. Toxicol. 146, 111831.

Hourihane, J.O'.B., Allen, K.J., Shreffler, W.G., DunnGalvin, G., Nordlee, J.A., Zurzolo, G.A., DunnGalvin, A., Gurrin, L.C., Baumert, J.L., Taylor, S.L., 2017. Peanut allergen threshold study (PATS): novel single-dose oral food challenge study to validate eliciting doses in peanut allergic children. J. Allergy Clin. Immunol. 139, 1583–1590.

Kattan, J., 2016. The prevalence and natural history of food allergy. Curr. Allergy Asthma Rep. 16, 47.

Leonard, M.M., Sapone, A., Catassi, C., et al., 2017. Celiac disease and nonceliac gluten sensitivity: a review. JAMA 318 (7), 647–656.

Luzzatto, L., Arese, P., 2018. Favism and glucose-6-dehydrogenase deficiency. N. Engl. J. Med. 378, 60–71.

Lyons, S.A., Clausen, M., Knulst, A.C., Ballmer-Weber, B.K., Fernandez-Rivas, M., Barreales, L., Bieli, C., Dubakiene, R., Fernandez-Perez, C., Jedrzejczak-Czechowicz, M., Kowalski, M.L., Kralimarkova, T., Kummeling, I., Mustakov, T.B., Papadopoulos, N.G., Popov, T.A.,

Xepapadaki, P., Welsing, P.M.J., Potts, J., Mills, E.N.C., van Ree, R., Burney, P.G.J., Le, T.-W., 2020. Prevalence of food sensitization and food allergy in children across Europe. J. Allergy Clin. Immunol. Pract. 8 (8), 2736–2746.e9.

National Academies of Sciences, Engineering, and Medicine, 2017. Finding a Path to Safety in Food Allergy: Assessment of the Global Burden, Causes, Prevention, Management, and Public Policy. The National Academies Press, Washington, DC.

Price, A., Ramachandran, S., Smith, G., Stevenson, M.L., Pomeranz, M.K., Cohen, D.E., 2015. Oral allergy syndrome (pollen-food allergy syndrome). Dermatitis 26 (2), 78–88.

Remington, B.C., Krone, T., Koppelman, S.J., 2018. Quantitative risk reduction through peanut immunotherapy: safety benefits of an increased threshold in Europe. Pediatr. Allergy Immunol. 29, 762–772.

Remington, B.C., Krone, T., Kim, E.H., Bird, J.A., Green, T.D., Lack, G., Fleischer, D.M., Koppelman, S.J., 2019. Estimated risk reduction to packaged food reactions by epicutaneous immunotherapy (EPIT) for peanut allergy. Ann. Allergy Asthma Immunol. 123 (5), 488–493.e2.

Remington, B.C., Westerhout, J., Meima, M.Y., et al., 2020. Updated population minimal eliciting dose distributions for use in risk assessment of 14 priority allergens. Food Chem. Toxicol. 139, 111259.

Sampson, H.A., 2016. Food allergy: past, present and future. Allergol. Int. 65, 363–369.

Sampson, H.A., O'Mahony, L., Burks, A.W., et al., 2018. Mechanisms of food allergy. J. Allergy Clin. Immunol. 141 (1), 11–19.

Santos, A.F., Kulis, M.D., Sampson, H.A., 2022. Bringing the next generation of food allergy diagnostics into the clinic. J. Allergy Clin. Immunol. Pract. 10 (1), 1–9.

Savage, J., Johns, C.B., 2015. Food allergy: epidemiology and natural history. Immunol. Allergy Clin. North Am. 35 (1), 45–49.

Sicherer, S.H., Abrams, E.M., Wegryzn, A.N., Hourihane, J.O.'.B., 2022. Managing food allergy when the patient is not highly allergic. J. Allergy Clin. Immunol. Pract. 10 (1), 46–55.

Suárez-Fariñas, M., Suprun, M., Kearney, P., Getts, R., Grishina, G., et al., 2021. Accurate and reproducible diagnosis of peanut allergy using epitope mapping. Allergy Eur. J. Allergy Clin. Immunol. 76 (12), 3789–3797.

Taylor, S.L., Baumert, J.L., Kruizinga, A.G., Remington, B.C., Crevel, R.W.R., et al., 2014. Establishment of reference doses for residues of allergenic foods: report of the VITAL expert panel. Food Chem. Toxicol. 63, 9–17.

Trendelenburg, V., Dolle-Bierke, S., Unterleider, N., Alexiou, A., Kalb, B., et al., 2022. Tolerance induction through non-avoidance to prevent persistent food allergy (TINA) in children and adults with peanut or tree nut allergy: rationale, study design and methods of a randomized controlled trial and observational cohort study. Trials 23, 236.

Tuck, C.J., Biesiekierski, J.R., Schmid-Grendelmeier, P., Pohl, D., 2019. Food intolerances. Nutrients 11 (7), 1684.

Turner, P.J., Baumert, J.L., Beyer, K., et al., 2016. Can we identify patients at risk of life-threatening allergic reactions to foods? Allergy 71 (9), 1241–1255.

Upton, J., Nowak-Wegrzyn, A., 2018. The impact of baked egg and baked milk diets on IgE- and non-IgE-mediated allergy. Clin Rev Allergy Immunol 55, 118–138.

Webber, C.M., England, R.W., 2010. Oral allergy syndrome: a clinical, diagnostic, and therapeutic challenge. Ann. Allergy Asthma Immunol. 104 (2), 101–108.

Westerhout, J., Baumert, J.L., Blom, W.M., et al., 2019. Deriving individual threshold doses from clinical food challenge data for population risk assessment of food allergens. J. Allergy Clin. Immunol. 144 (5), 1290–1309.

Wood, R.L., 2003. The natural history of food allergy. Pediatrics 111 (6), 1631–1637.

CHAPTER 7

Genetically modified organisms (GMO) for food use

Richard E. Goodman
Department of Food Science, Food Allergy Research and Resource Program,
University of Nebraska-Lincoln, Lincoln, NE, United States

Introduction

Agricultural productivity and food availability face many challenges. Advances in plant genetics and farming practices over centuries have increased productivity and enhanced food product quality. But they have not been able to overcome many obstacles including specific bacterial, fungal, and viral diseases; insect infestation, soil, and nutrient limitations; or sustained production with global warming sufficient to feed the growing human population. While research scientists in plant breeding and agronomy have developed highly varied plant genotypes and phenotypes that help tremendously, there are limits in the ability to overcome many of these obstacles. Time and expense of developing new varieties of plants are also factors in determining limitations. Using biotechnology, scientists have developed many useful and safe transgenic traits and crops in a few years since the first approval in 1994 to overcome some shortcomings and to improve characteristics of the crop output. The new GM varieties must be bred into plant varieties appropriate for different geographies, soil types, moisture, and temperature regimes to be useful. Examples will be discussed here where genes from other organisms provide some rapid solutions. It is important to review progress made through genetic engineering and to consider the costs and uncertainties of tests that are unlikely to provide absolute assurances of the safety of these or any crop developed using different technologies.

A compendium of genetically engineered or genetically modified events approved anywhere in the world is available at the website http://www.isaaa.org/gmapprovaldatabase. Information about the complete DNA insert with regulatory elements and markers is usually included in the descriptions. Information on some approved events is not available in the database

History of Food and Nutrition Toxicology
https://doi.org/10.1016/B978-0-12-821261-5.00004-0
141

but event numbers are listed for many, and other resource data are usually available. Although genetics and agronomy practices usually overlap, some countries accept new events for cultivation and consumption, while other countries have only approved consumption of specific GM products grown in other countries, usually with restrictions on importation. And some countries reject any GM event.

Development of a regulatory system for GM approvals began in the 1980s as outlined for the United States Food and Drug Administration, Environmental Protection Agency and the Department of Agriculture worked to establish a regulatory framework for the safety evaluation of these new food sources (Federal Register notice 49 FR 50856, 1984). The International Food Biotechnology Council (IFBC) conducted an extensive review of food safety questions and issues that might be related to genetically modified foods recognizing that current developments were to make minor modifications to extensively used food crops. The IFBC review included recommendations for compositional analysis of foods, nutrients, microorganisms, and toxicants and was published in the journal *Regulatory Toxicology and Pharmacology*, 1990, volume 12. It suggested that current US laws and regulations for food safety are sufficient for evaluating the questions of human, animal health, and environmental protection for such products. The US government agencies responsible for food safety considered methods of evaluation and sought scientific and public opinion and have used existing food safety laws and regulations to effectively manage new GM events. The final rule for the United States was announced in the Federal Register notice 5,722,984–23,005, May 29, 1992. Other countries including those in the European Union adopted their own policies and the EU directive 258/97/EC of 27 January 1997 defined the process in the EU. Similar regulations have been developed and are evolving in most countries. International scientific consultations have continued through consultations held by the FAO/WHO organization that produced an outline assessment in 2001 (FAO/WHO, 2001) with extensive additional testing recommendations and then an overarching guideline by the CODEX Alimentarius organization in 2003 (CODEX, 2003). The record of safety of GM events should be considered along with questions of the safety of new products produced by other methods and without demonstrated scientific evidence of increased food allergy, food toxicity, or environmental damage (Anderson et al., 2021).

DNA transfer to plants to develop each GM event has been accomplished initially using either DNA-coated biolistic particles to carry the new DNA into plant cells where they can incorporate into breaks in the chromosome or a modified crown–gall bacterial transmission plasmid from *Agrobacterium tumefaciens* that mimic natural plant infections (Fig. 1). Those methods introduce DNA randomly into the chromosomes or plastids of the plant cells and these are then selected by functional growth and measured physical characteristics while discarding thousands of poorly performing insertion events. Selection is based on plant growth, reproduction, DNA insertion characteristics, and plant phenotypic properties. In addition to the useful DNA sequence (trait), regulatory sequences for gene expression and marker genes including selected antibiotic resistance genes or other markers are included for selection. Markers including a green fluorescence protein or enzymes such as phosphomannose isomerase, phosphinothricin *N*-acetyltransferase (PAT), or herbicide resistance genes such as CP4 EPSPS have been used to allow rapid and efficient selection of successfully transformed plants. In all cases, the safety of the inserted gene, protein or RNA product, and marker genes has been evaluated before a GM plant will be accepted for commercial production as described in a later chapter. A variety of events have been made and selected for commercial plant improvements as described here.

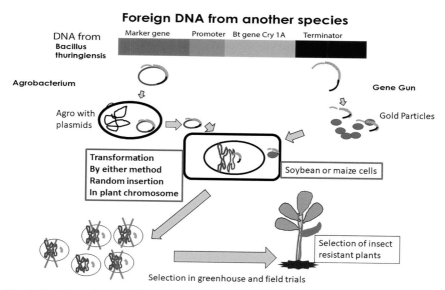

Fig. 1 Creation of a GM plant by two possible transformation methods to put foreign DNA of another organism into the chromosome of current commercial variety used for food. Agrobacterium or gene gun transfer of DNA into the plant cell, then selection and finally testing. *(Credit: MMG 2332014 Genetics & Genomics Wiki-Fandom.)*

Early in 1994, the first GM food crop authorized for food use was a delayed ripening tomato, FLAVR SAVR, designed to delay ripening of the fruit on the plant to facilitate machine harvesting and increase fruit preservation. However, that product was not particularly accepted by consumers or food companies. Many other traits followed quickly, including insect-resistant, viral-resistant, and herbicide-tolerant plants, to reduce chemical pesticide use and increase crop yields.

Insect-resistant traits

The first insect-resistant traits used in crop plants relied on proteins expressed by genes in various bacterial strains of *Bacillus thuringiensis* (Bt) that have been used as commercial organic pesticides since approximately 1927. The Bt bacterium was first discovered in 1902 in Japan as a problem that causes the death of cultivated silkworms. Scientists eventually identified the genes and proteins that can provide a useful trait against specific insects. Specific Bt crystal proteins have been identified and one was transformed into tobacco plants by Plant Genetic Systems (PGS) of Belgium and tested for protection from insect pests. Organic farmers and companies had been using whole microbial Bt populations to produce strains to protect some vegetable crops since the early 1900s and in the 1980s genes were considered for transfer in GM plants (Nester et al., 2002). Certain strains of *B. thuringiensis* were superior at stopping the growth and maturation of selected insect pests. Soon after, the Monsanto Company introduced different genes from *B. thuringiensis* proteins including the gene encoding the Cry3A protein which was transferred into the potato to control Colorado Potato beetles, a Coleopteran insect. Other genes encoding the Cry1Ab protein in maize to control the Lepidopteran (moth) pests European corn borer and by insertion of the gene encoding the Cry1Ac in cotton to control pink bollworm. The transgenic versions of plants that incorporate the genes and expressed those proteins were characterized and tested in the greenhouse and in field studies before being approved by regulators between 1994 and 1996 in the United States and later in other countries. Other similar products were approved soon after using different genes and proteins such as Cry1F and Vip3A to control Lepidopteran pests (introduced by Pioneer and Syngenta, respectively) in maize.

The gene expressing the Cry9C protein was introduced in maize by PGS, which was purchased by Aventis Agrosciences, Inc. It was registered for cultivation in the United States to be used as an animal feed in 1998 but was not approved for food use, primarily because the protein was found to be stable to digestion in a pepsin test tube assay recommended for food safety evaluations. In 2000 the product was recalled as a nonapproved food crop as it was not accepted by the FDA for food use due to stability of the protein in a pepsin test tube assay that suggested possible risks of food allergy. It was a rapid food and commodity recall stimulated by complaints of 120 consumers who alleged allergic responses following consumption of taco shells or corn chips that may have contained StarLink corn. Since the event had not been approved for food use, regulators in the United States rapidly investigated the complaints using field officers and clinical experts from the Centers for Disease Control and Prevention and the FDA. Many of those consumers voluntarily complied and provided blood samples to test for IgE antibodies specific to Cry9C. About half did not give samples. The symptoms and cooccurrence of symptoms in multiple family members are uncommon for food allergy. None of the subjects showed clear IgE binding to Cry9C, which would have demonstrated probable allergy, and no evidence of clinical reactivity to the protein was proven (Raybourne et al., 2003; Diaz et al., 2002; Bucchini and Goldman, 2002). The Cry9C was present at 50 to 80 ppm in corn grain, well below typical levels of allergens in foods that cause food-allergic reactions to allergenic proteins such as peanut, tree nuts, milk, or eggs. Questions had been raised regarding possible airway exposure to Cry1 proteins in farmworkers in Ohio who applied organic Bt sprays (Bernstein et al., 2003). However, the protein extracts in the Bernstein tests in 2003 would not have contained the crystal proteins, and the soluble proteins that were used were not proven to be a causative allergenic agent for the few farmworkers with symptoms of asthma. Furthermore, that data were not about risks of foods, it was instead about potential risks to farmworkers who already have to use precautions to protect their health. Questions raised by the FAO/WHO, 2001 scientific panel (FAO/WHO, 2001) and the public outcry stimulated regulators from the United States, UK, Japan, Canada, and other countries to evaluate preapproval processes for allergenicity risks in a meeting in September 2001 in Vancouver, BC, in Canada. The final approval process was finished after full review and publication of the CODEX Alimentarius Commission Guidelines in 2003 (CODEX, 2003). The CODEX guidelines helped to clarify much of the allergenicity risk assessment process for GM crops, microbes, and animals; potential risks of celiac disease; toxicity; and nutrient and antinutrient content of new GM crops (CODEX Alimentarius, 2003/2009).

Since StarLink was originally grown on more than 300,000 acres for animal feed, the EPA and Aventis Agroscience, Inc. undertook a program to remove seeds and grain from seed producers, grain handlers, farms, and food and feed companies. All of the seeds and products were removed from the market as reported by the EPA as being completed by 2008 (EPA-HQ-OPP-2007-0822-003). However, the disruption to food supplies, seeds, and foods cost between $500 million and USD 1 billion to companies ranging from seed companies, farm cooperatives, and food and agricultural commodity companies, becoming a major issue for accepting new GM crops for foods (en.wikipedia.org/wiki/StarLink_corn_recall).

Other scientists have studied the genes and proteins of the *Bacillus thuringiensis* bacterium which includes approximately 5463 genes and proteins (Fu et al., 2017). Genes for many crystal proteins and some vegetative proteins have been individually tested or used to control specific insect pests including moths, flies, beetles, sucking insects, ants, and snails as well as some human cancer cells (Palma et al., 2014). Toxicity is usually quite specific for the toxin to the organism affected and the mechanisms of toxicity are generally scientifically understood. Specific insect-resistant traits listed in the ISAAA database have been registered for cotton (*Gossypium hirsutum*, 50 events), cowpea (*Vigna unguiculata*, 1 event), eggplant (*Solanum melongena*, 1 event), maize (*Zea mays*, 208 events), poplar tree (*Populus sp.*, 2 events), potato (*Solanum tuberosum*, 30 events), soybean (*Glycine* max, 6 events), sugarcane (*Saccharum sp.*, 3 events), and tomato (*Lycopersicon esculentum*, 1 event). The database includes multiple approved events that have been combined by traditional breeding techniques and shown to be genetically stable over several breeding cycles.

Most of these traits have been produced by a small number of large commercial companies with a few by government-funded researchers. Most have been approved for cultivation in the United States, but a few such as Bt cowpea are approved for growing only in Nigeria and Bt brinjal or eggplant only for Bangladesh and the Philippines. Some of the listed events have not been registered for cultivation in any country or they may not be cultivated at this time. Regulators in the United States have considered potential food risks for Golden Rice and some other GM crops in case they are produced and come into the United States through international trade.

Herbicide-tolerant traits

Chemical herbicides have been used for decades to improve the farmer's ability to reduce weeds that compete with crop species for a variety of crops. Herbicide-tolerant crops have been transformed with an enzyme that is resistant to specific herbicides that can then be safely sprayed on the GM crop without harming the plants while controlling weeds. Many crops and ornamental plants (alfalfa, Argentine canola, carnations, chicory, cotton, creeping bent grass, flax, maize, Polish canola, potato, rice, soybean, sugar beet, tobacco, and wheat) have been made tolerant to specific herbicides by inserting genes encoding proteins that are not susceptible to those herbicides. The specific herbicides that are approved depend on the enzyme or transformation genes and regulatory approvals vary by country (Reddy and Nandula, 2012). The majority of herbicide-tolerant (HT) crops resist glyphosate or glufosinate, some are resistant to dicamba or HPPD, and some to 2,4-D. There are a few nontransgenic herbicide-tolerant crops that have been found following mutagenesis or natural mutations in some individual plant species.

The most useful GM events include those resistant to glyphosate, which became the primary HT phenotype in commercial agriculture (Reddy and Nandula, 2012). Resistance to glyphosate has been primarily created by introducing a bacterial homolog of the commonly conserved plant enzyme, 5-enolpyruvylshikame-3-phosphate synthase (EPSPS). The bacterial protein, known as CP4-EPSPS, was resistant to the herbicide while the protein in most plants binds glyphosate and is inactivated by it. The enzyme in plants is an important metabolic enzyme that produces a precursor to aromatic amino acids and other secondary metabolites. Blocking the production of the single metabolite blocks production of aromatic amino acids as well as some metabolites. Since glyphosate inactivates the enzyme of most plant varieties, the plant would normally die within days when sprayed with this herbicide. Transformed glyphosate-tolerant plants include soybeans, maize, cotton, and canola, allowing the plants to grow normally in the presence of glyphosate. GM soybean and maize crops transformed with this enzyme were approved in 1995 and 1996 and are important in weed control and plant production and were tested and found to be nutritionally as safe and useful as nontransgenic soybeans and maize (Padgette et al., 1995, 1996; Sidhu et al., 2000). Food and feed safety studies and nutritional evaluations are performed on each GM crop before they are approved for cultivation or consumption in the United States and many other countries. The safety studies are usually published in peer-reviewed journals, and many are listed on the ISAAA website. Other important HT traits include glufosinate-resistant crops and early on, a few bromoxynil-resistant crops although the ability of bromoxynil to kill a variety of weeds has limited their utility (Reddy and Nandula, 2012).

A primary environmental concern is the overuse of specific herbicides which provides pressure for weeds to evolve with resistance to the herbicide. The development of herbicide-resistant varieties of weeds has occurred before GM events were available due to the overuse of preemergent herbicides and several resistant weeds have been identified after their introduction, limiting to some degree the useful life of specific herbicides (Kumar et al., 2020). There is a clear need to be vigilant in the development of herbicide-tolerant weeds around the world and take actions based on the herbicides, the crops, and farming practices (Peterson et al., 2018). Some stacked GM varieties of plants are being developed that include tolerance to specific herbicides as well as resistance to insects and plant diseases and their durability must also be monitored and protected (Chuanxu et al., 2020).

Viral-resistant traits

Plant viruses are major pests in specific crops. One of the first crops to be transformed to escape viral infection was zucchini or crooked neck squash that was transformed with two viral constructs (ZW20) to avoid the yellow mosaic virus and the watermelon mosaic virus and a second transformed squash with three viral constructs (CZW3) to resist cucumber mosaic virus, zucchini yellow mosaic potyvirus, and watermelon mosaic potyvirus. The transformation was accomplished with Agrobacterium-mediated transformation (www.isaaa.org/gmapprovaldatabase). These plants were transformed with vectors including part of the viral genes by the Asgrow Company which was purchased by Monsanto Company and by Seminis Vegetable Seeds, Inc. One was approved in 1995 and the other in 1997 for consumption in the United States, but these are only approved for cultivation in the United States. These events are specific as there are natural RNAse enzyme pathways that will disable or cut double-stranded RNA and inactivate the viruses. The traits are quite specific due to sequence differences among viruses of similar types.

The papaya industry in Hawaii was saved from the papaya ringspot virus by inserting part of the viral gene that acted via RNA interference (Gonsalves, 1998; Ferreira et al., 2002). It was approved in 1997–1998 and is still grown there. A similar construct was developed in other strains of papaya in other geographies to stop genetically distinct viruses in China and SE Asia and approved for growth in China in 2006. The events are resistant to only a few viral strains, meaning new events are typically needed in different lines of plants. However, attempts to use this approach in Thailand were unsuccessful to a large extent because of pressure from an NGO, Greenpeace International, who worked the civil and political system well to stop the acceptance of a nonprofit horticultural tool (Davidson, 2008). Viral types in countries including Bangladesh show the genetic variation that may require newer transgenic constructs to control this insect-borne disease (Akhter et al., 2013).

Another important viral-resistant crop was the NewLeaf Russet Burbank potato that was transformed by Monsanto to be resistant to the Colorado potato beetle through the insertion of a Bt gene Cry 3 (approved in 1995) and resistant to potato Leaf Roll virus (plrv) of the family Solemoviridae and the "Y" virus of family Closteriviridae by insertion of RNA-expressing genes from both viruses with approvals in 1998 in the United States. Both viruses are frequently transferred into susceptible plants of these crops by sucking insects including aphids and mealybugs that feed on healthy plants after feeding on infected plants. The GM plants were able to slow or stop the damage caused by the specific viruses. Initially, the mechanism of action of the virus protection was not understood, but it became clear that RNA inhibition or RNA digestion mechanisms were the primary mechanisms of disruption of infection. The GM NewLeaf-viral protected potatoes had a significant reduction in crop losses from field trials. Even though these events were approved for cultivation in the United States in 1995 and 1998, the backlash of some consumers regarding GM crop acceptability was an important driver for retail fast food markets and food producers including MacDonald's and McCain Foodservices to not use these potatoes. They pressured Monsanto and the company sold the GM potato business as Nature Mark. But that was not a commercial success. Clearly, consumer preferences can drive business and regulatory decisions despite scientific data that show no evidence of risk or harm, and despite clear benefits of reduced plant damage.

Bacterial-resistant traits

Bacterial plant pathogens are often spread to uninfected plants from nearby infected plants by sucking insects including leafhoppers, aphids, and mealybugs, or by farmer's tools. Citrus Greening Disease (CGD) which is also known as Huanglongbing has been known since the early 1990s although it has been in Asia and Africa for more than 50 years (da Graca, 1991; Garnier and Bove, 1993). It is caused by a bacterium-like organism that is a gram-negative proteobacterium that invades phloem in the trees and reduces ripening. It causes the decline and death of the trees within a few years. The organism, *Candidatus* Liberibacter *asiaticus*, can infect most citrus genotypes (McCollum et al., 2016). The insect vector spreading the disease in Africa is *Trioza erytreae*, and in Asia it is *Diaphorina citri* (Garnier and Bove, 1993). One of the main vectors (*D. citri*) was discovered in Florida in the United States as a vector of CGD and the assessment predicted expanded citrus tree decline and decimation of the orange and citrus industry unless controls can be identified (Halbert and Manjunath, 2004). Importantly the insect vectors have become resistant to the chemical pesticides that were successful in controlling the spread of the disease which decreased orange production by 74% in 2019 and has spread to most citrus-growing areas in the world (Singerman and Rogers, 2020). Part of the lack of control of CGD is also due to the farmers' behavior as many did not remove and burn their infected trees and many did not use an effective chemical control plan as recommended by the USDA (www.aphis.usda.gov/aphis/ourfocus/planthealth/plant-pest-and-disease-programs-and-citrus/citrus-greening). Active programs are searching for solutions using genetic engineering to CGD. One option currently under extensive field trials is the introduction of genes encoding multiple very small spinach defensin proteins that can be inserted as transgenic graphs on rootstock or as an infection of trees with viruses containing similar spinach defensin proteins (USDA Application). One method that was being tested is by grafting shoots of a transgenic citrus tree onto native rootstock. The other potential control mechanism is by the use of a retrovirus that will infect the orange trees and provide protection very early, before the decline of the trees. The USDA APHIS, Southern Gardens Citrus Nursery, LLC obtained Permit 17–044-101r to release genetically engineered *Citrus tristeza* virus containing the spinach defensin proteins. In 2018 my laboratory performed preliminary testing of the spinach defensin proteins using bioinformatics and by testing the stability of the proteins in pepsin. These proteins do not represent a risk of food allergy even if they are expressed in orange fruits. However, the effectiveness of the approach needs to be demonstrated while the industry in the United States faces significant competition from Mexican and Brazilian citrus producers who probably still rely on the use of chemical pesticides.

Another citrus disease is canker, caused by a *Xanthomonas citri* bacterium (Islam et al., 2019). The canker bacteria are spread by wind and water, with transmission distances depending on the weather. In Florida with hurricanes, transmission can be extensive within a grove and to neighboring groves (Bock et al., 2010). Genetic modification and gene editing products designed for use in combating this disease are being considered to combat several diseases including citrus canker and citrus greening disease as well as fungal and viral diseases (Sun et al., 2019). Gene editing methods use CRISPR and Cas9 to provide tools for making the trees resistant or less susceptible to these diseases. One real challenge for genetic engineering is the life cycle length for the reproduction of citrus trees.

Sun et al. (2019) discussed the issues of differences in accepting different GM products and gene-edited crops between the United States and the EU, especially the difference in decision processes for gene editing. Interestingly, Sun et al. (2019) do not discuss the process in China, a country that has been very hesitant to openly accept GM products.

Fungal-resistant traits

Potatoes are susceptible to a variety of specific diseases including late blight disease which is caused by a water mold, *Phytophthora infestans*. This organism was responsible for the Irish potato famine and is still common in the United States and many other countries. *P. infestans* also attacks tomatoes and other Solanaceous plants (Fig. 2). The disease is still a major global problem that requires the use of a variety of toxic chemical pesticides to keep it in check with implications for environmental and farmer safety. Potatoes transformed with three genes from wild-type potato species are resistant to this organism (Ghislain et al., 2019). The first *P. infestans*-resistant potatoes were developed at the University of Wisconsin-Madison. Michigan State University, JR Simplot scientists at the International Potato Center (Nairobi Kenya), and associated collaborators have been working to develop genetically engineered potatoes resistant to this organism since 2005. The International Potato Center collaboration has two transgenic African potato lines transformed with three resistance genes and the ntpII kanamycin marker gene was selected and characterized and tested for resistance to *P. infestans*. Production in greenhouse experiments and confined field trials have been conducted in Uganda. The transformed Victoria potato line was chosen for additional field trials and regulatory submission. Based on data from early field trials, this GM potato should improve tuber quality and potato yields in many regions in Africa that have *P. infestans* as a significant potato pathogen (Ghislain et al., 2019).

Cereal crops around the world are affected by a variety of fungal diseases. Various Fusarium species infect wheat, causing head blight, which introduces food toxins in the grain (Wang et al., 2020; Kazan and Gardiner,

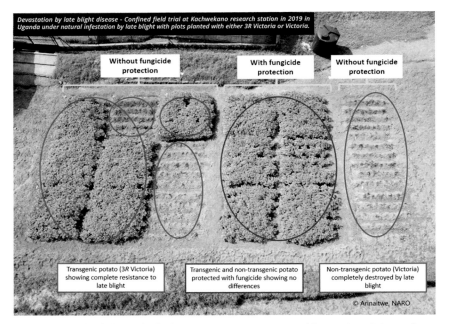

Fig. 2 Successful field trial of African GM potato protected from *Phytophthora infestans.* Potato researchers in Africa transformed and selected a Victoria variety of potato commonly grown in parts of Africa using three genes from wild potato varieties, then performing field trials with controls as marked in this picture. (Credit: National Agricultural Research Organization in Uganda and the International Potato Center (CIP) of Kenya.)

2018). Understanding the disease-causing organism in wheat, barley, and rye can help identify methods that may help in stopping the production of toxins and the loss of grains.

Nutritional quality traits

Golden Rice was developed to provide the precursor of vitamin A to diets of humans who are at risk of vitamin A deficiency (Beyer et al., 2002; Paine et al., 2005). Vitamin A deficiency affects as many as 100 million people in cultures with rice as the dominant food component. Vitamin A is important for maintaining an adequate immune system and for vision. Certainly, vitamin A-deficient diets cause night blindness but also increase the vulnerability to malaria and other diseases. Supplementation with vitamin A is limited as too much intake is toxic. Golden Rice expresses enzymes that produce beta-carotene, then enzymes in the consumer can convert the beta-carotene to vitamin A. The initial transformed versions of rice were created by insertion of phytoene synthase and lycopene beta-cyclase from *Narcissus pseudonarcissus* and a bacterial phytoene desaturase from *Erwinia uredovora* (Beyer et al., 2002). Production of beta-carotene was not as high as hoped and it was determined that genes from other common plant varieties might be more suitable, including a phytoene synthase from maize in place of the daffodil proteins. The maize psy (phytoene synthase) and crtI (carotene desaturase) genes were used in another transformation (Paine et al., 2005). A few transformed events were developed and characterized. Finally, the GR2E event was tested for total compositional analysis and utility (Swamy et al., 2019) and has now been accepted by the Government of the Philippines (www.isaaa.org/kc/cropbiotechupdate/article/defaults. asp?ID-18916).

Other nutritionally improved crop varieties have been in development during the last 15 years, including iron and zinc fortification and improved beta-carotene levels in other plants and increased vitamin E for cassava as well as a reduction in cyanide in cassava, and reduction in glutens for celiac disease and possible reduction in allergens in peanuts. However, none of these have received government approvals, yet.

Gene editing

Newer methods of modifying native DNA in plants and animals include the use of newly discovered gene-editing methods available with Zinc-Finger-mediated edits, TALEN-mediated, and CRISPR/Cas9 to modify endogenous gene sequences rather than introducing new genes. Most events are deletions of a segment of DNA and repair of the DNA backbone, as happens in natural mutations but that occur at targeted sequences. The technology allows specific gene targeting nucleotide changes, deletions and specifically designed edits, insertion of DNA for control, or whole new genes in the third type of editing (Kumar et al., 2020). Controlled sequence insertion by guide RNA tags rather than random insertion occurs using biolistics or Agro-mediated transformation. Directed transformation has been done to correct rare genetic diseases in humans, including cycle cell anemia and a few other genetic problems. Recently genome editing using CRISPR-Cas9 has been used in monocots and dicots to reduce plant virus susceptibility, to enhance yield, quality of the grain, and nutritional performance (El-Mounadi et al., 2020). Other advances in plant and animal genetics will be happening in the coming years. Some countries have made conscious decisions to not regulate gene-edited organisms by the same methods used for genetically modified organisms. The USDA does not classify gene-edited varieties as GMOs. However, the European Commission and the European Food Safety Authority treat gene-edited organisms as they do GM events. For insertions of new genes, it makes sense to request data on possible allergenicity or toxicity from inserted genes. Maybe the US regulators will change, for instance, where direct gene insertion is being done or when changes are made to intentionally alter nutrient content. But for simple nucleotide replacements, that does not seem reasonable as each new event could well represent a simple, natural mutation.

Conclusions for the future

Marketing forces in the United States and many countries continue to dictate market preferences that should be driven by farmers, economists, and scientific decisions about efficacy, safety, and costs. But as climate change is happening and the population continues to grow, it seems relevant to consider efficiencies, improvements, and costs. Why is the human food industry pushing non-GMO labels and products? Why has the dog food industry in the US market joined with "non-GMO" as a major labeling feature on high-end retail dog food brands? Dogs that commonly consume carrion and other dogs' feces when allowed to do so do not read labels and unless the feces contain parasites or infections agents, it does not seem to harm the dogs. When issues like vitamin A insufficiency occur for millions of consumers and when citrus greening disease reduces the ability to eat nutritious foods, it seems sensible for consumers to consider accepting the technology that has developed over decades where changes can be documented and benefits are clear and economically viable. It seems that otherwise, we are losing the benefits of technology that our scientific community has invested in and developed.

References

Akhter, M.S., Basavaraj, Y.B., Akanda, A.M., Mandal, B., Jain, R.K., 2013. Genetic diversity based on coat protein of papaya ringspot virus (Pathotype P) isolates from Bangladesh. Indian J. Virol. 24 (1), 70–73.

Anderson, J.A., Herman, R.A., Carlson, A., Mathesius, C., et al., 2021. Hypothesis-based food, feed and environmental safety assessment of GM crops: a case study using maize event DP-2-2216-6. GM Crops Food 12 (1), 282–291.

Bernstein, J.A., Bernstein, I.L., Buchini, L., Goldman, L.R., Hamilton, R.G., Lehrer, S., Rubin, C., Sampson, H.A., 2003. Clinical and laboratory investigation of allergy to genetically modified foods. Environ. Health Perspect. 111 (8), 1114–1121.

Beyer, P., Al-Babili, S., Ye, X., Lucca, P., Scshaub, P., Welsch, R., Potrykus, I., 2002. Golden Rice: introducing the beta-carotene biosynthesis pathway into rice endosperm by genetic engineering to defeat vitamin A deficiency. J. Nutr. 132 (3), 506S–510S.

Bock, C.H., Graham, J.H., Gottwald, T.R., Cook, A.Z., Parker, P.E., 2010. Wind speed effects on the quantity of *Xanthomonas citri* spsp. *citri* dispersed downwind from canopies of grapefruit trees infected with citrus canker. Plant Dis. 94, 725–736.

Bucchini, L., Goldman, L.R., 2002. Starlink corn: a risk analysis. Environ. Health Perspect. 110, 5–13.

Chuanxu, L., Zhang, J., Ren, Z., Xie, R., et al., 2020. Development of multiresistance rice by an assembly of herbicide, insect and disease resistance genes with transgene stacking system. Pest Manag. Sci. 77 (3), 1536–1547.

CODEX Alimentarius, 2003/2009. Foods Derived from Modern Biotechnology. World Health Organization and Food and Agriculture Organization of the United Nations, Rome, Italy.

da Graca, J.V., 1991. Citrus greening disease. Annu. Rev. Phytopathol. 29, 109–136.

Davidson, S.N., 2008. Forbidden fruit: transgenic papaya in Thailand. Plant Physiol. 147 (2), 487–493.

Diaz, C., Fernandez, C., McDonald, R., Yeung, J.M., 2002. Determination of cry 9C protein in processed foods made with StarLink corn. J. AOAC Int. 85 (5), 1070–1076.

El-Mounadi, K., Morales-Floriano, M.L., Garcia-Ruiz, H., 2020. Principles, applications, and biosafety of plant genome editing using CRISPR-Cas9. Front. Plant Sci. https://doi.org/10.3389/fpls.2020.00056.

FAO/WHO, 2001. Evaluation of Allergenicity of Genetically Modified Foods. Report of a Joint FAO/WHO Expert Consultation on Allergenicity of Foods Derived from Biotechnology, 22–25 January 2001, Rome, Italy.

Ferreira, S.A., Pitz, K.Y., Manshardt, R., Zee, F., et al., 2002. Virus coat protein transgenic papaya provides practical control of papaya ringspot virus in Hawaii. Plant Dis. 86 (2), 101–105.

Fu, Y., Wu, Y., Yuan, Y., Gao, M., 2017. Complete genome sequence of bacillus thuringiensis Serovar rongseni reference strain SCG04-02, a strain toxic to *Plutella xylostella*. Am. Soc. Microbiol. 5 (39), e00691-17.

Garnier, M., Bove, J.-M., 1993. Citrus greening disease and the green bacterium. In: International Organization of Citrus Virologists Conference Proceedings (1957–2010).

Ghislain, M., Byarugaba, A.A., Magembe, E., Njoroge, A., Riverra, C., et al., 2019. Stacking three late blight resistance genes from wild species directly into African highland potato varieties confers complete field resistance to local blight races. Plant Biotechnol. J. 17 (6), 1119–1129.

Gonsalves, D., 1998. Control of papaya ringspot virus in papay: a case study. Annu. Rev. Phytopathol. 36, 415–437.

Halbert, S.E., Manjunath, K.L., 2004. Asian citrus psyllids (Sternorrhyncha: Psyllidae) and greening disease of citrus: a literature review and assessment of risk in Florida. Fla. Entomol. 87 (3), 330–353.

Islam, M.N., Ali, M.S., Choi, S.-J., Hyun, J.-W., Baek, K.-H., 2019. Biocontrol of citrus canker disease caused by *Xanthomonas citri* subsp. *citri* using an endophytic *Bacillus thuringiensis*. Plant Pathol. J. 35 (5), 486–497.

Kazan, K., Gardiner, D.M., 2018. Fusarium crown rot caused by *Fusarium pseudograminearum* in cereal crops: recent progress and future prospects. Mol. Plant Pathol. 19 (7), 1547–1562.

Kumar, K., Gambhir, G., Dass, A., Tripathi, A.K., Singh, A., Jha, A.K., et al., 2020. Genetically modified crops: current status and future prospects. Planta 251, 91. https://doi.org/10.1007/soo425-020-03372-8.

McCollum, G., Hilf, M., Irey, M., Luo, W., Gottwald, T., 2016. Susceptibility of sixteen citrus genotypes to 'Candidatus Liberibacter *asiaticus*'. Plant Dis. 100 (6), 1080–1086.

Nester, E.W., Thomashow, L.S., Metz, M., Gordon, M., 2002. 100 Years of *Bacillus thuringiensis*: A Critical Scientific Assessment. American Society for Microbiology, Washington, DC, USA.

Padgette, S.R., Kolacz, K.H., Delannay, D.B., Re, J.B., et al., 1995. Development, identification and characterization of glyphosate-tolerant soybean line. Crop. Sci. 35, 1451–1461.

Padgette, S.R., Taylor, N.B., Nida, D.L., Bailey, M.R., et al., 1996. The composition of glyphosate-tolerant soybean seeds is equivalent to that of conventional soybeans. J. Nutr. 126, 702–716.

Paine, J.A., Shipton, C.A., Chaggar, S., Howells, R.M., Kennedy, M.J., Vernon, G., Wright, S.Y., Hinchliffe, E., Adams, J.L., Silverstone, A.L., Drake, R., 2005. Improving the nutritional value of Golden Rice through increased pro-vitamin A content. Nat. Biotechnol. 23, 482–487.

Palma, L., Munoz, D., Berry, C., Murillo, J., Caballero, P., 2014. *Bacillus thuringiensis* toxins: an overview of their biocidal activity. Toxins 6 (12), 3296–32325.

Peterson, M.A., Collavo, A., Overjero, R., Shivram, V., Walsh, M., 2018. The challenge of herbicide resistance around the world. Current summary. Pest Manag. Sci. 74 (10), 2246–2259.

Raybourne, R.B., Williams, K.M., Vogt, R., Reissman, D.B., Winterton, B.S., Rubin, C., 2003. Development and use of an ELISA test to detect IgE antibody to Cry9C following possible exposure to bioengineered corn. Int. Arch. Allergy Immunol. 132 (4), 322–328.

Reddy, K.N., Nandula, V.K., 2012. Herbicide resistant crops: history, development and current technologies. Indian J. Agron. 57 (1), 1–7.

Sidhu, R.S., Hammond, B.G., Fuchs, R.L., Mutz, J., et al., 2000. Glyphosate-tolerant corn: the composition and feeding value of grain from glyphosate-tolerant corn is equivalent to that of conventional corn (*Zea mays* L.). J. Agric. Food Chem. 48, 2305–2312.

Singerman, A., Rogers, M., 2020. The economic challenges of dealing with citrus greening: the case of Florida. J. Integr. Pest Manag. 11 (1), 1–7.

Sun, L., Nasrullah, K.F., Nie, Z., Wang, P., Xu, J., 2019. Citrus genetic engineering for disease resistance: past, present and future. Int. J. Mol. Sci. 20, 5256. https://doi.org/10.3390/ijms20215256. MDPI.

Swamy, B.P.M., Samia, M., Boncodin, R., Marundan, S., Rebong, D.B., Ordonio, R.L., Miranda, R.T., Rebong, A.T.O., Alibuyog, A.Y., Adeva, C.C., Reinke, R., MacKenzie, D.J., 2019. Compositional analysis of genetically engineered GR2E "Goden Rice" in comparison to that of conventional rice. J. Agric. Food Chem. 67 (28), 7986–7994.

Wang, H., Sun, S., Ge, W., Zhao, L., Hou, B., Wang, K., Lyu, Z., et al., 2020. Horizontal gene transfer of Fhb7 from fungus underlies fusarium head blight resistance in wheat. Science 368 (6493). https://doi.org/10.1126/science.aba5435.

CHAPTER 8

Dietary supplements

Cynthia V. Rider

Division of Translational Toxicology, National Institute of Environmental Health Sciences, Research Triangle Park, NC, United States

Introduction

The use of dietary supplements in the United States is widespread and growing, with 57.6% of adults reporting any dietary supplement use in the latest National Health and Nutrition Examination Survey (NHANES) analysis (2017–2018) (Mishra et al., 2021). Notable patterns from NHANES data included women reporting greater use of dietary supplements than men, dietary supplement use increasing with age, and a sizeable portion of adults taking multiple dietary supplements (e.g., approximately 25% of adults 60 and over reported using four or more dietary supplements) (Mishra et al., 2021). The safety of dietary supplements is an important public health concern due to the large population of dietary supplement users, the potential for use by vulnerable populations (e.g., pregnant women, the elderly, and people with preexisting conditions), and the high recommended doses (100–1000 s mg per day).

While the origins of individual dietary supplement ingredients are disparate and stretch into the distant past, the formal definition of dietary supplements was established less than 30 years ago in the 1994 Dietary Supplement Health and Education Act (DSHEA), which amended the Federal Food, Drug, and Cosmetic Act of 1938 (FD&C Act). According to DSHEA, dietary supplements are products (other than tobacco) that are intended to supplement the diet and contain one or more vitamin, mineral, botanical, amino acid, or other dietary substance, or a concentrate, metabolite, constituent, extract, or combination of such (Table 1). Furthermore, only products intended for ingestion are dietary supplements. Dietary supplements can come in many forms including tablets, capsules, powders, tinctures, gummies, or energy bars. They cannot be represented as conventional food and must be labeled as a dietary supplement. While a dietary supplement ingredient can be developed into a drug, a substance that is first

History of Food and Nutrition Toxicology
https://doi.org/10.1016/B978-0-12-821261-5.00006-4

157

Table 1 Dietary supplements.

Category	Examples
Vitamin	Vitamins A, B (thiamine, riboflavin, niacin, pantothenic acid, biotin, B6, B12, and folate), C, D, E, and K
Mineral	Cobalt, copper, fluoride, iodine, iron, manganese, selenium, zinc
Herb or other botanical	*Aloe vera*, ashwagandha, black cohosh, echinacea, elderberry, fenugreek, garlic, ginkgo, ginseng, horehound, saw palmetto, turmeric, yohimbe
Amino acid	Branched-chain amino acids (leucine, isoleucine, valine), L-carnitine, L-tryptophan
Other	Bee pollen, deer velvet, beta-ecdysterone, diatomaceous earth, fish oil, probiotics
Concentrate	Chlorophyll concentrate, cranberry juice concentrate
Metabolite	Creatine, coenzyme Q10, phosphocreatine, nicotinamide ribonucleoside
Constituent	Berberine, caffeine, quercetin, resveratrol
Extract	Grapefruit extract, green tea extract, pine bark extract, spinach extract
Combination	Multivitamins, echinacea + goldenseal, multiingredient weight loss supplements (e.g., Hydroxycut, OxyElitePro), multiingredient sexual enhancement supplements (e.g., Black Stallion, Stag Fuel), multiingredient muscle building supplements (Jack3d, Insane Veinz)

approved as a drug or authorized for investigation as a new drug cannot later be marketed as a dietary supplement.

Despite the definition of dietary supplements provided in DSHEA, the terminology used to describe related products can be confusing. Both dietary supplements and functional foods can be referred to as nutraceuticals. The term "nutraceutical" does not have regulatory significance but refers generally to food-related products that claim to have health benefits (Phillips and Rimmer, 2013). Functional foods are foods that have been enriched or fortified to provide health benefits beyond those of the original food (e.g., iron- and folate-fortified cereal). Unlike functional foods, dietary supplements do not resemble conventional food and cannot provide a complete diet. However, depending on the claims associated with the functional food, it could be regulated as a food or as a dietary supplement (Phillips and Rimmer, 2013).

The dietary supplement industry has grown exponentially over the past several decades. At the time of the passage of DSHEA, there were an estimated 4000 dietary supplements produced by approximately 600 manufacturers in the United States. Currently, the Dietary Supplement Label Database maintained by the Office of Dietary Supplements within the National Institutes of Health contains label information for approximately 76,000 products available in the market (https://dsld.od.nih.gov/). The industry has grown from $4 billion in annual sales in 1994 to an estimated $46 billion in 2020 (Global Industry Analysts, 2021).

Historical roots of dietary supplements

The dietary supplement definition articulated in DSHEA contains a broad range of substances (Table 1) with correspondingly diverse origins and safety issues. While vitamins and minerals are relatively simple entities with known active compounds, botanicals can contain thousands of constituents often with a large unidentified fraction and little information linking specific constituents to purported biological activity (Shipkowski et al., 2018). To understand the safety issues associated with dietary supplements, it is important to look back at their history of use.

The most common dietary supplement across age groups is the multivitamin-mineral (Mishra et al., 2021). The origin story of vitamin supplements involves discoveries motivated by diseases resulting from dietary deficiencies such as scurvy, pellagra, beriberi, and rickets (Rosenfeld, 1997). The term vitamin was originally vitamine, coined by Casimir Funk in 1912 to describe the vital-to-life amine that Funk isolated from rice bran and believed was responsible for restoring health in pigeons suffering from polyneuritis due to nutritional deficiency (Rosenfeld, 1997). A lack of evidence supporting the presence of amines in these substances led to a modification of the term vitamine to vitamin (the "in" ending indicating "a neutral substance of undefined composition") and was then applied to multiple substances, such as vitamins A, B, and C (Rosenfeld, 1997). In an illustrative example of vitamin deficiency research, Smithells et al. (1976) describe findings from the Leeds Pregnancy and Nutrition Study. Researchers measured vitamin levels (folate in red blood cells, serum folate, vitamin C in white blood cells, riboflavin, and serum vitamin A) in a cohort of pregnant women and evaluated the correlation of vitamin levels with social class and the occurrence of central nervous system defects (e.g., neural tube defects). They found more satisfactory levels of the measured vitamins in the two higher classes and significantly lower levels of folate in red blood cells and vitamin C in white blood cells in women who gave birth to children with central nervous system defects (Smithells et al., 1976). The recommendation for folate-containing multivitamin supplementation during pregnancy, which continues today, emerged from studies such as the one described here.

In contrast to vitamins, the history of herbal or botanical dietary supplements is difficult to untangle from ancient origins rooted in both food and medicinal use of plants. Archaeological evidence suggests the use of medicinal plants by Neanderthals 60,000–80,000 years ago (Hardy et al., 2012; Lietava, 1992). Written evidence of the medicinal use of plants is recorded in the earliest written language preserved on Sumerian tablets (around 2100 BCE), where cuneiform impressions describe instructions for preparing plant-based remedies (Janick, 2003). These ancient applications of plants to treat ailments evolved in different regions into rich systems of practice such as Traditional Chinese Medicine; Ayurveda in India; Kampo in Japan; Traditional Korean Medicine; and Unani, a Greco-Arabic plant-based medicinal practice that remains popular in India (Yuan et al., 2016). Traditional healers in the Americas and Africa continue to rely on medicinal plants today (Aumeeruddy and Mahomoodally, 2021). Importantly, plant use in these traditional medicinal practices was expressly for the treatment of disease with a clear understanding that some plant-based treatments are not without toxicity, but the cost-benefit calculation is critical (Bao, 2017; Cai et al., 2019; Lu and Lu, 2014). Experts in Traditional Chinese Medicine point out the fallacy that people often assume natural equals safe (Bao, 2017). Additionally, the preparation and use pattern of Traditional Chinese Medicine differs significantly from that of dietary supplements. Traditional Chinese Medicines often involve multiple botanical ingredients simmered over hours to prepare a decoction with a short duration of prescribed use in the treatment of a specific ailment. Whereas dietary supplements can contain isolated compounds or concentrated plant extracts and can be used for a prolonged period as a prophylactic without the guidance of medical professionals. These differences have raised concerns that the lack of appropriate context could lead to toxicity (Lu and Lu, 2014). Some plants, like cranberry and green tea, have been used as both food and medicine. However, their application in botanical dietary supplements can differ from either food or traditional medicinal practices that use whole plants or plant parts. For example, some green tea extract supplements can be highly concentrated compared to the traditional green tea beverage (Oketch-Rabah et al., 2020).

The exploitation of probiotics for their health benefits far preceded the coining of the term by Werner Kollath in 1953, which derives from the Latin "pro" and the Greek "βιοσ" meaning "for life" (Gasbarrini et al., 2016). Probiotics have ancient beginnings in fermented milk products, such as the traditional yak milk yogurt consumed by Tibetan nomads, which is high in *Lactobacillus fermentum* and *Lactobacillus casei* (Guo et al., 2014; McFarland, 2015). The first discovery of the connection between bacteria and health benefits is attributed to Elie Metchnikoff of the Pasteur Institute chronicled in the 1908 book *The Prolongation of Life: Optimistic Studies* (Metchnikoff, 1908). Subsequent studies demonstrated improvements in patients suffering from various ailments (e.g., diarrhea, constipation, eczema, mental disease) following treatment with *Lactobacillus acidophilus* (Kopeloff et al., 1932; Rettger and Cheplin, 1922). The next boom in probiotic research focused on screening different strains, evaluating the ability of strains to colonize the human gut, and exploring mechanisms of action (McFarland, 2015).

Two steps forward, one step back: The history of dietary supplement regulation in the United States

The passage of DSHEA represented a critical inflection point in the push and pull between accessibility and safety of dietary supplements. Before their definition in DSHEA, dietary supplements suffered from an identity crisis, existing somewhere between food and drugs. The point of divergence between the regulatory paths for food and drugs can be traced to the early 20th century. Both food and drugs were subject to rampant adulteration and deceptive marketing practices before the passage of the Pure Food and Drug Act in 1906 (Borchers et al., 2007). Shocking examples included ground lice sold as brown sugar and tonics marketed as cure-alls with patented, undisclosed formulas containing cocaine or opium in addition to various herbs and minerals (Borchers et al., 2007). The landmark Pure Food and Drug Act legislation hastened the establishment of the Food and Drug Administration as the first consumer protection agency in the United States (Swann, 2016). It also delineated drugs as substances used to cure, mitigate, or prevent disease with required standards for strength, quality, and purity, and food as any article for food, drink, confectionary, or condiment (Swann, 2016). A major focus of the legislation was improving the accuracy and truth in labeling of food and drug products with the intent of allowing consumers to make informed decisions. Certain substances (e.g., acetanilide, alcohol, chloral hydrate, chloroform, cocaine, eucaine, marijuana, morphine, and opium) were required to be listed on the labels for either food or drug products (Borchers et al., 2007). Additionally, labels were prohibited from containing false or misleading statements (Borchers et al., 2007).

Obstacles to fully realizing the potential of the Pure Food and Drug Act included a lack of adequate funding for enforcement, the burden of proving intentional mislabeling, and loopholes that continued to allow for fraudulent claims in advertising (Borchers et al., 2007). The FD&C Act replaced the Pure Food and Drug Act and represented a vast improvement in consumer protection. In particular, it required safety testing prior to bringing drugs to the market (Borchers et al., 2007). Regarding supplements, the FD&C Act expanded the definition of a drug to include nonfood articles intended to affect structure or function in humans or animals. The discussion in Congress surrounding this provision made clear that the intended use of a substance was the critical determinant of whether it was classified as a food or drug (Swann, 2016). Furthermore, the law introduced misbranding provisions that required foods claiming to have special dietary use to indicate the vitamin, mineral, or other dietary properties on the label (Swann, 2016). These provisions led the FDA to establish minimum daily requirements of vitamins and minerals. Labeling requirements included qualification about the lack of evidence that the substance is needed, the quantity of each ingredient, and directions for its use (Swann, 2016). Finally, the legislation brought labeling and advertising under consistent directives (Swann, 2016).

In the decades following the passage of the FD&C Act, the FDA pursued violations of the labeling requirements and fraudulent claims (Swann, 2016). During this time, the public sentiment surrounding health and wellness was one of looking outside of the constraints of the traditional patient-doctor structure, exploring alternative health practices, and taking their health into their own hands (Swann, 2016). An update to regulations pertaining to vitamins and minerals was proposed in 1973. The most consequential piece was a proposed cap on the allowable level of nutrients in supplements (Swann, 2016). The rule stated that supplements containing vitamins or minerals at greater than 150% of the US Recommended Daily Allowance would be treated as over-the-counter drugs (Swann, 2016). This rule change was met with unprecedented backlash from the public, trade associations, and manufacturers (Swann, 2016). This was followed by the passage of the Vitamin-Mineral Amendment, also known as the Proxmire Amendment, of 1976, which prohibited the FDA from both classifying vitamins and minerals as drugs and limiting combinations of vitamins, minerals, and food ingredients (Swann, 2016).

The Nutrition Labeling and Education Act was passed in 1990 to clarify the widespread confusion around labeling of food and dietary supplements. Regarding supplements, the legislation mandated validation of specific health claims (Swann, 2016). During this period, the FDA regarded supplement ingredients as unapproved substances falling under the category of either drug or food additive (Porter, 2002). The Nutrition Labeling and Education Act catalyzed another wave of public outcry against potential limits to dietary supplement accessibility. The Dietary Supplement Act followed in 1992 and prohibited the implementation of most of the provisions of the New Labeling Education Act that affected dietary supplements, although requirements for health claims stood (Porter, 2002). Additionally, the Dietary Supplement Act commissioned multiple reports aimed at investigating whether the FDA was applying disproportionate regulatory pressure on supplements and what could be learned from supplement regulatory frameworks in other countries (Porter, 2002).

Fearing that FDA would ban supplements containing ingredients without sufficient evidence of efficacy or require prescriptions for access, a campaign for dietary supplement legislation was waged by retailers (Porter, 2002). The campaign against restrictive regulation of dietary supplements was unparalleled—resulting in more letters to Congress than the Watergate scandal (Swann, 2016). The frenzied response can probably best be illustrated by a 1990s commercial featuring a fully armed SWAT team raiding Mel Gibson's home to stop him from taking vitamin C. The message of the advertisement was clear: the FDA was trying to take away your vitamins and only public mobilization could stop them. Passage of DSHEA was a legislative response to the public outcry. The bill was championed by Orrin Hatch, a Republican senator representing Utah, a state with a significant number of dietary supplement manufacturers (Pray, 2012).

The motivation driving passage of DSHEA is clear from the wording in the legislation. The introductory (i.e., Congressional findings) section emphasizes the potential health benefits of dietary supplements, protecting consumer access to them, and their importance in the US economy. In defining dietary supplements, as described in the introduction, DSHEA created a separate regulatory category for these substances. While definitively placing them under the umbrella of food as opposed to drugs, DSHEA specified that they were distinct from both conventional foods and food additives. This distinction from drugs and food additives is particularly stark in consideration of premarket approval. Unlike drugs and food additives, which require premarket approval by the FDA, dietary supplement ingredients that were on the market prior to the passage of DSHEA are assumed to be safe and do not require premarket approval. The burden of proving harm from a dietary supplement rests on the FDA and relies on postmarket surveillance of adverse events. Stated another way, the FDA is only permitted to act when a dietary supplement product is found to be unsafe, adulterated, or misbranded (O'Dwyer and Vegiraju, 2020).

Another important part of the DSHEA legislation deals with clarification of label claims. There are four permitted categories of label claims under DSHEA that apply to both foods and dietary supplements: health claims, qualified health claims, structure/function claims, and nutrient content claims (Wallace, 2015). Health claims, established under the Nutrition Labeling and Education Act, require FDA review and approval based on significant scientific agreement; approved health claims (e.g., calcium and osteoporosis) are listed on the FDA website (Wallace, 2015). A challenge to the Nutrition Labeling and Education Act in 1999 arose from the US Court of Appeals, which struck down the FDA's requirement for significant scientific agreement on health claims in *Pearson v. Shalala* and led to the creation of qualified health claims (Vladeck, 2000). Qualified health claims have some scientific support but do not rise to the standard for significant scientific agreement and, therefore, require a disclaimer (Wallace, 2015). Structure/function claims are intended to describe the role of the supplement ingredient in maintaining the structure or function of the body (e.g., echinacea supports the immune system) and represent the majority of claims used in supplement advertising (O'Dwyer and Vegiraju, 2020). Finally, nutrient claims are intended to characterize the level of nutrients present in the product. For dietary supplements, nutrient claims typically describe the percentage of a dietary ingredient in the supplement (https://www.fda.gov/food/food-labeling-nutrition/label-claims-conventional-foods-and-dietary-supplements).

Perhaps the most important piece of the DSHEA legislation in terms of dietary supplement safety is the specification that dietary supplements are considered adulterated if they are not produced under current good manufacturing practices (cGMP). The cGMP guidelines are intended to establish that dietary supplement products contain the ingredients listed on the label at the specified purity, strength, and composition (Bailey, 2020). FDA published a final rule on June 25, 2007, that established cGMPs for manufacturing, labeling, and holding operations for dietary supplements (Pawar and Grundel, 2017). A dietary supplement is considered to be adulterated if it is not prepared, packaged, and held under conditions specified by the cGMPs.

While the cGMP rules provide an important enforcement authority for the FDA, the FDA lacks adequate budget and staff to inspect and monitor existing facilities (Bailey, 2020).

The DSHEA legislation makes a clear distinction between dietary supplement ingredients in the marketplace prior to 1994 and new dietary ingredients (i.e., ingredients that have not been in the food supply as a food or dietary supplement). While ingredients on the market before 1994 do not require premarket approval, new dietary ingredients require submission of a premarket safety notification to FDA at least 75 days prior to their introduction into interstate commerce. Draft guidance for the industry was released by FDA in 2011 and updated in 2016 to clarify the new dietary ingredient notification requirements and process (FDA, 2016a). New dietary ingredient notifications should contain a complete description of the identity and composition of the ingredient and supplement, an explanation of why the ingredient is considered a new dietary ingredient, a description of the supplement's recommended conditions of use, and history of use for the ingredient or other evidence of safety supporting a conclusion of a reasonable expectation of safety (FDA, 2016a).

The final action mandated by DSHEA was to establish the Office of Dietary Supplements within the National Institutes of Health (Costello and Coates, 2001). The mission of the Office of Dietary Supplements is to increase our scientific understanding of dietary supplements and their role in health (Kuszak et al., 2016). Additionally, the Director of the Office of Dietary Supplements was tasked with serving as an advisor to the National Institutes of Health, the Centers for Disease Control and Prevention, and the FDA on dietary supplement issues. Finally, the Office of Dietary Supplements was instructed through the legislation to compile a database of research on dietary supplements.

Following the passage of DSHEA, many experts expressed concern that the lack of premarket approval for dietary supplements and widespread availability of products with little safety data expose the public to undue harm (Bryan et al., 2001; Kroll, 2004; Nesheim, 1999). In 2004 the American Society of Health System Pharmacists published a statement asserting that the regulatory framework established by DSHEA did not provide consumers or healthcare workers with sufficient information on the safety and efficacy of dietary supplements and that product quality standards were inadequate (Kroll, 2004). The statement included recommendations for three changes to the dietary supplement regulatory structure: (1) FDA approval for safety and efficacy evidence; (2) more rigorous standards for identity, strength, quality, purity, packaging, and labeling of supplements; and (3) mandatory postmarket adverse event reporting with particular emphasis on supplement–drug interactions (Kroll, 2004). While the basic regulatory structure imposed by DSHEA has remained in place, there have been a few additions that have helped strengthen the system for reporting adverse events and enforcement of quality issues.

The Dietary Supplement and Nonprescription Drug Consumer Protection Act of 2006 required manufacturers to report serious adverse events to the FDA. The law was motivated by findings that manufacturers failed to report significant cardiac events in consumers following the use of ephedra-containing supplements to the FDA, thereby inhibiting FDA action (Porter, 2007). Serious adverse events were defined as death, life-threatening experience, hospitalization, persistent or significant disability or incapacity, congenital anomaly or birth defect, or requiring medical or surgical intervention (Porter, 2007). While the Food Safety Modernization Act purportedly strengthened FDA's authority to preemptively act against misbranded or adulterated foods and dietary supplements, dietary supplements were notably excluded from much of the legislation (Sax, 2015). Recommendations for strengthening the regulatory framework for dietary supplements moving forward include increasing enforcement efforts of existing cGMP regulations with particular attention to adulteration, strengthening scientific evidence requirements for efficacy and safety, and improving adverse event reporting (Brown, 2017; Sax, 2015; Wallace, 2015).

Toxicity of dietary supplements

Throughout the history of dietary supplement use, there have been notable instances of toxicity with certain ingredients or products. As noted in the previous section, dietary supplements do not require premarket safety evaluation and approval by the FDA but rely on postmarket adverse event reporting for identifying safety concerns. Therefore it can be difficult to observe patterns of toxicity across populations and to causally link adverse events to harmful dietary supplements. This effort is further complicated when people take multiple dietary supplements (Maiello et al., 2019) or when they do not report use of dietary supplements to their healthcare providers.

There are many possible ways to organize information on the toxicity of dietary supplements (e.g., by ingredient type, by organ system). In the following discussion, historically important examples of dietary supplement toxicity are presented with a focus on the following broad categories: toxicity elicited by the ingredient itself, the toxicity of an adulterant, toxicity due to contamination, and toxicity due to interactions between a dietary supplement and other substances. Here, adulteration refers to the intentional addition of unlabeled substances either for economic (i.e., use of cheaper material) or functional (i.e., use of potent chemicals) purposes and contamination refers to unintentional addition of unlabeled substances either through poor quality source material or inadequate manufacturing practices.

Toxicity elicited by dietary supplement ingredients

Many of the dietary supplement ingredients that have been found to elicit significant toxicity come from the botanical category. Ironically, people often perceive botanical supplements to be safe because they are considered to be "natural" and come from plants (Snyder et al., 2009). Additional rationale for perceiving botanicals as safe is applicable to all dietary supplements and includes their availability without a prescription and ubiquity in the marketplace (Snyder et al., 2009). Despite a perception of safety, it is not surprising that botanical ingredients can display toxicity, especially considering their historical use as medicines with recognized margins of safety. The use of botanical ingredients in dietary supplements involves their removal from the traditional medicinal context (i.e., prescribed use under the care of a trained practitioner for treatment of specific ailments) and introduction into the self-guided personal health and wellness setting with its inherent assumptions of safety and that if some is good, more is better.

The National Toxicology Program (NTP) recognized the need for research into the toxicity of commonly used botanical ingredients and initiated a testing program in the 1990s (Matthews et al., 1999). In the decades since, the NTP has evaluated the toxicity of numerous botanical ingredients in short- and long-term rodent toxicity assays including aloe vera extract (Boudreau et al., 2013; NTP 2013), black cohosh extract (Mercado-Feliciano et al., 2012), ephedra (Dunnick et al., 2007), *Ginkgo biloba* extract (NTP, 2013b), ginseng (NTP, 2011a), green tea extract (NTP, 2016), goldenseal root powder (NTP, 2010), gum guggul extract (NTP, 2020), kava kava extract (NTP, 2012b), milk thistle extract (NTP, 2011b), and senna (NTP, 2012a). More recent studies have been aimed at providing methods for comparing across complex botanical products using both chemical and biological activity data (Catlin et al., 2018b; Ryan et al., 2019).

Ephedra

A clear example of toxicity elicited by a dietary supplement ingredient can be found with ephedra. Ephedra, from several species in the Ephedraceae family (most notably *Ephedra sinica*), is referred to as Ma Huang in Traditional Chinese Medicine where it has been used for centuries to treat respiratory symptoms (Mehendale et al., 2004). Isolated ephedra alkaloids, such as (−)-ephedrine and (+)-pseudoephedrine, have been used in Western medicine as bronchodilators and stimulants based on their beta-adrenergic agonism and sympathomimetic activity (Tye et al., 1967). In 1972 Dr. Erikson, a general practitioner in Elsinore, Denmark, prescribed a compound containing ephedrine, caffeine, and phenobarbital to asthma patients and observed unintentional weight loss (Malchowmoller et al., 1981). Rumors of an effective weight loss pill, the holy grail of pharmaceuticals, spread like wildfire. Side effects, in the form of skin rashes, were attributed to phenobarbital and led to a reconstitution of the treatment known as the "Elsinore Pill" with only ephedrine and caffeine (Greenway, 2001). In the United States, ephedra-containing supplements, either with or without caffeine, claiming to aid in weight loss and/or boost energy were widely available in the marketplace (e.g., Natural Trim, Metabolife, Herbal Ecstacy, Ripped Fuel) following the passage of DSHEA (Gurley et al., 2000). As with other botanical dietary supplements, discrepancies were observed between the levels of ephedra specified on labels and measured levels (Gurley et al., 2000).

During the height of ephedra dietary supplement use, the FDA received numerous adverse event reports involving ephedra-containing products and requested an independent review of these reports. The review, published in 2000, found that 31% of the 140 adverse events reported between June 1, 1997, and March 31, 1999, were definitely or probably associated with the use of ephedra supplements, and 31% were possibly related (Haller and Benowitz, 2000). The types of adverse events that were definitely, probably, or possibly associated with ephedra use included hypertension, palpitations and/or tachycardia, stroke, and/or seizures, with 10 events resulting in death and 13 in permanent disability (Haller and Benowitz, 2000). Another review of adverse events reported between 1995 and 1997 concluded that the use of ephedra was temporally related to serious cardiovascular events including stroke, myocardial infarction, and sudden death; that underlying cardiovascular disease was not a prerequisite for these events; and that massive doses were not required to elicit cardiovascular effects (Samenuk et al., 2002). Toxicological research in animal models replicated the cardiotoxic effects seen in humans and provided dose-response information on the joint effects of ephedra and caffeine (Dunnick et al., 2007).

In response to the evidence indicating significant risk associated with the use of ephedra, the FDA first proposed a rule limiting the amount of ephedrine alkaloids in dietary supplements (FDA, 1997). However, further evidence from adverse event analyses led FDA to reconsider the proposed rule and instead issue a final regulation that declared dietary supplements containing any amount of ephedrine alkaloids adulterated under the FD&C Act (FDA, 2004). A recent study of dietary supplements available online found that approximately 11% of ephedra product labels indicated potential violations of the ephedra alkaloid ban, highlighting the challenges in the enforcement of dietary supplement legislation (Lai et al., 2021).

Pyrrolizidine alkaloids in botanical dietary supplements

Prior to the first isolation of pyrrolizidine alkaloids from *Senecio latifolius* in 1909 (Watt, 1909), it was known that several members of the *Senecio* genus, commonly known as ragwort, could be toxic to grazing animals, such as horses and cattle. The toxicity manifested as acute cirrhosis of the liver, followed by death (Cushny, 1911; Watt, 1909). Following Watt's identification of the pyrrolizidine alkaloids, senecifoline and senecidolidine, Cushny embarked on a series of experiments in a wide range of animal subjects (i.e., frogs, rabbits, rats, and cats) to evaluate the toxicity of these compounds. Cushny characterized their hepatotoxicity using descriptive toxicology and pathological examination, confirming that the pyrrolizidine alkaloids were indeed the toxic constituents (Cushny, 1911). While these studies focused on shorter-term exposures and acute effects, Cook et al. (1950) demonstrated that long-term exposure to pyrrolizidine alkaloids isolated from *Senecio jacobaea* L. could induce liver tumors in albino rats.

Despite this early knowledge, the use of plant species containing pyrrolizidine alkaloids in teas, herbal medicines, and dietary supplements continued. Comfrey (*Symphytum officinale* L., Boraginaceae), for example, is known to contain pyrrolizidine alkaloids and has had a long history of use as a medicinal plant to soothe gastrointestinal distress (Betz et al., 1994). While widespread episodes of pyrrolizidine alkaloid poisoning resulting from contamination of food have taken place in countries such as Afghanistan (Mohabbat et al., 1976) and India (Tandon et al., 1976), the typical scenario in the United States involved more isolated incidences of adverse events, such as veno-occlusive disease, associated with the use of pyrrolizidine-containing dietary supplements or teas. For example, Ridker et al. (1985) described an incidence of veno-occlusive disease in a 49-year-old woman who took an herbal tea and a "comfrey-pepsin" capsule containing comfrey root powder. Both products were found to contain pyrrolizidine alkaloids and her exposure level was estimated at approximately 15 μg/kg per day over several months (Ridker et al., 1985).

In response to cases such as the one described before, the FDA sent a letter to dietary supplement manufacturers in 2001, advising them to remove products containing comfrey from the market (FDA, 2001). The FDA stated that products containing comfrey or other sources of pyrrolizidine alkaloids would be considered adulterated under the FD&C Act, as amended by DSHEA. In coordination with the FDA, the Federal Trade Commission took several enforcement actions against firms marketing comfrey products for internal use on the web (FDA, 2001). However, pyrrolizidine alkaloids continue to be detected in products available in the market (Avula et al., 2015).

Multicomponent weight loss supplements

In some of the most egregious cases of dietary supplement toxicity, the exact ingredient responsible for the toxicity is difficult to identify due to the multicomponent nature of the product and changing formulations. Two examples of this phenomenon can be found in the histories of Hydroxycut and OxyELITE Pro, which contain multiple ingredients in formulations that have changed over time. Both examples involve liver toxicity. Dietary supplements have increasingly been associated with liver injury (Navarro et al., 2014). Hillman et al. (2016) found that the fraction of acute liver injury and acute liver failure cases attributed to complementary and alternative medicines (i.e., dietary supplements and herbal medicines) increased from 12% in the 1998–2007 period to 21% in the 2007–2015 period.

Soon after Hydroxycut entered the market as a "fat-burning" weight loss supplement in 2002, the FDA started to receive adverse event reports of hepatotoxicity associated with its use (Dara et al., 2008; Fong et al., 2010). In a detailed case series report, Fong et al. (2010) describe 17 patients with severe hepatotoxicity following Hydroxycut use, with three requiring liver transplants, and the death of a 20-year-old male patient. In general, patients presented with nausea, lethargy, jaundice, elevated aminotransferase levels, and hepatocellular injury (Fong et al., 2010). Fifteen cases were deemed to be probably, likely, or definitely linked to Hydroxycut use, while only two cases were possibly related (Fong et al., 2010). The FDA released a warning letter urging consumers to stop using Hydroxycut in 2009 after receiving 23 reports of hepatotoxicity through the Center for Food and Safety and Applied Nutrition (CFSAN) Adverse Event Reporting System

(CAERS). Following the warning letter, the manufacturer Iovate (Oakville, Ontario, Canada) voluntarily recalled Hydroxycut products from the market. However, numerous Hydroxycut products (e.g., Hydroxycut Hardcore Elite, Black Onyx Hydroxycut, Hydroxycut Platinum) with variable ingredients continue to be widely available. The ingredient responsible for the hepatotoxicity remains to be identified. Prior to the 2004 FDA ephedra ban, ephedra was included in Hydroxycut formulations and was implicated as the ingredient responsible for observed hepatotoxicity (Neff et al., 2004). Following reformulation of Hydroxycut, ingredients such as *Garcinia gummi-gutta*, chromium, and green tea extract were suggested to be potential drivers of hepatotoxicity (Dara et al., 2008).

OxyELITE Pro offers a second example of a multicomponent weight loss supplement with changing formulations eliciting hepatotoxicity. OxyELITE Pro (USPlabs LLC, Dallas, TX) was marketed as a weight loss and muscle building supplement beginning around 2009. The original OxyELITE Pro formulation contained caffeine, yohimbe bark extract, *Bauhinia purpurea* extract, *Bacopa monnieri* extract, *Cirsium oligophyllum* extract, and the synthetic compound 1,3-dimethylamylamine HCl, known commonly as DMAA (Johnston et al., 2016). DMAA is a synthetic amphetamine derivative that does not meet the standards laid out in the DSHEA legislation for being a dietary ingredient. Therefore, beginning in 2012, the FDA issued warning letters to manufacturers of dietary supplements containing DMAA, including the makers of OxyELITE Pro. In response, the manufacturer reformulated the product, replacing DMAA with aegeline, an alkaloid isolated from the plant *Aegle marmelos* (Johnston et al., 2016). Notably, reports of cardiovascular events following the use of DMAA-containing supplements represented the primary concern (Karnatovskaia et al., 2015). Around the time that the reformulated products entered the market, multiple reports described severe liver disease following use of OxyELITE Pro, with some cases requiring liver transplants (Foley et al., 2014; Klontz et al., 2015; Roytman et al., 2014). Interestingly, some cases reported liver toxicity with the use of the old formulation (containing DMAA) (Foley et al., 2014), while others noted the use of the new formulation (containing aegeline) (Roytman et al., 2014). A pocket of cases was identified in Hawaii and was thoroughly investigated (Johnston et al., 2016). A representative subset of samples was screened for known hepatotoxicants such as pyrrolizidine alkaloids and usnic acid, but researchers found that the contents reflected ingredients on the label (Johnston et al., 2016). In October 2013, the FDA sent another warning letter to the manufacturer regarding the use of aegeline in dietary supplements. As with DMAA, aegeline was determined to not qualify as a dietary ingredient, and all products containing aegeline are adulterated according to the FDA.

Vinpocetine

Vinpocetine has been marketed as a dietary supplement for improving mental acuity. Due to a lack of evidence for vinpocetine being in the diet or used as a dietary supplement prior to the 1994 passage of DSHEA, manufacturers were required to submit new dietary ingredient notices to the FDA. Multiple new dietary ingredient notices were filed for vinpocetine during the 1990s (FDA, 2016b). While vinpocetine advertising suggested that it was a natural constituent of the periwinkle plant (*Vinca minor* L.), it is in fact a synthetic compound that is derived from plant alkaloids (e.g., vincamine, tabersonine). In 2016 the FDA tentatively concluded that vinpocetine did not meet the dietary ingredient definition and could not be included in dietary supplements (FDA, 2016b). Shortly after, studies at the NTP showed that treatment of pregnant animals with vinpocetine resulted in increased fetal loss in rat dams and increased incidences of malformations in their offspring with similar effects noted in the rabbit at higher doses (Catlin et al., 2018a). Based on these studies, the FDA released a warning for women of childbearing age about risks from vinpocetine-containing dietary supplements (FDA, 2019).

Adulterated dietary supplements

According to the FD&C Act of 1938 (21 U.S. Code § 342), a food (or dietary supplement) "shall be deemed to be adulterated—(a) if it bears or contains any poisonous or deleterious substance which may render it injurious to health... [or] (b) if any valuable constituent has been in whole or in part omitted or abstracted therefrom." As discussed in the introduction, issues with the adulteration of dietary supplements date back to their inception. There are two broad categories of adulteration: functional and economic. Functional adulteration refers to the addition of a known active ingredient that is either not permitted under the law (e.g., ephedra) and/or that is not included on the label (e.g., an undeclared pharmaceutical compound) to boost the pharmacological effect of a supplement. Economic adulteration refers to the addition of cheaper material to a dietary supplement. A few notable examples of adulteration of dietary supplements that resulted in toxicity are highlighted as follows.

Pharmaceutical compounds or their analogs in dietary supplements

Anabolic steroids have a long history of use for improving muscle growth and enhancing athletic performance. The first reported use of anabolic steroids in athletes dates back to the 1954 Olympics, where a US team physician reported that Russian athletes were receiving doses of testosterone (Wade, 1972). Anabolic steroids were added to the list of banned substances by the Olympics in 1975. The use of prohormones (precursors that can be converted to anabolic steroids in the body) to enhance athletic performance first drew public attention when in 1998 Mark McGwire, then the reigning Major League Baseball home run record holder, received extensive media attention for his use of androstenedione (Brown et al., 2003). Prohormones continued to be popular ingredients in performance-enhancing dietary supplements until they were banned by the 2004 Anabolic Steroid Control Act.

Adulteration of performance-enhancing dietary supplements with anabolic steroids was first reported in 1999 in connection with the detection of a prohormone in a positive doping case (Geyer et al., 2008). Since that time, there have been numerous examples of undeclared anabolic steroids detected in dietary supplements (Rocha et al., 2016). While some cases likely reflected low level contamination of dietary supplements with prohormones (e.g., androstenedione, androstenediol, dehydroepiandrosterone) which were legally marketed as dietary supplements in the United States until 2004, other cases continue to reflect intentional adulteration of dietary supplements with high levels of anabolic androgenic steroids (e.g., metandienone, stanozolol, oxandrolone) (Geyer et al., 2008). There are many well-known health effects associated with the use of anabolic androgenic steroids, including cardiovascular disease, liver toxicity, and reproductive effects (Albano et al., 2021). It stands to reason that dietary supplements containing anabolic steroid adulterants would also elicit adverse effects. In fact, body building supplements are the category most commonly implicated in reported cases of hepatotoxicity associated with the use of dietary supplements (Navarro et al., 2014).

Dietary supplements marketed to enhance sexual performance represent another category that has been frequently adulterated with pharmaceutical compounds or their analogs. The FDA found that in the period of 2007–2016 sexual enhancement supplements were the category most frequently adulterated, with sildenafil (a phosphodiesterase-5 inhibitor and the active compound in Viagra) identified as the most common adulterant in those supplements (Tucker et al., 2018).

Dietary supplements contaminated with toxic substances

Many of the regulations pertaining to dietary supplements (Table 2) recognized the dangers posed by contamination of dietary supplements with harmful substances (e.g., heavy metals, mycotoxins, microbes, pesticides, and herbicides). Unlike the cases of intentional adulteration outlined before, contamination of dietary supplements tends to result from a lack of good manufacturing practices or quality issues along the supply chain. It is particularly difficult to link contaminants in specific products to the development of diseases that have long latencies, such as cancer. Cases of acute toxicity due to contamination are more likely to be identified.

Aristolochia fangchi

One flagrant case of contaminated dietary supplements linked to life-threatening toxicity can be found in a case of mistaken plant identity. In 1992 two women under 50 presented with rapidly progressing kidney failure at a nephrology center in Belgium (Vanherweghem et al., 1993). Both women had received a weight loss regimen from a medical clinic consisting of weekly injections of artichoke extract and euphyllin, a small dose of amphetamines, and a multiingredient dietary supplement (Vanherweghem et al., 1993). Multiple additional cases followed the first two. The dietary supplement was reformulated in 1990; specifically, pancreas powder, laminaria powder, and fucus extract were removed, and belladonna extract and powders from two Chinese herbs, *Stephania tetrandra* and *Magnolia officinalis,* were added. Researchers noted that all the women presenting with kidney disease had taken the new dietary supplement formulation. They embarked on an epidemiological assessment of women who attended the clinic from 1990 to 1991 and were able to pinpoint the period of poisoning to May–December 1990 (Vanherweghem et al., 1993). Analysis of dietary supplement samples using thin-layer chromatography revealed that marker constituents for *Stephania tetrandra* were not present, but aristolochic acids were, implicating the known nephrotoxic plant species *Aristolochia fangchi* (Vanhaelen et al., 1994). Both *Stephania tetrandra* and *Aristolochia fangchi* are used in Traditional Chinese Medicine and are part of the same "Fang Ji" family of therapeutics (Nortier and Vanherweghem, 2007). Therefore the mix up is not surprising and should serve as a warning to producers and consumers (Nortier and Vanherweghem, 2007).

Table 2 Dietary supplement legislative milestones in the United States.

Year	Title	Description
1906	Pure Food and Drug Act	Improved the accuracy and truth in labeling of food and drug products
1938	Food, Drug, and Cosmetic Act	Replaced the Pure Food and Drug Act with greater consumer protections
1976	Vitamin-Mineral (Proxmire) Amendment to the Food, Drug, and Cosmetic Act	Prohibited the FDA from regulating the potency of vitamins and minerals in dietary supplements and from classifying dietary supplements as drugs
1990	Nutrition Labeling and Education Act	Clarified labeling of food and dietary supplements
1994	Dietary Supplement Health and Education Act	Defined dietary supplements, clarified label claims, imposed good manufacturing practices, and established the Office of Dietary Supplements
1999	*Pearson v. Shalala*	Struck down health claim requirement of significant scientific evidence and gave rise to qualified health claim option
2003	Launch of the CFSAN Adverse Event Reporting System (CAERS)	Supported CFSAN's safety surveillance program to monitor adverse events and product complaint reports
2004	Anabolic Steroid Control Act	Banned the inclusion of anabolic steroids or prohormones in dietary supplements
2006	Dietary Supplement and Nonprescription Drug Consumer Protection Act	Required reporting of serious adverse events for dietary supplements and over-the-counter drugs
2007	Final Rule on Good Manufacturing Practices	Established minimum current good manufacturing practices necessary for manufacturing, packaging, labeling, or holding dietary supplements to ensure quality
2011	Food Safety Modernization Act	Strengthened FDA's authority to act when foods are misbranded or adulterated, but excluded dietary supplements from application of the law; allowed for Drug Enforcement Authority notification of anabolic steroids in dietary supplements
2016	Draft Guidance for Industry on New Dietary Ingredient Notifications and Related Issues	Clarified new dietary ingredient notification requirements

Drug-supplement interactions

The potential for drug-drug interactions is carefully considered by doctors when they prescribe medications. Unlike drugs, dietary supplements require no prescription, and the use of dietary supplements is not always disclosed to medical professionals, thereby opening the door for possible drug-supplement interactions. In these cases, the dietary supplement could be free of toxic effects when taken individually but could change the pharmacokinetic profile of a drug with a small therapeutic window and cause toxicity indirectly. Alternatively, dietary supplements could decrease the efficacy of life-saving medications leading to disease progression.

St. John's Wort

Many botanical ingredients found in dietary supplements have been implicated in drug-supplement interactions (Fugh-Berman, 2000). Perhaps the most well-studied example of a botanical ingredient interacting with drugs is St. John's Wort (*Hypericum perforatum*). St. John's Wort is marketed as a dietary supplement to support mental and emotional health. A review of clinical trials in the 1990s revealed that St. John's Wort compared favorably with available antidepressants in treating mild to moderate depression (Linde et al., 1996), and it has been a widely used dietary supplement in the years since. However, a significant body of research has indicated that St. John's Wort is a potent inducer of the metabolizing enzyme cytochrome P450 3A4 and the drug efflux transporter p-glycoprotein (Zhou et al., 2004). Studies have shown that St. John's Wort decreased the blood concentration of numerous drugs (e.g., digoxin, midazolam, warfarin) and decreased the efficacy of birth control medication (Zhou et al., 2004). Finally, multiple incidences of serotonin syndrome have been reported in patients taking both St. John's Wort and selective serotonin reuptake inhibitors (Barbenel et al., 2000; Lantz et al., 1999; Parker et al., 2001). While some manufacturers do provide a warning about potential drug interactions, St. John's Wort continues to be widely available as an over-the-counter dietary supplement.

Conclusions

The nature of medicine and wellness has undergone tremendous changes over the course of modern history. However, a review of the path leading from the snake oil sales of the past to the present domination of dietary supplements in the wellness marketplace indicates that many challenges remain. The regulatory pendulum has swung back and forth between facilitating unencumbered access to dietary supplements and attempting to protect public health and rein in bad actors, with the current system trying to strike a balance between the two. As in the past, it is often a dramatic episode of conspicuous toxicity or even death that leads to changes in the system and brings about additional safeguards. Issues with quality and consistency of dietary supplements continue to be a problem with examples of adulteration and contamination leading to toxicity. On the other side of the coin, advances in chemical analysis and toxicity testing have improved our ability to identify and characterize hazards associated with dietary supplements.

Acknowledgments

This work was supported by the Intramural Research Program of the National Institutes of Health (NIH), National Institute of Environmental Health Sciences (NIEHS), and Intramural Research project ZIA ES103316-04.

References

Albano, G.D., Amico, F., Cocimano, G., Liberto, A., Maglietta, F., Esposito, M., Rosi, G.L., Di Nunno, N., Salerno, M., Montana, A., 2021. Adverse effects of anabolic-androgenic steroids: a literature review. Healthcare 9, 97. https://doi.org/10.3390/healthcare9010097.

Aumeeruddy, M.Z., Mahomoodally, M.F., 2021. Global documentation of traditionally used medicinal plants in cancer management: a systematic review. S. Afr. J. Bot. 138, 424–494.

Avula, B., Sagi, S., Wang, Y.H., Zweigenbaum, J., Wang, M., Khan, I.A., 2015. Characterization and screening of pyrrolizidine alkaloids and N-oxides from botanicals and dietary supplements using UHPLC-high resolution mass spectrometry. Food Chem. 178, 136–148.

Bailey, R.L., 2020. Current regulatory guidelines and resources to support research of dietary supplements in the United States. Crit. Rev. Food Sci. 60, 298–309.

Bao, K., 2017. Non-scientific classification of Chinese herbal medicine as dietary supplement. Chin. J. Integr. Med. 23, 166–169.

Barbenel, D.M., Yusufi, B., O'Shea, D., Bench, C.J., 2000. Mania in a patient receiving testosterone replacement postorchidectomy taking St John's wort and sertraline. J. Psychopharmacol. 14, 84–86.

Betz, J.M., Eppley, R.M., Taylor, W.C., Andrezejewski, D., 1994. Determination of pyrrolizidine alkaloids in commercial comfrey products (Sympthytum Sp). J. Pharm. Sci. 83, 649–653.

Borchers, A.T., Hagie, F., Keen, C.L., Gershwin, M.E., 2007. The history and contemporary challenges of the US Food and Drug Administration. Clin. Ther. 29, 1–16.

Boudreau, M.D., Mellick, P.W., Olson, G.R., Felton, R.P., Thorn, B.T., Beland, F.A., 2013. Clear evidence of carcinogenic activity by a whole-leaf extract of *Aloe barbadensis* miller (aloe vera) in F344/N rats. Toxicol. Sci. 131, 26–39.

Brown, A.C., 2017. An overview of herb and dietary supplement efficacy, safety and government regulations in the United States with suggested improvements. Part 1 of 5 series. Food Chem. Toxicol. 107, 449–471.

Brown, W.J., Basil, M.D., Bocarnea, M.C., 2003. The influence of famous athletes on health beliefs and practices: mark McGwire, child abuse prevention, and androstenedione. J. Health Commun. 8, 41–57.

Bryan, Q., Coleman, L.K., Meisberger, S.M., Copmann, T., 2001. Issues in the regulation of dietary supplements. Drug Inf. J. 35, 529–538.

Cai, P.P., Qiu, H., Qi, F.H., Zhang, X.Y., 2019. The toxicity and safety of traditional Chinese medicines: please treat with rationality. Biosci. Trends 13, 367–373.

Catlin, N., Waidyanatha, S., Mylchreest, E., Miller-Pinsler, L., Cunny, H., Foster, P., Sutherland, V., McIntyre, B., 2018a. Embryo-fetal development studies with the dietary supplement vinpocetine in the rat and rabbit. Birth Defects Res. 110, 883–896.

Catlin, N.R., Collins, B.J., Auerbach, S.S., Ferguson, S.S., Harnly, J.M., Gennings, C., Waidyanatha, S., Rice, G.E., Smith-Roe, S.L., Witt, K.L., Rider, C.V., 2018b. How similar is similar enough? A sufficient similarity case study with *Ginkgo biloba* extract. Food Chem. Toxicol. 118, 328–339.

Cook, J.W., Duffy, E., Schoental, R., 1950. Primary liver Tumours in rats following feeding with alkaloids of Senecio-Jacobaea. Br. J. Cancer 4, 405–410.

Costello, R.B., Coates, P., 2001. In the midst of confusion lies opportunity: fostering quality science in dietary supplement research. J. Am. Coll. Nutr. 20, 21–25.

Cushny, A.R., 1911. On the action of senecio alkaloids and the causation of the hepatic cirrhosis of cattle (Pictou, Molteno, or Winton disease). J. Pharmacol. Exp. Ther. 2, 531–548.

Dara, L., Hewett, J., Lim, J.K., 2008. Hydroxycut hepatotoxicity: a case series and review of liver toxicity from herbal weight loss supplements. World J. Gastroenterol. 14, 6999–7004.

Dunnick, J.K., Kissling, G., Gerken, D.K., Vallant, M.A., Nyska, A., 2007. Cardiotoxicity of Ma Huang/caffeine or ephedrine/caffeine in a rodent model system. Toxicol. Pathol. 35, 657–664.

FDA, 1997. Dietary supplements containing ephedrine alkaloids; proposed rule. 21 CFR Part 111 Federal Register.

FDA, 2001. FDA advises dietary supplement manufacturers to remove comfrey products from the market.

FDA, 2004. Final rule declaring dietary supplements containing ephedrine alkaloids adulterated because they present an unreasonable risk. In: 21 CFR Part 119.

FDA, 2016a. Dietary supplements: new dietary ingredient notifications and related issues: guidance for industry. In: Draft Guidance. 81 FR 68434.

FDA, 2016b. Request for comment on the status of vinpocetine. In: Federal Register.

FDA, 2019. Statement on warning for women of childbearing age about possible safety risks of dietary supplements containing vinpocetine.

Foley, S., Butlin, E., Shields, W., Lacey, B., 2014. Experience with OxyELITE pro and acute liver injury in active duty service members. Dig. Dis. Sci. 59, 3117–3121.

Fong, T.L., Klontz, K.C., Canas-Coto, A., Casper, S.J., Durazo, F.A., Davern, T.J., Hayashi, P., Lee, W.M., Seeff, L.B., 2010. Hepatotoxicity due to Hydroxycut: a case series. Am. J. Gastroenterol. 105, 1561–1566.

Fugh-Berman, A., 2000. Herb-drug interactions. Lancet 355, 134–138.

Gasbarrini, G., Bonvicini, F., Gramenzi, A., 2016. Probiotics history. J. Clin. Gastroenterol. 50, S116–S119.

Geyer, H., Parr, M.K., Koehler, K., Mareck, U., Schanzer, W., Thevis, M., 2008. Nutritional supplements cross-contaminated and faked with doping substances. J. Mass Spectrom. 43, 892–902.

Global Industry Analysts, 2021. Global Dietary Supplements Industry, Market Report.

Greenway, F.L., 2001. The safety and efficacy of pharmaceutical and herbal caffeine and ephedrine use as a weight loss agent. Obes. Rev. 2, 199–211.

Guo, X.S., Long, R.J., Kreuzer, M., Ding, L.M., Shang, Z.H., Zhang, Y., Yang, Y., Cui, G.X., 2014. Importance of functional ingredients in yak Milk-derived food on health of Tibetan nomads living under high-altitude stress: a review. Crit. Rev. Food Sci. 54, 292–302.

Gurley, B.J., Gardner, S.F., Hubbard, M.A., 2000. Content versus label claims in ephedra-containing dietary supplements. Am. J. Health Syst. Pharm. 57, 963–969.

Haller, C.A., Benowitz, N.L., 2000. Adverse cardiovascular and central nervous system events associated with dietary supplements containing ephedra alkaloids. N. Engl. J. Med. 343, 1833–1838.

Hardy, K., Buckley, S., Collins, M.J., Estalrrich, A., Brothwell, D., Copeland, L., Garcia-Tabernero, A., Garcia-Vargas, S., de la Rasilla, M., Lalueza-Fox, C., Huguet, R., Bastir, M., Santamaria, D., Madella, M., Wilson, J., Cortes, A.F., Rosas, A., 2012. Neanderthal medics? Evidence for food, cooking, and medicinal plants entrapped in dental calculus. Naturwissenschaften 99, 617–626.

Hillman, L., Gottfried, M., Whitsett, M., Rakela, J., Schilsky, M., Lee, W.M., Ganger, D., 2016. Clinical features and outcomes of complementary and alternative medicine induced acute liver failure and injury. Am. J. Gastroenterol. 111, 958–965.

Janick, J., 2003. Herbals: the connection between horticulture and medicine. Hort. Technology 13, 229–238.

Johnston, D.I., Chang, A., Viray, M., Chatham-Stephens, K., He, H., Taylor, E., Wong, L.L., Schier, J., Martin, C., Fabricant, D., Salter, M., Lewis, L., Park, S.Y., 2016. Hepatotoxicity associated with the dietary supplement OxyELITE pro (TM) Hawaii, 2013. Drug Test. Anal. 8, 319–327.

Karnatovskaia, L.V., Leoni, J.C., Freeman, M.L., 2015. Cardiac arrest in a 21-year-old man after ingestion of 1,3-DMAA-containing workout supplement. Clin. J. Sport Med. 25, E23–E25.

Klontz, K.C., DeBeck, H.J., LeBlanc, P., Mogen, K.M., Wolpert, B.J., Sabo, J.L., Salter, M., Seelman, S.L., Lance, S.E., Monahan, C., Steigman, D.S., Gensheimer, K., 2015. The role of adverse event reporting in the FDA response to a multistate outbreak of liver disease associated with a dietary supplement. Public Health Rep. 130, 526–532.

Kopeloff, N., Blackman, N., McGinn, B., 1932. The incidence of *Lactobacillus acidophilus* in adults. J Infect Dis 50, 426–429.

Kroll, D.J., 2004. ASHP statement on the use of dietary supplements. Am. J. Health-Syst. Pharm. 61, 1707–1711.

Kuszak, A.J., Hopp, D.C., Williamson, J.S., Betz, J.M., Sorkin, B.C., 2016. Approaches by the US National Institutes of Health to support rigorous scientific research on dietary supplements and natural products. Drug Test. Anal. 8, 413–417.

Lai, S., Yu, C., Dennehy, C.E., Tsourounis, C., Lee, K.P., 2021. Online marketing of Ephedra weight loss supplements: labeling and marketing compliance with the U.S. Food and Drug Administration ban on Ephedra. J. Altern. Complement. Med.

Lantz, M.S., Buchalter, E., Giambanco, V., 1999. St. John's wort and antidepressant drug interactions in the elderly. J. Geriatr. Psychiatry Neurol. 12, 7–10.

Lietava, J., 1992. Medicinal-plants in a middle Paleolithic grave Shanidar-Iv. J. Ethnopharmacol. 35, 263–266.

Linde, K., Ramirez, G., Mulrow, C.D., Pauls, A., Weidenhammer, W., Melchart, D., 1996. St John's wort for depression- -an overview and meta-analysis of randomised clinical trials. BMJ 313, 253–258.

Lu, W.I., Lu, D.P., 2014. Impact of Chinese herbal medicine on American society and health care system: perspective and concern. Evid. Based Complement. Alternat. Med. 2014, 251891.

Maiello, M., Carbone, M.G., Dell'Osso, L., Simoncini, M., Miniati, M., 2019. Acute cognitive and psychomotor impairment in a patient taking forty different herbal products and dietary supplements: a case report. J. Psychopathol. 25, 231–235.

Malchowmoller, A., Larsen, S., Hey, H., Stokholm, K.H., Juhl, E., Quaade, F., 1981. Ephedrine as an anorectic - the story of the Elsinore pill. Int. J. Obes. (Lond) 5, 183–187.

Matthews, H.B., Lucier, G.W., Fisher, K.D., 1999. Medicinal herbs in the United States: research needs. Environ. Health Perspect. 107, 773–778.

McFarland, L.V., 2015. From yaks to yogurt: the history, development, and current use of probiotics. Clin. Infect. Dis. 60, S85–S90.

Mehendale, S.R., Bauer, B.A., Yuan, C.S., 2004. Ephedra-containing dietary supplements in the US versus ephedra as a Chinese medicine. Am. J. Chin. Med. 32, 1–10.

Mercado-Feliciano, M., Cora, M.C., Witt, K.L., Granville, C.A., Hejtmancik, M.R., Fomby, L., Knostman, K.A., Ryan, M.J., Newbold, R., Smith, C., Foster, P.M., Vallant, M.K., Stout, M.D., 2012. An ethanolic extract of black cohosh causes hematological changes but not estrogenic effects in female rodents. Toxicol. Appl. Pharmacol. 263, 138–147.

Metchnikoff, E., 1908. Lactic acid as inhibiting intestinal putrifaction. In: Mitchell, P.C. (Ed.), The Prolongation of Life: Optimistic Studies. G.P. Putnam's Sons, New York, pp. 161–183.

Mishra, S., Stierman, B., Gahche, J.J., Potischman, N., 2021. Dietary Supplement Use Among Adults: United States, 2017–2018. NCHS Data Brief, No. 399. National Center for Health Statistics, Hyattsville, MD, https://doi.org/10.15620/cdc:101131.

Mohabbat, O., Srivastava, R.N., Younos, M.S., Merzad, A.A., Sediq, G.G., Aram, G.N., 1976. Outbreak of hepatic Veno-occlusive disease in northwestern Afghanistan. Lancet 2, 269–271.

Navarro, V.J., Barnhart, H., Bonkovsky, H.L., Davern, T., Fontana, R.J., Grant, L., Reddy, K.R., Seeff, L.B., Serrano, J., Sherker, A.H., Stolz, A., Talwalkar, J., Vega, M., Vuppalanchi, R., 2014. Liver injury from herbals and dietary supplements in the U.S. Drug-induced liver injury network. Hepatology 60, 1399–1408.

Neff, G.W., Reddy, K.R., Durazo, F.A., Meyer, D., Marrero, R., Kaplowitz, N., 2004. Severe hepatotoxicity associated with the use of weight loss diet supplements containing ma huang or usnic acid. J. Hepatol. 41, 1062–1064.

Nesheim, M.C., 1999. What is the research base for the use of dietary supplements? Public Health Nutr. 2, 35–38.

Nortier, J.L., Vanherweghem, J.L., 2007. For patients taking herbal therapy- -lessons from aristolochic acid nephropathy. Nephrol. Dial. Transplant. 22, 1512–1517.

NTP, 2010. NTP technical report on the toxicology and carcinogenesis studies of goldenseal rootpowder (HydrastisCanadensis) in F344/N rats and B6C3F1 mice (feed studies). In: Technical Report Series. National Institutes of Health Public Health Service, U.S. Department of Health and Human Services. Research Triangle Park, NC.

NTP, 2011a. NTP technical report on the toxicology and carcinogenesis studies of ginseng (Cas no. 50647-08-0) in F344/N rats and B6C3F1 mice (gavage studies). In: Technical Report Series. National Institutes of Health Public Health Service, U.S. Department of Health and Human Services. Research Triangle Park, NC.

NTP, 2011b. NTP technical report on the toxicology and carcinogenesis studies of Milk thistle extract in F344/N rats and B6C3F1 mice (feed studies). In: Technical Report Series. National Institutes of Health Public Health Service, U.S. Department of Health and Human Services. Research Triangle Park, NC.

NTP, 2012a. NTP report on the toxicology studies of Senna (CAS no. 8013-11-4) in C57BL/6NTac mice and toxicology and carcinogenesis study of senna in genetically modified C3B6.129F1/Tac-Trp53tm1Brd N12 haploinsufficient mice (feed studies). In: Genetically Modified Model (GMM) Report Series. National Institutes of Health Public Health Service, U.S. Department of Health and Human Services. Research Triangle Park, NC.

NTP, 2012b. NTP technical report on the toxicology and carcinogenesis studies of kava kava extract (CAS no. 9000-38-8) in F344/N rats and B6C3F1 mice (gavage studies). In: Technical Report Series. National Institutes of Health Public Health Service, U.S. Department of Health and Human Services. Research Triangle Park, NC.

NTP, 2013a. NTP technical report on the toxicology and carcinogenesis studies of a nonde-colorized whole leaf extract of *Aloe Barbadensis* Miller (*Aloe Vera*) in F344/N Rats and B6C3F1 Mice (Drinking Water Studies). In: Technical Report Series. National Institutes of Health Public Health Service, U.S. Department of Health and Human Services. Research Triangle Park, NC.

NTP, 2013b. NTP technical report on the toxicology and carcinogenesis studies of *Ginkgo biloba* extract (CAS No. 90045-36-6) in F344/N rats and B6C3F1/N Mice (Gavage Studies). In: Technical Report Series. NIEHS/NTP. Research Triangle Park.

NTP, 2016. NTP technical report on the toxicology studies of green tea extract in F344/NTac Rats and B6C3F1/N mice and toxicology and carcinogenesis studies of green tea extract in Wistar Han [Crl:WI(Han)] Rats and B6C3F1/N Mice (Gavage Studies). In: Technical Report Series. National Institutes of Health Public Health Service, U.S. Department of Health and Human Services. Research Triangle Park, NC.

NTP, 2020. NTP technical report on the toxicity studies of a gum guggul extract formulation administered by gavage to sprague dawley (Hsd:Sprague Dawley® SD®) Rats and B6C3F1/N Mice. In: Toxicity Report Series. National Institutes of Health Public Health Service, U.S. Department of Health and Human Services. Research Triangle Park, NC.

O'Dwyer, D.D., Vegiraju, S., 2020. Navigating the maze of dietary supplements regulation and safety. Top. Clin. Nutr. 35, 248–263.

Oketch-Rabah, H.A., Roe, A.L., Rider, C.V., Bonkovsky, H.L., Giancaspro, G.I., Navarro, V., Paine, M.F., Betz, J.M., Marles, R.J., Casper, S., Gurley, B., Jordan, S.A., He, K., Kapoor, M.P., Rao, T.P., Sherker, A.H., Fontana, R.J., Rossi, S., Vuppalanchi, R., Seeff, L.B., Stolz, A., Ahmad, J., Koh, C., Serrano, J., Low Dog, T., Ko, R., 2020. United States Pharmacopeia (USP) comprehensive review of the hepatotoxicity of green tea extracts. Toxicol. Rep. 7, 386–402.

Parker, V., Wong, A.H., Boon, H.S., Seeman, M.V., 2001. Adverse reactions to St John's wort. Can. J. Psychiatry 46, 77–79.

Pawar, R.S., Grundel, E., 2017. Overview of regulation of dietary supplements in the USA and issues of adulteration with phenethylamines (PEAs). Drug Test. Anal. 9, 500–517.

Phillips, M.M., Rimmer, C.A., 2013. Functional foods and dietary supplements. Anal. Bioanal. Chem. 405, 4323–4324.

Porter, D.V., 2002. Dietary Supplements: Legislative and Regulatory Status, Report for Congress. Congressional Research Service, Library of Congress.

Porter, D.V., 2007. Dietary supplement and Nonprescription Drug Consumer Protection Act (P.L. 109-462), Report for Congress. Congressional Research Service, Library of Congress.

Pray, W.S., 2012. Orrin hatch and the dietary supplement health and education act: Pandora's box revisited. J. Child Neurol. 27, 561–563.

Rettger, L.F., Cheplin, H.A., 1922. Bacillus acidophilus and its therapeutic application. Arch. Intern. Med. 29, 357–367.

Ridker, P.M., Ohkuma, S., Mcdermott, W.V., Trey, C., Huxtable, R.J., 1985. Hepatic Venocclusive disease associated with the consumption of pyrrolizidine-containing dietary-supplements. Gastroenterology 88, 1050–1054.

Rocha, T., Amaral, J.S., Oliveira, M.B.P.P., 2016. Adulteration of dietary supplements by the illegal addition of synthetic drugs: a review. Compr. Rev. Food Sci. Food Saf. 15, 43–62.

Rosenfeld, L., 1997. Vitamine-vitamin. The early years of discovery. Clin. Chem. 43, 680–685.

Roytman, M.M., Porzgen, P., Lee, C.L., Huddleston, L., Kuo, T.T., Bryant-Greenwood, P., Wong, L.L., Tsai, N., 2014. Outbreak of severe hepatitis linked to weight-loss supplement OxyELITE Pro. Am. J. Gastroenterol. 109, 1296–1298.

Ryan, K.R., Huang, M.C., Ferguson, S.S., Waidyanatha, S., Ramaiahgari, S., Rice, J.R., Dunlap, P.E., Auerbach, S.S., Mutlu, E., Cristy, T., Peirfelice, J., DeVito, M.J., Smith-Roe, S.L., Rider, C.V., 2019. Evaluating sufficient similarity of botanical dietary supplements: combining chemical and in vitro biological data. Toxicol. Sci. 172, 316–329.

Samenuk, D., Link, M.S., Homoud, M.K., Contreras, R., Theoharides, T.C., Wang, P.J., Estes 3rd, N.A., 2002. Adverse cardiovascular events temporally associated with ma huang, an herbal source of ephedrine. Mayo Clin. Proc. 77, 12–16.

Sax, J.K., 2015. Dietary supplements are not all safe and not all food: how the Low cost of dietary supplements preys on the consumer. Am. J. Law Med. 41, 374–394.

Shipkowski, K.A., Betz, J.M., Birnbaum, L.S., Bucher, J.R., Coates, P.M., Hopp, D.C., MacKay, D., Oketch-Rabah, H., Walker, N.J., Welch, C., Rider, C.V., 2018. Naturally complex: perspectives and challenges associated with botanical dietary supplement safety assessment. Food Chem. Toxicol. 118, 963–971.

Smithells, R.W., Sheppard, S., Schorah, C.J., 1976. Vitamin deficiencies and neural tube defects. Arch. Dis. Child. 51, 944–950.

Snyder, F.J., Dundas, M.L., Kirkpatrick, C., Neill, K.S., 2009. Use and safety perceptions regarding herbal supplements: a study of older persons in Southeast Idaho. J. Nutr. Elder. 28, 81–95.

Swann, J.P., 2016. The history of efforts to regulate dietary supplements in the USA. Drug Test. Anal. 8, 271–282.

Tandon, B.N., Tandon, R.K., Tandon, H.D., Narndranathan, M., Joshi, Y.K., 1976. Epidemic of Veno-occlusive disease of liver in Central India. Lancet 2, 271–272.

Tucker, J., Fischer, T., Upjohn, L., Mazzera, D., Kumar, M., 2018. Unapproved pharmaceutical ingredients included in dietary supplements associated with US Food and Drug Administration warnings. JAMA Netw. Open 1, e183337.

Tye, A., Patil, P.N., Lapidus, J.B., 1967. Steric aspects of adrenergic drugs. 3. Sensitization by cocaine to isomers of sympathomimetic amines. J. Pharmacol. Exp. Ther. 155, 24.

Vanhaelen, M., Vanhaelen-Fastre, R., But, P., Vanherweghem, J.L., 1994. Identification of aristolochic acid in Chinese herbs. Lancet 343, 174.

Vanherweghem, J.L., Depierreux, M., Tielemans, C., Abramowicz, D., Dratwa, M., Jadoul, M., Richard, C., Vandervelde, D., Verbeelen, D., Vanhaelen-Fastre, R., et al., 1993. Rapidly progressive interstitial renal fibrosis in young women: association with slimming regimen including Chinese herbs. Lancet 341, 387–391.

Vladeck, D.C., 2000. Truth and consequences: the perils of half-truths and unsubstantiated health claims for dietary supplements. J. Public Policy Mark. 19, 132–138.

Wade, N., 1972. Anabolic steroids - doctors denounce them, but athletes Arent listening. Science 176, 1399.

Wallace, T.C., 2015. Twenty years of the dietary supplement health and education act-how should dietary supplements be regulated? J. Nutr. 145, 1683–1686.

Watt, H.E., 1909. The alkaliods of Senecio latifolius. J. Chem. Soc. 95, 466–477.

Yuan, H.D., Ma, Q.Q., Ye, L., Piao, G.C., 2016. The traditional medicine and modern medicine from natural products. Molecules 21, 559.

Zhou, S., Chan, E., Pan, S.Q., Huang, M., Lee, E.J., 2004. Pharmacokinetic interactions of drugs with St John's wort. J. Psychopharmacol. 18, 262–276.

CHAPTER 9

A historical overview of food regulations in the United States

David Tonucci
Regulatory and Toxicology, SCiFi Foods, San Leandro, CA, United States

Historical background

Due to the increase in globally available information and media sources, it may seem like there is a recent increase in incidence for foodborne illnesses, even within the United States. However, significant numbers of people have died due to disease from foodborne illnesses since the beginning of human presence. The lifespan of people living before the time of cooking and preserving foods was significantly shorter than it is today largely in part due to sanitation, foodborne illnesses, and inadequate nutrition (Lásztity et al., 2009). Historical accounts of foodborne illness date back to antiquity. The first suggested documented case of a known foodborne illness dates to 323 BCE According to historians who studied historical accounts of Alexander the Great's symptoms and death, the ancient ruler is believed to have died from typhoid fever, which was caused by *Salmonella typhi* (Cunha, 2004).

This relationship between food quality, purity, and public health was realized by those living centuries ago. There are several examples of laws from early civilizations that attempted to control food standards of identity and purity. For example, Mosaic and Egyptian laws included provisions to prevent the contamination of meat (Lásztity et al., 2009). More than 2000 years ago, India had regulations prohibiting the adulteration of grains and edible fats. Books of the Old Testament prohibited the consumption of meat from animals that died from other than slaughter. The Egyptians, Romans, Greeks, Chinese, and others also regulated weights and measures in foods and other commodities. The Roman state enacted laws to control food supplies and to protect against bad food quality and fraud. Documentation relating to the first century CE describes the falsification of olive oil by a

History of Food and Nutrition Toxicology
https://doi.org/10.1016/B978-0-12-821261-5.00011-8

product made from wood, leaves, and berries of trees, and the falsification of wine by a substance made from a variety of plants (Foster, 2011). Probably this is the origin of the term "made wine," which is used in the common nomenclature that classifies products for customs purposes (Lasztity, 2009). Food safety did ebb and waned throughout history with the economic and social conditions of countries, regions, and territories. For example, after the fall of the Roman Empire in the West, the plague ran rampant in Europe, largely due to the lack of sanitary food and health conditions of the population. With the industrial revolution and the enlightenment in the West, there were attempts to improve food purity and sanitation. The efforts in the West had parallel issues and efforts in the East realized by the major empires and countries, including Japan and China.

Global influence: US history

It would be wrong to suggest that during the period before and during the industrial revolution the United States led the global development of food safety and purity laws. As advances were being made in chemistry and manufacturing, motivated "entrepreneurs" found very creative ways to increase profits at the expense of consumers. The principle "caveat emptor" or "buyer beware" was enthusiastically practiced in the United States and Europe during the 18th and 19th centuries. As a result, there are multiple cases of new chemicals and substances being used by manufacturers to enhance poor products, salvage waste, and/or deceive consumers. In both Europe and the United States, heavy metal salts were being used to color confectionaries, formaldehyde used to "preserve" spoiled milk, honey made of colored salts and corn syrup, and coffee grounds made of mostly sawdust (Blum, 2018).

Similarly, in Europe, there were several notable cases of children dying from lead and arsenic poising, and the use of clay in candy was a common practice. In 1820 Frederick Accum published the results of his analysis of foods and drinks from local shops in London (Accum, 1820). Although there is some disagreement on how much of what Accum published was his own work, the work of others, or pure embellishment, his work was the first to identify widespread adulteration of foods in London at the time. Accum's work did garnish brief support, but he was forced to flee the UK for unrelated legal issues resulting in a loss of momentum for his work. Years later, others continued Accum's work and confirmed his results. Fifty to 100% of the examined food in the UK was adulterated. In the early

1850s, Dr. Thomas Wakley (creator of *The Lancet*) established the Analytical Sanitary Commission in London. The commission supported research to examine contamination in foods in London. In 1855 two of Wakley's experts, Drs. Arthur Hill and Henry Letheby, published their results that confirmed Accum's earlier conclusions. This led to public outcry that resulted in the passing of the Sale of Foods and Drugs Act in 1875. These new regulations established food purity guidelines and required foods to be unadulterated. Unfortunately, there were only civil penalties for breaking these laws, and even those penalties were meager. Nonetheless, England was the first major country to enact civil penalties for food adulteration during the industrial revolution.

This change did not take place as quickly in the United States as industrialists and business leaders had a firm influential grip on the Federal government. Although there were similar public health disasters and outcries in the United States, they fell on deaf ears in the US Congress. Multiple attempts were made to develop a national framework for food purity standards. Most notably, Wisconsin Senator Robert La Follette commented on the adulteration of foods in the US Senate in 1886. Yet no one else in Congress felt it worthy to pursue national food purity laws (Blum, 2018). Even with the first National Pure Food and Drug Congress of 1898 held in Washington, DC, attendees were unable to move Congress to enact meaningful regulations at the time (Anon, n.d.-a).

Food and Drug Administration
1800–1906 history

It is difficult to come up with a single timeline of events that led to the development of the first food regulations in the United States. This is largely due to the political perspective and bias of those telling the story. According to the Food and Drug Administration's website (Anon, n.d.-a), the FDA started as part of the US Patent Office. According to the FDA Archives, "Today's position of Commissioner of Food and Drugs perhaps can be traced back to Lewis Caleb Beck, hired around 1848 to conduct chemical investigations for the agricultural division in the Patent Office of the Department of Interior. In 1846 Professor Beck, M.D., then of Rutgers College and Albany Medical College, published the first American treatise on the adulteration of food and drugs. Two years later, at the request of Patent Commissioner Edmund Burke, Congress appropriated $1000 for the Commissioner of Patents to conduct chemical analyses of "vegetable substances produced and used for the food of man and animals in the United States." Commissioner Burke recruited Dr. Beck to do this work for the Patent Office. Dr. Beck submitted his Report on the Breadstuffs of the United States in 1849 and a second report in 1850" (Hutt, 1990). Here we see the beginnings of an interest in developing standards for foods but food safety itself was not important enough to create a specific agency or entity to manage it.

Not until 1862, was there a formal intent to examine the quality of foods. This is when President Lincoln appoints a chemist, Charles Wetherill, to serve in the Department of Agriculture to investigate the quality of specific foods. Initially, Dr. Wetherill focused on the wine industry and fertilizers, but soon he began investigating the adulteration of agricultural commodities. His small staff grew until in 1901 his team becomes the "Bureau of Chemistry" within the Department of Agriculture (Anon, n.d.–a).

Over the next 25 years, Dr. Wetherill and subsequent heads of the Bureau of Chemistry supported the introduction of over 100 bills in Congress to regulate the quality of foods due to the clear identification of adulterations. Unfortunately, Congress did not support creating additional laws giving the Department of Agriculture additional powers to regulate food quality. In response to this federal inactivity, several states enacted laws to protect their citizens. For example, North Dakota enacted a Pure Food Law in 1903 and California had begun enacting its laws in the late 1800s. Wisconsin, South Dakota, and Massachusetts also put into place food regulations to protect their citizens. These various and different state laws, while trying to protect local consumers, also had the unintended effect of making interstate trade difficult (Hutt, 1990).

A watershed moment occurs when Dr. Harvey Wiley became chief chemist and expands the Bureau of Chemistry's adulterations studies. Years before his appointment in the US government, Harvey Wiley was pursuing a career in chemistry as the first professor of chemistry at Purdue University. This was after obtaining a bachelor's and master's degree from Hanover College, a medical degree from Indiana Medical College, and a second bachelor's degree in chemistry from Harvard. In his early years at Purdue, Wiley developed a reputation for his ability to identify substances in food. To further his skills in analytical chemistry Dr. Wiley went to Germany in 1878 and came back to build the leading food chemistry laboratories in the country. President Lincoln later recognized his accomplishments and appointed Dr. Wiley to head the Chemistry Section of the Department of Agriculture in 1883. From this position, Wiley studied dozens of foods for adulteration. What he found was similar to Wetherill before him. Many of the processed foods Wiley examined contained some sort of adulteration meant to enhance a product or deceive the consumer regarding the originality or purity of a product (Hutt, 1990).

Dr. Wiley eventually became known as the "Crusading Chemist" and the "Father of the Pure Food and Drug Acts." During his time at the Department of Agriculture, he created the "hygienic table trials" later to be called the "Poison Squad." Dr. Wiley used the "Poison Squad" to examine the deleterious effects of food additives in volunteers drawn largely from fellow employees at the Department of Agriculture.

Dr. Wiley's studies demonstrated widespread cases of adulteration and drew public concern. These studies also drew public support for the creation of federal laws to protect consumers.

The history and accomplishments of the "Poison Squad" are a valuable and critical component to the development of the US Food Safety laws. An excellent history of Dr. Wiley and the Poison Squad and their findings is elegantly described in Deborah Blum's book *The Poison Squad* (Blum, 2018).

1906–1950 history

Largely due to public criticism and pressure brought on the federal government by Dr. Wiley's activities, the original Pure Food and Drug Act (PFDA) was passed by Congress on June 30, 1906, and signed into law that year by President Theodore Roosevelt. This act prohibited interstate commerce of misbranded and adulterated foods, drinks, and drugs. At this time, the authority to enforce the Food and Drug Act was still held within the US Department of Agriculture. The FDA is not officially born until years later.

When examining the history of regulatory sciences in the food industry, it is critical to understand why regulations are promulgated and what they are designed to accomplish. The Food and Drug Act and the Meat Inspection Act are the foundations in this regard within the United States. The principles laid out in these two landmark federal laws are that food is safe (e.g., not adulterated) and that food is correctly labeled, providing true, factual information for the consumer (e.g., not misbranded). These concepts are the underpinnings of all food regulations in the United States and around the world. Is it safe? Is the consumer misled? These concepts are critical to reaching correct regulatory assessments for any concerns within the food industry. Added to these two critical ideals is the establishment of a level playing field, where competitors cannot obtain an unfair advantage due to false or misleading advertising.

1906 Pure Food and Drug Act

This act, which the USDA Bureau of Chemistry was charged to administer, prohibited the interstate transport of unlawful food and drugs under penalty of seizure of the questionable products and/or prosecution of the responsible parties. The basis of the law rested on the regulation of product labeling rather than premarket approval. Foods were not defined according to standards, but the law prohibited the addition of any ingredients that would substitute for the food, conceal the damage, pose a health hazard, or constitute a filthy or decomposed substance. Also, the food label could not be false or misleading, and the presence and amount of 11 dangerous ingredients, including alcohol, heroin, and cocaine, had to be clearly identified. Interpretations of the food provisions in the law led to many, sometimes protracted, court battles. If the manufacturer opted to list the weight or measure of a food, this had to be accurate (Swann, 2006).

Amendments and revisions of the original Food, Drug, and Cosmetic Act authorized the Food and Drug Administration (FDA) to provide inspection services for all livestock and poultry species not listed in the Federal Meat Inspection Act (FMIA) or the Poultry Products Inspection Act (PPIA), including venison and buffalo. The Agricultural Marketing Act authorizes the USDA to offer voluntary, fee-for-service inspection services for these same species (Anon, n.d.-b). The history and development of the USDA food regulations are discussed in more detail later in the chapter.

Other important regulations passed by Congress involving the FDA or USDA from 1906 through 1938 include:

- Certified Colors Regulations of 1907 approved the use of seven colors for use in foods. The burden of proving that a food or drug was adulterated or misbranded was placed on the Bureau of Chemistry in the US Department of Agriculture (USDA). In 1907 USDA published a list of seven synthetic organic dyes considered to be safe for use in food. This list was based on a study of 80 dyes then in use in food. These were the first "approved" color additives, and four of the seven dyes are still permitted today (Anon, n.d.-c).
- Gould Amendment of 1913 [sponsored by Rep Samuel Gould (Maine)] required food package contents to be plainly and conspicuously on the outside of the package to contain the weight, measure, or numerical count (62nd U.S. Congress, 1913).
- US Supreme Court decision in the US vs. *Lexington Mill and Elevator Company* of 1914 ruling on food additives. This ruling was in favor of the Lexington Mill Company in that it required the government to

prove that the addition of nitrite to flour was unsafe. The court ruled that the mere presence of an additive did not render the food product unsafe. This ruling was eventually reversed in subsequent cases where the concept of recognized safety for any food additive must be demonstrated before its commercial use (Anon, n.d.-d).

- *US vs Barrels Alleged Apple Cider Vinegar* ruling of 1924. The Supreme Court ruled that the Food and Drug Act condemns every statement, design, or device on a product label that misleads the consumer, even if the statement is technically true. This broad expansion of the terms misbranding is a significant change from the positions and opinions of prior courts supporting "Caveat Emptor" or "Buyer Beware" to one where truth and transparency are of prime concern (Anon, n.d.-e).
- The 1930 McNary-Mapes Amendment authorized the FDA to establish standards for the canned foods industry. The so-called Canner's Amendment authorized FDA standards of quality and fill of container for canned food, excluding meat and milk products. These standards of identity were the first of hundreds currently published by the FDA and USDA (Anon, n.d.-f).
- In 1933 the FDA encouraged Congress to revise the obsolete 1906 Food and Drug Act.

The organization and lines of authority also evolved for the FDA during this time and into the next decade. The following is a brief outline of the movement of responsibilities for food oversight within the US government agencies (Anon, n.d.-f):

- In 1927 USDA's Bureau of Chemistry was reorganized and renamed the Food, Drug, and Insecticide Administration.
- In 1931 it was renamed the Food and Drug Administration (FDA).
- In 1938 Congress passed the Federal Food, Drug, and Cosmetic Act, which gave the FDA the authority to issue food safety standards, among other authorities.
- In 1940 the FDA was moved from USDA to the Federal Security Agency, which in 1953 became the Department of Health, Education, and Welfare—now the Department of Health and Human Services.

Federal Food, Drug, and Cosmetics Act of 1938

In 1938 the Federal Food, Drug, and Cosmetic (FDC) Act (Anon, n.d.-f) was passed by Congress and replaced the earlier Pure Food and Drug Act of 1906. The introduction of this act was influenced by the death of more than

100 patients due to a sulfanilamide medication where diethylene glycol was used to dissolve the drug and make a liquid form (ref. elixir sulfanilamide disaster). This act contains new provisions related to proper drug safety and labeling of food, the establishment of food standards, false statements about food items, imitation foods, misleading containers, and other items related to misrepresentation. In addition, it regulates the safety and labeling of cosmetics for the first time at the national level.

The following is a list of substantial changes related to food from the previous 1906 law:

- The addition of poisonous substances to foods was prohibited except where unavoidable or required in production. Safe tolerances were authorized for residues of such substances like pesticides.
- Specific authority was provided for factory inspections.
- Food standards were required to be set up when needed "to promote honesty and fair dealing in the interest of consumers."
- Federal court injunctions against violations were added to the previous legal remedies of product seizures and criminal prosecutions.

Around this same time, the Wheeler-Lea Act (Anon, n.d.-g) amended the current authority of the Federal Trade Commission to include the regulation of food advertising separate from food labeling. Entirely new sections were added by Congress to the act to implement the commission with definite and specific power over the dissemination of the advertising of food, drugs, devices, and cosmetics.

The amendments made it unlawful and an unfair or deceptive act or practice, to disseminate, or cause to be disseminated, by the United States mails, any false advertisement for the purpose of inducing, or which is likely to induce, directly or indirectly, the purchase of food, drugs, devices, or cosmetics. It was likewise made unlawful to disseminate, by any means, a false advertisement for the purpose or with the likelihood of inducing the purchase in interstate commerce of food, drugs, devices, and cosmetics. These changes were a major step in providing transparency and honest product advertising for consumers. Initial FTC regulations only protected against unfair competitive advertising practices between companies (Anon, n.d.-h).

In 1940 the FDA is transferred from the Department of Agriculture to the Federal Security Agency, with Walter G. Campbell appointed as the first commissioner. Walter G. Campbell, born in Kentucky, received his BA in 1902 and in 1906, received a law degree from the University of Louisville (1905) and began practicing law. In 1907 Campbell took the first Civil Service examination for inspectors to enforce the federal Pure Food and Drugs Act of 1906. Wiley personally selected Campbell as the agency's chief inspector over others who scored higher on the analyst exam because he discerned Campbell's great skills as a leader. During the earliest days of enforcement under the new law, Campbell was determined to take action against rectified whiskey, which he deemed adulterated, and when the district attorney did not know how to proceed, Campbell prepared the first libel for seizure under the law. He also drafted the first inspectors' manual. During the first decade and a half under the law, some 60 food products warranted special investigations, including milk, eggs, vinegar, oysters, olive oil, and tomato products. Many outrageous patent medicines were removed from the marketplace, and crises involving canned salmon and ripe olives contaminated with a toxin causing botulism were resolved. Following Wiley's retirement, Campbell refused appointment as chief of the bureau, believing that a chemist should hold this post and arguing that law enforcement and chemical research did not belong in the same organization. In 1927 Campbell became chief of the Food, Drug, and Insecticide Administration. He also continued as director of regulatory work for the Department of Agriculture from 1923 to 1933. In 1930 the FDIA became the Food and Drug Administration (FDA), and in 1940 was transferred from Agriculture to the Federal Security Agency. Campbell then became commissioner of Food and Drugs (Anon, n.d.-a).

According to FDA archives, "Campbell was considered a consummate administrator who 'commanded the respect of all who knew him'." Campbell recognized inadequacies in the 1906 law from the beginning of his career in the Bureau of Chemistry, and during the 1920s fought off many attempts to weaken it further. With the arrival of the New Deal, Campbell directed the strategy in the five-year campaign for a more adequate statute, leading to the ultimate passage of the 1938 Food, Drug, and Cosmetic Act. Campbell's greatest disappointment in the new law was the provision granting jurisdiction over food and drug advertising and labeling to the Federal Trade Commission. Nonetheless, the new law was a vast improvement over the outdated Wiley Act, and as one observer expressed it, "Mr. Campbell was to the Federal Food, Drug, and Cosmetic Act of 1938 what Dr. Wiley was to the 1906 law." He worked closely with Congress and was an especially effective committee witness, presenting convincing testimony that finally resulted in a better consumer protection law.

Upon Campbell's retirement, *Business Week* noted that Campbell's greatest achievement seemed to be "the amount of public protection he could squeeze out of the small appropriations which Congress gave him."

With influence from the retired Campbell, the FDA publishes the first guidance to industry in 1949. This guidance, "Procedures for the Appraisal of the Toxicity of Chemicals in Foods," came to be known as the "black book." This is the first in a now common practice where the agency can influence the activities of an industry without having to mandate specific regulations or standards. As "guidance" they also allow for a more flexible and fluid mechanism for the agency to adapt to advances in science and technology, ensuring that consumers are protected as the food industry and food technology advances (Lehman et al., 1949).

1950–2000 history

With the enactment of the 1938 Food, Drug, and Cosmetic Act, the new FDA had a significant amount of work ahead of it and there were only a few major laws passed until the Food Safety Modernization Act described later in this chapter. This is not to say that the FDA did not move regulations and guidance forward on many fronts.

Poultry Products Inspection Act of 1957 and the Egg Products Inspection Act of 1970

Enacted by Congress on August 28, 1957 (as amended in 1968), the Poultry Products Inspection Act (PPIA) requires the USDA to regulate poultry products, processing, and transportation in interstate or foreign commerce, to remove from commerce poultry products that are injurious to the public, adulterated, and improperly labeled and packaged poultry products. Further specific details about this act can be found on the USDA website (Anon, n.d.-i).

On December 19, 1970, Congress enacted the Egg Products Inspection Act (EPIA) to protect consumers from adulterated, contaminated, or spoiled egg products. The act was amended in 1989 to require specific temperatures during storage and transportation to reduce the development of bacterial contamination (Anon, n.d.-j).

Food Additive Amendment of 1958

This amendment was a major step forward in regulating and ensuring the safety of food additives. In the amendment, food additives are defined as any substance, the intended use of which results or may reasonably be expected to result, directly or indirectly, in its becoming a component or otherwise affecting the characteristics of any food (including any substance intended for use in producing, manufacturing, packing, processing, preparing, treating, packaging, transporting, or holding food, and including any source of radiation intended for any such use) (Anon, n.d.-k).

Food additives need to be specifically preauthorized before commercialization. Food additives must be referenced in the FDA regulations prior to use and will identify specifications and conditions of use and common and usual name for the ingredient. The approved food additives and color additives are found in 21CFR21 Parts 170–199 for food additives and Parts 73 and 74 for color additives. The FDA has identified specific toxicology, chemistry, and use data that are required for the application to be reviewed. Once successfully approved, the regulations are updated and the additive may be commercialized. The FDA provides extensive guidance on this procedure (Guidance for Industry: Questions and Answers About the Food Additive or Color Additive Petition Process | FDA). This process is often cited as more transparent and comprehensive than the GRAS process discussed as follows. However, due to the need to update current CFR regulations, the process to obtain approval for a food additive petition can take years.

As mentioned before, the 1958 amendment (under sections 201(s) and 409) also introduced the concept of Generally Recognized As Safe (GRAS) as a type of food additive that is generally recognized, among experts qualified by scientific training and experience to evaluate its safety, as having been adequately shown through scientific procedures (or, in the case of a substance used in food prior to January 1, 1958, through either scientific procedures or experience based on common use in food) to be safe under the conditions of its intended use. The notable exceptions to the GRAS classification are pesticides and colors used in foods which must be approved separately. What GRAS provides is a legal process to commercialize food additives that have not received direct FDA review and precommercialization approval (81 FR 54960—August 17, 2016).

The concept of GRAS has been a very useful and appropriate tool for commercializing hundreds of useful and safe food additives (Anon, n.d.-l). Unfortunately, it has also been misused and abused by food manufacturers to skirt FDA or public review of many food additives. The reason for this dichotomy lay in the specific language within the 1958 law. According to the 1958 amendment regarding food additives:

If such substance is not generally recognized, among experts qualified by scientific training and experience to evaluate its safety, as having been adequately shown through scientific procedures (or, in the case of a substance used in food prior to January 1, 1958, through either scientific procedures or experience based on common use in food) to be safe under the conditions of its intended use.

This provides for the classification of substances that are classified as safe among experts qualified by scientific training and experience to evaluate the safety of additives that can be marketed without food additive petitions. The issue is what are the specific criteria of GRAS? Well, that is really in the eye of the beholder. According to the final rule published by the FDA in addition to documents produced by several industry and nonindustry groups, GRAS has several components:

(1) The data required for GRAS use versus a Food Additive petition is the same. The toxicological, chemical, and use condition data needed to reach a GRAS determination and a Food Additive petition approval is identical. The primary difference is that for a food additive petition data submitted to the FDA may be held confidential.

(2) For a GRAS determination, there must be publicly available data to establish a sound safety review by any qualified expert. The data required is identical to the data required for a food additive petition and is mandatory.

(3) There must be stated use levels based on the available safety data for the additive.

(4) As a food additive approval, the classification of GRAS is specific to the substances' intended use, meaning what type of foods is the additive permitted to be included in. Therefore the stated use levels must be identified specifically for each food category (i.e., nonalcoholic beverages, cereals, soups, sauces, etc.).

From the late 1960s until 1997, the FDA reviewed GRAS applications and issue GRAS Affirmation determinations. After 1997 the FDA determined that it no longer had the resources to keep up with reviewing all GRAS substances. At this time the GRAS process moved to a voluntary affirmation process where the FDA would review voluntary applications and issue a "No further questions at this time" document, essentially agreeing with the independent GRAS assessment. This allowed for private GRAS determinations where there was no FDA notification nor public awareness of what materials were considered GRAS by the food industry.

Public concern over the "private GRAS" process led to the FDA updating its regulations and issuing a final rule in 2016. The final rule did not substantially change the process for obtaining voluntary GRAS affirmations but did explicitly outline how the FDA defines the GRAS process and what data are needed to determine a substance is GRAS.

Food Safety and Modernization Act (FSMA)

The FDA and USDA have stated that the Food Safety Modernization Act (FSMA) is the most significant regulatory improvement in food safety since the initial Food and Drug Act of 1938 (Anon, n.d.-m). This law, signed into law by President Obama in 2011, provides for better control and enforcement capabilities by the FDA and USDA to protect public health by improving the safety of the food supply, farm to fork. It allows the federal government to focus more on preventing food safety problems rather than relying primarily on reacting to problems after they occur. The law also gives FDA important new tools to hold imported foods to the same standards as domestic foods and directs FDA to build an integrated national food safety system in partnership with state and local authorities.

The following are among FDA's key new authorities and mandates. Due to the extensive impact and complexity of the new regulatory framework, the FDA gradually introduced these new regulations over several years starting in 2013 through 2020. The following areas are those directly impacted by FSMA.

Prevention (HACCP)

The FDA requires comprehensive, science-based preventive controls across the food supply, including:
- All food facilities are required to implement a written preventive controls plan. This is commonly referred to as a HACCP plan. A **Hazard Analysis** and **Critical Control Points** plan involves:
  - evaluating the hazards that could affect food safety,
  - specifying what preventive steps, or controls, will be put in place to significantly minimize or prevent the hazards,
  - specifying how the facility will monitor these controls to ensure they are working through regular monitoring,
  - specifying what actions the facility will take to correct problems that arise.
  The FDA maintains current guidance on developing a HACCP plan at *Hazard Analysis Critical Control Point (HACCP) | FDA.*

Mandatory produce safety standards

The FDA established science-based minimum standards for the safe production and harvesting of fruits and vegetables. Those standards consider naturally occurring hazards, as well as those that may be introduced either unintentionally or intentionally, and must address hygiene, packaging, temperature controls, animals in the growing area, and water. (Final regulation due about 2 years following enactment.)

Authority to prevent intentional contamination

The FDA has issued regulations to protect against the intentional adulteration of food, including the establishment of science-based mitigation strategies to prepare and protect the food supply chain at specific vulnerable points. (Final rule due 18 months following enactment.)

Inspection and compliance

An important improvement in the FSMA regulations is increased oversight and penalties for noncompliance. The FSMA establishes a mandated inspection frequency, based on risk, for food facilities and requires the frequency of inspection to increase immediately if warranted. Specific requirements of the classification of high- and low-risk facilities, as well as inspection frequency, are identified in guidance issued by the FDA (CFSAN, 2020).

To deal with noncompliance or safety issues, FSMA provides FDA with the authority to issue a mandatory recall when a company fails to voluntarily recall unsafe food after being asked by FDA. This is a major change from the prior regulations that limited the FDA's ability to require a manufacture to issue a food recall.

Finally, FDA can suspend the registration of a facility if it determines that the food poses a reasonable probability of serious adverse health consequences or death.

In the area of importation of food products, the FSMA gives FDA authority to:

— Require importers to verify they have HACCP equivalent plans and procedures in place in their foreign facility.
— Establishes a program through which qualified third parties can certify that foreign food facilities comply with US food safety standards.
— FDA has the authority to require that high-risk imported foods be accompanied by a credible third-party certification or other assurance of compliance as a condition of entry into the United States.

- FDA must establish a voluntary program for importers that provides for expedited review and entry of foods from participating importers. Eligibility is limited to, among other things, importers offering food from certified facilities.
- FDA can refuse entry into the United States of food from a foreign facility if FDA is denied access by the facility or the country in which the facility is located.

US Food Safety Inspection Service (FSIS) and the Department of Agriculture (USDA)

Like the FDA, the FSIS was not created during the early history of the USDA. In fact, authority to regulate livestock was not initially given to the USDA.

In 1865 USDA secretary Isaac Newton urged Congress to enact legislation providing for the quarantine Animal Diseases and Interstate Commerce Act to become law, under the jurisdiction of the Treasury Department. Since the Treasury Department was not equipped to enforce the new law, little preventive action was taken and diseased animals continued to be imported. Consequently, individual states attempted to control or eradicate livestock diseases, but the inconsistencies in state requirements and enforcement were problematic (Anon, n.d.-n).

In May 1884, President Chester Arthur signed an act establishing the USDA Bureau of Animal Industry (BAI), charged with preventing diseased animals from being used as food (Anon, n.d.-o). This transferred responsibility from the Treasury Department to the newly created BAI within the USDA. In 1886 the Supreme Court ruled in the Wabash case that only the federal government could regulate interstate commerce.

However, these laws only required inspection of imported livestock and did not control or regulate local livestock. These were still regulated at the local level.

In parallel to increased import inspections, exported meat products came under more foreign food safety scrutiny. This resulted in the loss of foreign business by US farmers due to the inability to pass foreign meat inspections. Therefore the meat producers and packer industry requested that the federal government establish inspection capabilities to ensure US exported products would meet import requirements. On August 30, 1890, the first law requiring inspection of exported meat products was enacted. The Foreign Trade and Meat Inspection law required that USDA, through the Bureau of Animal Industry, inspect salted pork and bacon intended for exportation. In 1891 this law was amended to require the inspection and certification of all live cattle and beef intended for exportation.

The focus only on imported and exported meat is interesting. The industry was able to get Congress and the federal government to respond to their needs to protect their business, but no one was interested in protecting the consumer. There was still resistance to local control of meat production to protect the US population.

The book entitled *The Jungle* by Upton Sinclair (Sinclair, 1905), published in 1905, vividly articulates the horrific living and working conditions of the poor in the Chicago meat processing industry. Sinclair, an avid supporter of social reform, identified how laborers were abused, disfigured, and literally worked to the bone. The author describes butchers without thumbs, skinners without nails, and children working with raw chemicals. Not only were the workers treated poorly, but consumers also fared no better. Sinclair tells a woeful tale of Jurgis and his family trying to find work and a life in Packingtown. Although meant to be more of a socialist manifesto, it highlights the awful working conditions of the meatpacking and processing industry of the 19th century. For example, Jurgis tells the story of workers in the pickling plant. Where people who had cuts and scrapes would become infected due to likely microbial contamination and suffer horrible debilitating infections without treatment, to men who had their fingertips dissolved off over time due to the use of acids, and others who worked in cooking rooms that had high rates of tuberculosis infections. On the consumer side, owners of Packingtown food processing plants adulterated foods for the sole purpose of profiting from every last scrap of rotting food. Sinclair describes spoiled meat being chopped up and used in sausage, pickled rotten meat covered in soda ash to be sold for fresh meat given away at free counters. In addition to pickling and chemical treatment to hide rancid foods, there were examples of how food was colored with metal salts to change the color from gray to pink.

This book led to public outcry and was a significant motivating factor for the passing of the Meat Inspection Act in 1906, at the same time as the Pure Food and Drug Act (PDFA). Like the initial PFDA, the Meat Inspection Act fell under the authority of the USDA. The timing of the publication of Sinclair's novel and the passing of the Food and Drug Act as well as the Meat Inspections Act are coincidental. The additional impact of these two federal laws was the preemption of federal law over existing state laws. This provided a more consistent regulatory landscape for food manufacturers as many producers were very much involved with interstate commerce.

The USDA Bureau of Animal Industry, the forerunner of the USDA Food Safety and Inspection Service (FSIS), was established in 1884 to prevent diseased animals from being used as food. This will be discussed more fully in the following section.

1906 Meat Inspection Act

The Federal Meat Inspection Act of 1906 (FMIA) made it illegal to adulterate or misbrand meat and meat products sold as food and ensured that meat and meat products are slaughtered and processed under regulated sanitary conditions. These requirements also applied to imported meat products, which must be inspected under equivalent foreign standards. The FMIA mandated the US Department of Agriculture (USDA) inspection of meat processing plants that conducted business across state lines, thus creating the FSIS (Federal Meat Inspection Act of 1906, 2017).

The Poultry Products Inspection Act (PPIA) of 1957 added the requirement for the US Department of Agriculture (USDA) to inspect poultry (Anon, n.d.-p).

The four primary requirements of the Meat Inspection Act of 1906 were as follows:

(1) Mandatory inspection of livestock before slaughter (cattle, sheep, goats, equines, and swine);
(2) Mandatory postmortem inspection of every carcass;
(3) Sanitary standards established for slaughterhouses and meat processing plants; and
(4) Authorized US Department of Agriculture ongoing monitoring and inspection of slaughter and processing operations.

The USDA was also pressured to ensure that animals were slaughtered using humane procedures. In 1958 after a three-year campaign by animal advocacy groups, the Humane Methods of Slaughter Act (HMSA) was signed into law (Anon, n.d.-q). It required that the government only purchase livestock that had been slaughtered humanely. However, due to the influence of industry groups, the new law did not directly require it of industry. It was not until the 1978 amendment was passed to the HMSA requiring that all meat inspected by FSIS for use as human food be produced from livestock slaughtered by humane methods.

In 1953 the Eisenhower administration inaugurated sweeping organizational changes at USDA. Scientific bureaus, including the Bureau of Animal Industry and the Bureau of Dairy Industry, were abolished and their functions were transferred to the newly established Agricultural Research Service (ARS).

In 1967 and 1968, respectively, the Wholesome Meat Act and the Wholesome Poultry Act amended the FMIA and the PPIA (Anon, n.d.–r). These changes were enacted to ensure that state agencies, who were inspecting local meat and poultry facilities on behalf of the USDA, maintained programs equivalent to the federal requirements.

In 1965 the sections responsible for meat and poultry inspections of the USDA were reorganized, merging federal meat and poultry inspection into one program.

In 1972 all of the meat and poultry inspection functions of ARS' Consumer and Marketing Service were transferred to the newly created Animal and Plant Health Service (APHIS). Today, USDA-ARS focuses on research programs. According to the ARS 2020 Annual Report (ARS Annual Report on Science FY 2020.pdf, 2020):

Research of the ARS Animal Production and Protection National Programs improves the health, well-being, and efficiency of livestock, poultry, and aquatic food animals to ensure a productive and safe food supply. These research programs provide the scientific information and tools to support US food animal industries as they supply the nutritious animal products required by the nation, compete successfully in worldwide trade, and contribute toward global food security. The program also addresses the many veterinary problems created by arthropod pests and vectors and zoonotic diseases, producing solutions to protect the health and well-being of American citizens.

In 1977 the Food Safety and Quality Service (FSQS) was created to perform meat and poultry grading, as well as inspection activities, instead of APHIS. In 1981 FSQS was reorganized and renamed the Food Safety and Inspection Service (FSIS).

Food allergies

The importance and impact of food allergies have developed into a significant topic for public health and regulatory guidance. Due to the potentially life-threatening outcomes related to exposure to certain foods, the FDA has spent significant time and resources to ensure that the public is informed and protected to the extent possible. Food allergies and other types of food hypersensitivities affect millions of Americans and their families. Food-allergic reactions vary in severity from mild symptoms involving hives and lip swelling to severe, life-threatening symptoms, anaphylaxis, that may involve fatal respiratory problems and shock and death.

One mechanism the FDA uses to inform susceptible individuals is to require the clear listing of all ingredients contained within a food on the package label. For foods or foods that contain substances that cause allergies or other hypersensitivity reactions, the FDA requires specific label identifiers.

The FDA also conducts inspections and sampling to check that major food allergens are properly labeled on products and to determine whether food facilities implement controls to prevent allergen cross-contact (the inadvertent introduction of a major food allergen into a product) and labeling controls to prevent undeclared allergens during manufacturing and packaging.

Major food allergens

Congress passed the Food Allergen Labeling and Consumer Protection Act of 2004 (FALCPA) (Anon, n.d.-s). This law identified eight foods as major food allergens: milk, eggs, fish, shellfish, tree nuts, peanuts, wheat, and soybean. On April 23, 2021, the Food Allergy Safety, Treatment, Education, and Research (FASTER) Act was signed into law, declaring "sesame" as the 9th major food allergen recognized by the United States (Anon, n.d.-t). This change will become effective on January 1, 2023, so labeling of sesame as an allergen will not be required until that time.

At the time of FALCPA's passage, the eight major allergens accounted for 90% of food allergies and serious allergic reactions in the US FALCPA require that foods or ingredients that contain a "major food allergen" be specifically labeled with the name of the allergen source. The FDA enforces the provisions of this law in most packaged food products. This includes dietary supplements but does not include meat, poultry, and egg products (which are regulated by the US Department of Agriculture); alcoholic beverages subject to Alcohol and Tobacco Tax and Trade Bureau labeling regulations; raw agricultural commodities; drugs; cosmetics; and most foods sold at retail or food service establishments that are not prepackaged with a label.

Other allergens or allergenic substances

More than 160 foods have been identified to cause food allergies in sensitive individuals. Several food ingredients cause nonallergic hypersensitivity reactions in sensitive individuals that require specific labeling. For example, in addition to the eight major food allergens identified by law, the FDA monitors the food supply to determine if other allergens, food ingredients, or food additives pose a significant health risk and acts accordingly. Gluten, certain additives (e.g., yellow 5, carmine, sulfites), and other food allergens for which new science has emerged are examples of other substances the FDA monitors and, in some cases, require specific labeling for (Anon, n.d.-u).

Gluten

Gluten describes a group of proteins found in certain grains (e.g., wheat, barley, and rye). In people with celiac disease, foods that contain gluten trigger an immune response that attacks and damages the lining of the small intestine. Such damage may not only limit the ability of celiac disease patients to absorb nutrients, leading to problems such as iron deficiency anemia, osteoporosis, and malnutrition, but it puts them at increased risk for potentially serious health problems, including intestinal cancers and autoimmune diseases such as diabetes. On August 2, 2013, the FDA issued a final rule defining "gluten-free" for food labeling, which helps consumers, especially those living with celiac disease, be confident that items labeled "gluten-free" meet a defined standard for gluten content (Anon, n.d.-v). The regulation requires labeling any food product that contains greater than 20 ppm. On August 12, 2020, the FDA issued a final rule to establish compliance requirements for fermented and hydrolyzed foods, or foods that contain fermented or hydrolyzed ingredients, bearing the "gluten-free" claim. Foods that are labeled gluten-free, according to the Food and Drug Administration rules, must have fewer than 20 ppm of gluten (Anon, n.d.-w).

Color and food additives

Some individuals may have hypersensitivity reactions to a color additive. The FDA requires all products containing FD&C Yellow No. 5 to be identified on the label. Color additives made from cochineal extract and carmine, which are derived from insects, have been identified as allergenic substances that must be declared on the label of all food and cosmetic products. The FDA also conducts ongoing surveillance, taking regulatory actions when appropriate. The FDA's "Current Good Manufacturing Practice, Hazard Analysis, and Risk-Based Preventive Controls for Human Food" rule (CGMP and PC rule, 21 CFR part 117) includes requirements for allergen preventive controls to prevent allergen cross-contact in manufacturing and packaging and to prevent undeclared allergens.

Testing

The FDA conducts periodic surveys and sampling assignments to gather information about specific foods. For example, in 2013 and 2014, the FDA conducted a survey to estimate the prevalence of undeclared milk allergens in dark chocolate products. A second survey of samples collected in 2018 and 2019 was conducted to understand the extent to which dark chocolate bars and dark chocolate chips labeled as "dairy-free" contained levels of milk that would be potentially hazardous to consumers with milk allergies (Anon, n.d.-x). In 2015 and 2016 the FDA conducted sampling of a variety of foods to determine compliance with "gluten-free" labeling requirements.

Dietary supplements

Currently, dietary supplements are regulated under the Dietary Supplement Health and Education Act (DSHEA), which is a statute of US Federal legislation enacted in 1994 that amended the Federal Food, Drug and Cosmetic Act (Anon, n.d.-y). DSHEA defines and regulates dietary supplements. Under the act, supplements are effectively regulated by the FDA for Good Manufacturing Practices under 21 CFR Part 111. DSHEA has two primary goals: to ensure continued consumer access to a wide variety of dietary supplements and to provide consumers with more information about the intended use of dietary supplements. It accomplished these goals without changing the fundamental regulatory status of dietary supplements as a category of foods.

Before DSHEA, dietary supplements were regulated under the 1938 Act with the addition of several regulations being issued by the FDA that limited the daily intake and controlled the labeling of dietary supplements. These limitations were based upon claims that several manufacturers were putting on dietary supplements. The new regulations were put in place by the FDA to ensure that there was a separation between drugs and foods. These new regulations also limited the combination of dietary supplements in single products.

In 1976, due to industry complaints about the FDA regulations regarding vitamin and mineral potency, Congress passed the Proxmire Amendment. The Proxmire Amendment prohibited the FDA from placing maximum limits of potency on vitamins or minerals within a food, invalidated the FDA's authority to classify a vitamin or mineral as a drug based on potency, and permitted vitamins and minerals to be sold within a food. After the Proxmire Amendment, the FDA attempted to regulate dietary supplements under the FDCA food additive provisions. However, in 1992, US courts of appeal rejected this theory at least regarding noncombination dietary supplements (Anon, n.d.-z).

DSHEA created a new structure for the regulation of dietary supplements by making dietary supplements a new category of regulation within the framework of food and apart from drugs. DSHEA enacted the following main provisions (Anon, n.d.-aa):

- created a new category of food and then defined this category by the inclusion of the specific dietary ingredients of vitamins, minerals, herbs or botanicals, amino acids, any substances consumed to supplement the diet, or concentrates, metabolites, constituents, extracts, or combinations;
- established dietary supplement safety provisions;
- exemptions for certain dietary supplement labeling;
- defined statements of nutritional support and labeling requirements;
- outlined regulations pertaining to new dietary ingredients;
- establishment of a commission on Dietary Supplement Labels;
- establishment of the Office of Dietary Supplements.

The most significant impact of DSHEA is the exclusion of dietary supplements from the FDCA food additive provision. Because dietary supplements are now excluded from the FDCA food additive provisions, dietary supplements cannot be deemed adulterated under the food additive provisions of the FDCA. All dietary supplements thus bypass the need to receive specific approval from the FDA for use as food additives. Dietary supplements also bypass the need to be Generally Recognized as Safe (GRAS) by the FDA or the food industry. And notably, by virtue of being excluded from the definition of food additives, dietary supplements do not have to comply with the Delaney Clause prohibiting the FDA from approving food additives that have been "found to induce cancer when ingested by man or animal." This has created a very "open" market for dietary supplements that has resulted in consumer confusion and cases of consumer injury (Starr, 2015).

Following the enactment of DSHEA, the FDA has worked to control the labeling of nutritional supplements and the introduction of new ingredients. In 1996 the FDA issued proposed rules establishing a premarket notification procedure for new dietary ingredients. And in 1997 the FDA issued final rules regarding new dietary ingredient premarket notification. These regulations apply only to a new dietary ingredient "that has not been present in the food supply as an article used for food in a form in which the food has not been chemically altered." This premarket notification includes the concentration of the new ingredient as well as the conditions of use. This is not the same as a premarket approval process though as the applicant may commercialize the new ingredient in the absence of a response by the FDA. This simply provides the FDA an opportunity to ban the new substance if it feels it is unsafe.

Under DSHEA, all claims are based on structure/function relationships established based on the nutritive value of the food. All health claims for nutritional supplements still require premarket approval under the Nutritional Labeling and Education Act (NLEA). Thus a dietary supplement may make a health claim by complying with the NLEA provisions regarding health claims for conventional foods.

In addition to the oversight by the FDA, the Federal Trade Commission ("FTC") is responsible for regulating advertising claims for all foods, including dietary supplements. Specifically, the FTC may prohibit the dissemination of false or misleading dietary supplement advertising. The FTC requires that dietary supplement advertising be truthful and not misleading and have adequate substantiation for all claims. The FTC tries to harmonize its enforcement of advertising claims with the FDA's enforcement of claims in food and dietary supplement labels.

A complete review of all relevant regulations and laws related to nutritional supplements is beyond the scope of this chapter. Additional resources providing additional detail on the DSHEA can be found on the FDA's website.

GMO

Three federal agencies within the US government work together to regulate most genetically modified organism (GMO) derived foods: the US Food and Drug Administration (FDA), the US Environmental Protection Agency (EPA), and the US Department of Agriculture (USDA). GMO foods include crops derived using molecular biology to alter the native species genome; proteins derived from plants, animals, or microorganisms through genetic modification; and biotechnology used to make substances from enzymatic or microbiological processes (Anon, n.d.-bb).

FDA regulates most human and animal food, including GMO foods. In doing so, FDA makes sure that foods that are GMO or have GMO ingredients meet the same strict safety standards as all other foods. In addition, the FDA reviews applications for new proteins to be used in the manufacture of food and food ingredients.

The US Environmental Protection Agency is responsible for protecting human health and the environment, which includes regulating pesticides. EPA regulates the safety of the substances that protect GMO plants, referred to as plant-incorporated protectants (PIPs) that are in some GMO plants to make them resistant to insects and disease. EPA also monitors all other types of pesticides that are used on crops, including on GMO and non-GMO crops.

The USDA Animal and Plant Health Inspection Service (APHIS) sets regulations to make sure GMO plants are not harmful to other plants, and the USDA's Biotechnology Regulatory Services implements these regulations.

FDA's plant biotechnology guidance

In 1992 the FDA provided guidance to industry on scientific and regulatory issues related to foods derived from genetically modified plants and animals (Anon, n.d.-cc). The 1992 policy applied to all foods derived from all new plant varieties, including varieties produced through traditional plant breeding as well as those developed using recombinant deoxyribonucleic acid (rDNA) technology. In 1996 the FDA provided a set of procedures for voluntary premarket food safety consultations with the FDA. These procedures are similar to the GRAS process but allow for ongoing dialogue with the FDA to ensure a complete assessment of the safety of the product during its development. The applicant meets with the agency to identify and discuss relevant safety, nutritional, or other regulatory issues regarding the food. The developer then submits to FDA a summary of its scientific and regulatory assessment of the food. The FDA evaluates the submission and responds to the developer by letter before marketing the product in commerce. In addition, new genetically modified foods with compositional differences that make them materially different from their traditional counterpart require labeling that identifies such differences.

In 2016 Congress passed the National Bioengineered (BE) Food Disclosure Standard Law, directing the US Department of Agriculture, Agricultural Marketing Service (USDA-AMS) to establish a national mandatory standard for disclosing bioengineered foods. The Standard defines bioengineered foods as those that contain detectable genetic material that has been modified through certain laboratory techniques and cannot be created through conventional breeding or found in nature. The implementation date of the Standard is January 1, 2020, except for small food manufacturers, whose implementation date is January 1, 2021. The mandatory compliance date is January 1, 2022.

The FDA has provided useful guidance and education documents on these topics on their website under the following headings: the "Consultation Programs on Food from New Plant Varieties" and the "Voluntary Plant Biotechnology Consultation Program Eases Pathway to Marketplace."

In 2017 the FDA published a notice titled "Genome Editing in New Plant Varieties Used for Foods" seeking public input to help inform its regulatory approach to human and animal foods derived from plants produced using genome editing (Anon, n.d.-dd). This request was in response to the development of new techniques to modify the deoxyribonucleic acid (DNA) sequences of plants and to characterize such modifications.

Emerging technologies: Cell-based or "cultivated" meats, poultry, and seafood

As of 2021, new technology is emerging that will require new regulations and guidelines to be issued by the USDA and FDA. Cultivated food products are being developed to supplement traditional nonmeat alternatives to beef, seafood, and chicken products (Anon, n.d.-ee). Vegetarian burgers and chicken nugget-type products have been available for some time. However, advances in molecular and cellular biology have resulted in the development of cell-based, cultivated meat and seafood products (I will collectively refer to all of these types of foods as "meats" for the remainder of the chapter). This is a technology that removes the need to raise livestock (that consumes huge amounts of environmental resources and produces more air pollution than the entire auto industry) from the equation to produce meat products. Essentially, small tissue samples from cows, chicken, pigs, fish, etc. are removed from a living donor and that tissue is grown to commercial volumes in an industrial setting much like beer and wine are fermented.

The discovery of stem cells and the ability to grow stem cells in in vitro cultures was the fundamental discovery that allowed for the development of cultivated or cell-cultured meat products. Stem cells are cells with the potential to develop into many different cells in the body. The process where a stem cell develops into another type of cell is called differentiation. This is a process where a stem cell becomes activated by signals generated within the body to differentiate into another type of cell. The final differentiated cell type no longer has the characteristics of a stem cell and cannot go backward in the process. Stem cells also have the potential to continually divide and produce more stem cells that can then develop into more differentiated cells. Most differentiated cells lose their ability to replicate and therefore require stem cells to serve as the body's main repair mechanism (Anon, n.d.-ff).

With the current understanding of how to force stem cells to develop into specific types of differentiated cells, it is now possible to theoretically produce all the cells necessary to produce a chicken breast, steak, or fish fillet. The remaining problems include how to organize these cells into structures that resemble actual tissues from animals and how to do this in an economically efficient way. These problems are not trivial, as today there are over 20 companies working on this problem and there is only one small commercially available product, a simple chicken nugget (Waltz, 2021).

To understand the complexity of this problem, one needs to understand the problems associated with selecting a stem cell, growing mammalian stem cells in large quantities, correctly differentiating these cells into the needed differentiated cell types, and then organizing them into the correct 3-dimensional structure that would be acceptable to the consumer. In addition to all of these problems, one also needs to produce a product that tastes good and is similar to the original meat. We will discuss these problems individually and then identify the regulatory hurdles that must be overcome to successfully commercialize these products (Specht et al., 2018).

The first problem that needs to be solved is selecting the proper stem cell. Embryonic stem cells (ESCs), also known as pluripotent stem cells, are a type of cell that can differentiate into any type of mammalian cell. Although these would be acceptable starting cells, it is obviously difficult to collect ESCs safely and humanely. In addition, there is no regulatory framework that supports the use of ESCs to produce foods. This makes ESCs a poor choice for the starting material for cultivated meats. Fortunately, there is another option. All basic tissue types have adult stem cells. For example, mesenchymal stem cells (MSCs) have limited differentiating capability and serve as the main local repair resource for bone, muscle, adipose, and cartilage repair. MSC resides in the adult tissue as dormant cells and can be activated when needed. If these types of stem cells are isolated from developed tissues, for example, muscle, they can be used as the starter cells for large-scale cell production as they have the capacity to replicate and then differentiate into muscle, fat, and other needed cells. The MSCs in muscle are readily available and are typically either myoblasts and fibroblasts. These myoblasts or fibroblasts typically serve as the starter cell for this type of meat production (Prockop et al., 2008).

After an appropriate myoblast or fibroblast is identified and isolated, it must be replicated in vast quantities to make products on a commercial scale. One parent must produce trillions of daughter cells in large scale bioreactors. Since myoblasts and fibroblasts have a robust ability to replicate where the final differentiated fat, muscle, and bone cells do not, most scientists are looking to develop processes where these cells are grown in large volumes, and then these cells can be differentiated after they grow to the needed volumes. Although myoblasts and fibroblasts have a significant ability to replicate, one typical MSC cannot normally produce trillions of cells. The average MSC can replicate 10–20 times. To make cells at the scale needed for commercial meat production, MSCs would need to replicate more than 40 times. This is at the very edge of replication capacity (the Hayflick limit of doublings) for mammalian cells. Therefore many companies are looking to genetically enhance these MSCs to replicate beyond the Hayflick limit to increase production efficiency. An second issue that must be addressed is the culture conditions needed to feasibly grow this volume of cells. Not only do you need huge bioreactors to grow this volume of cells, but you also need the media to allow these cells to grow differently. MSCs are used to growing on a surface such as a basement membrane or lamina. To grow the needed volume of cells on a surface need expansive bioreactors. Therefore many believe that growing cells in suspension is the most efficient way to produce cultivated meats. This requires tricking the cells to grow unattached. Another issue that must be addressed is the cost and contents of current culture media used to grow mammalian cells. Currently, mammalian cells are cultured in the presence of a host of growth hormones including Fetal Bovine Serum (FBS). FBS is serum taken from cow fetuses and is in extremely limited supply and is not ethically appropriate to use in food production. It does have current use in the production of some critical biologic pharmaceuticals and vaccines. Other growth hormones needed are also very expensive and in limited supply. Therefore many companies are focusing on reducing the costly components of current culture media. How these issues are going to be resolved is still under development, but this issue must be solved to make cultivated meats economically feasible. (Specht et al., 2018).

Once you have a good parent cell line and the right culture medium, you need to develop a huge bioreactor to produce your product. Currently, there are bioreactors up to 5000 L that are in commercial use. These are exclusively used by pharmaceutical companies. To make cultivated meat products you would need to develop bioreactors that are 10 times this size. The issue with bioreactor scale-up is not simply making a bigger bioreactor. The design has to ensure that all of the essential nutrients required by all of the cells are being delivered in a homogeneous process and that cellular metabolic wastes are removed. In addition, the continual addition of nutrients will be required as the cells replicate to the desired volume. Finally, after the myoblasts are present in the right quantity you may need to add differentiation factors to force the cells to become muscle or fat cells. This will require the ability to keep the cells alive and disperse the differentiating factors evenly in a huge bioreactor. Again, these technologies will require significant advances in engineering.

Finally, once you have all of the correct cells in the correct quantities many companies are looking to produce a product that resembles current chicken breasts, fish fillets, and/or steaks. This will require correctly organizing the cells at a microscopic level. There are currently a few options to do this. The two main approaches are to use a food-grade scaffolding that will provide a skeleton for the cells to attach themselves in the correct orientation. Another approach is to use the newly developed 3-D printing technology to "print" a steak. As none of these technologies currently exist, the first foods produced using cultivated meats are anticipated to be unstructured or hybrid products. For example, a chicken nugget could be easily produced where cultivated chicken cells are mixed with a binding component currently used to bind ground chicken. Another approach could be to combine cultivated beef cells with veggie-burger components to make a hybrid "cultivated" beef/veggie burger.

To ensure that these products are both safe and sanitary, the FDA and USDA have agreed to joint oversight of the approval on ongoing inspection of these products. Broadly speaking, the FDA is responsible for ensuring that food is not adulterated or misbranded, including regulating food ingredients used during the production of meat, poultry, and egg products. In addition to these responsibilities, the FDA conducts inspections of facilities that produce, process, and package these products. The USDA is similarly responsible for misbranding and adulteration of meat and poultry products and for inspecting the facilities where these products are processed and packaged. These facilities include a large number of meat and poultry slaughter and processing plants. On March 7, 2019, the USDA and FDA entered into a formal agreement for the purpose of outlining roles and responsibilities of each agency concerning the oversight of human foods produced using animal cell culture technology, derived from cell lines of USDA-amendable species and required to bear a USDA mark of inspection (Anon, n.d.-gg).

Under the agreement the FDA will be responsible for the following:

(1) Conduct premarket consultation processes with manufacturers to evaluate production materials, processes, and manufacturing controls, to include tissue collection, cell line, and cell banking, and all components and inputs used in the manufacture of the cell lines themselves.

(2) Oversee initial cell collection and the development and maintenance of qualified cell banks including regulations and guidance on inspections, as appropriate.

(3) Oversee cell proliferation and differentiation through the time of harvest, including the inspection of facilities involved in these activities. This will include ensuring GMPs and HACCP plans are developed and followed for cell production.

(4) Cooperate with and support activities to transfer oversight to the USDA at the time of cell harvesting.

Similarly, the USDA will be responsible for the following:

(1) Work with the FDA to determine that cells at the time of harvest are eligible to be processed into meat or poultry products that bear the USDA mark of inspection.

(2) Require each establishment that harvests cells cultured from livestock or poultry subject to FMIA or PPIA for the purpose of producing food required to bear the USDA mark of inspection to obtain a grant of inspection, as required by the FSIS regulations.

(3) Require that the labels of food products derived from cultured cells of livestock and poultry are preapproved and then verified through inspection.

(4) Ensure that all additional requirements to ensure safe and accurate labeling under FMIA and PPIA are identified, and new regulations or guidances are promulgated as needed.

(5) In order to facilitate the development of a new Labeling Rule for cell-cultured meat and poultry products, the USDA issued an advanced notice of proposed rulemaking (ANPR) on September 2, 2021. This ANPR sought input from stakeholders throughout the United States regarding the labeling of meat and poultry products. The USDA-FSIS stated they would use these comments to inform future regulatory requirements for labeling of products made using cultured cells derived from animals under FSIS jurisdiction.

At the time of this writing, there are no products that have been approved by both the USDA and FDA under this cooperative agreement. However, the agencies have met with several companies in the process of developing products, and it is anticipated that products will be on the market before the close of the current decade (e.g., 2029).

Summary

This chapter provides a historical overview of the development of food regulations within the United States and the events that motivated improvements in regulatory oversight by the federal government. It should not be viewed as an exhaustive summary of all food regulations within the United States, but an explanation of why certain regulations developed as they did and what are the main drivers of those regulations in existence today. The systematic abuse of consumers by greedy business owners before the establishment of the FDA and USDA cannot be underestimated. Private industry has been proven to be consumed by greed and heartlessness. This is not to say that the current private sector is without morals or integrity, but if left unchecked, there will always be those that will take advantage of a situation.

As a member of the private sector and one who has spent a career ensuring that products are safe for consumers, I hope this history serves to enlighten those to what could happen again and inspire us to be better than our predecessors. At the same time, I would ask that our current critics realize that overregulation and control do not improve consumer safety. It merely stifles innovation.

Today US regulations serve three main purposes, to ensure that food and food products are safe; that consumers are adequately informed about the ingredients and nutritional content, quality and benefits/risks of the foods they are eating; and finally, to ensure a level playing field for commercial competitors. Most people are aware of the first purpose, many are aware of the second, but few are aware of the third. However, ensuring a level playing field for food industry competitors ensures that no one party has an unfair advantage in the market. This last role is critical to ensure a fair and transparent market for consumers and competitors alike.

References

62nd U.S. Congress, 1913. Amendatory and Supplemental Enactments to the Federal Food and Drug Act of 1906. Gould Amendment, 37 Stat. 732. Public Law 59-384, U.S. Food and Drug Administration.

Accum, F., 1820. A Treatise on the Adulteration of Foods and Culinary Poisons. Longman, Hurst, Rees, Orme, and Brown, London.

Anon, n.d.-a https://www.fda.gov/about-fda/fda-history/fda-leadership-1907-today.

Anon, n.d.-b https://farmers.uslegal.com/federal-grain-inspection/agricultural-marketing-act/.

Anon, n.d.-c https://www.fda.gov/industry/color-additives/color-additives-history.

Anon, n.d.-d https://supreme.justia.com/cases/federal/us/232/399/.

Anon, n.d.-e https://www.law.cornell.edu/supremecourt/text/265/438.

Anon, n.d.-f https://www.fda.gov/about-fda/fda-history/milestones-us-food-and-drug-law.

Anon, n.d.-g https://www.ftc.gov/public-statements/1938/05/wheeler-lea-act.

Anon, n.d.-h https://www.ftc.gov/system/files/documents/public_statements/676351/19380517_freer_whe_wheeler-lea_act.pdf.

Anon, n.d.-i https://www.fsis.usda.gov/policy/food-safety-acts/poultry-products-inspection-act.

Anon, n.d.-j https://www.fsis.usda.gov/policy/food-safety-acts/egg-products-inspection-act.

Anon, n.d.-k https://www.govinfo.gov/content/pkg/STATUTE-72/pdf/STATUTE-72-Pg1784.pdf#page=1.

Anon, n.d.-l https://www.fda.gov/food/generally-recognized-safe-gras/fdas-approach-gras-provision-history-processes.

Anon, n.d.-m https://www.fda.gov/food/guidance-regulation-food-and-dietary-supplements/food-safety-modernization-act-fsma.

Anon, n.d.-n https://www.fsis.usda.gov/about-fsis/history.

Anon, n.d.-o https://ask.usda.gov/s/article/When-was-this-agency-formed.

Anon, n.d.-p https://www.animallaw.info/statute/us-poultry-products-inspection-act-ppia.

Anon, n.d.-q https://www.nal.usda.gov/legacy/awic/humane-methods-slaughter-act.

Anon, n.d.-r https://www.ncsl.org/documents/agri/foodsafetylaws.pdf.

Anon, n.d.-s https://www.fda.gov/food/food-allergensgluten-free-guidance-documents-regulatory-information/food-allergen-labeling-and-consumer-protection-act-2004-falcpa.

Anon, n.d.-t https://www.congress.gov/bill/117th-congress/senate-bill/578.

Anon, n.d.-u https://www.fda.gov/food/food-labeling-nutrition/food-allergies.

Anon, n.d.-v https://www.federalregister.gov/documents/2013/08/05/2013-18813/food-labeling-gluten-free-labeling-of-foods.

Anon, n.d.-w https://www.fda.gov/food/cfsan-constituent-updates/fda-issues-final-rule-gluten-free-labeling-fermented-and-hydrolyzed-foods.

Anon, n.d.-x https://www.fda.gov/food/sampling-protect-food-supply/fy1819-sample-collection-and-analysis-domestically-manufactured-dairy-free-dark-chocolate-products.

Anon, n.d.-y https://ods.od.nih.gov/About/DSHEA_Wording.aspx.

Anon, n.d.-z https://www.fdareview.org/issues/history-of-federal-regulation-1902-present/#p21.

Anon, n.d.-aa https://www.fda.gov/food/dietary-supplements.

Anon,n.d.-bb https://www.fda.gov/food/agricultural-biotechnology/how-gmos-are-regulated-food-and-plant-safety-united-states.

Anon, n.d.-cc https://www.fda.gov/safety/fdas-regulation-plant-and-animal-biotechnology-products.

Anon, n.d.-dd https://www.federalregister.gov/documents/2017/01/19/2017-00840/genome-editing-in-new-plant-varieties-used-for-foods-request-for-comments.

Anon, n.d.-ee https://gfi.org/science/the-science-of-cultivated-meat/.

Anon, n.d.-ff https://www.mayoclinic.org/tests-procedures/bone-marrow-transplant/in-depth/stem-cells/art-20048117.

Anon, n.d.-gg https://www.fsis.usda.gov/sites/default/files/media_file/2020-07/Formal-Agreement-FSIS-FDA.pdf.

ARS Annual Report on Science FY 2020.pdf, 2020. usda.gov.

Blum, D., 2018. The Poison Squad: One Chemist's Single-Minded Crusade for Food Safety at the Turn of the Twentieth Century. Penguin Press.

CFSAN, 2020. U.S. Agent Voluntary Identification System (VIS) for Food Facility Registration: Guidance for Industry. U.S. Department of Health and Human Services Food and Drug Administration Center for Food Safety and Applied Nutrition.

Cunha, B.A., 2004. The death of Alexander the Great: malaria or typhoid fever? Infect. Dis. Clin. N. Am. 18 (1), 53–63.

Federal Meat Inspection Act of 1906, 2017. as amended (21 U.S.C. 601 et seq.).

Foster, S., 2011. A Brief History of Adulteration of Herbs, Spices, and Botanical Drugs. 92 HerbalGram, pp. 42–57.

Hutt, P.B., 1990. Symposium on the history of fifty years of food regulation under the Federal Food, Drug, and Cosmetic Act: a historical introduction. Food Drug Cosmet. Law J. 45 (1), 17–19.

Lasztity, R., 2009. Chapter 3—history of the food quality standards. In: Lasztity, R., Petro-Turza, M., Foldesi, T., Accum, F.C. (Eds.), Food Quality Standards (UNESCO). Vol 3.

Lásztity, R., Petró-Turza, M., Földesi, T., 2009. Chapter 3. History of food quality standards. In: Lasztity, R. (Ed.), Food Quality and Standards.

Lehman, A.J., Laug, E.P., et al., 1949. Procedures for the appraisal of the toxicity of chemicals in foods. Food Drug Cosmet. Law Q 4 (3), 412–434.

Prockop, D.J., Bunnell, B.A., Phinney, D.G. (Eds.), 2008. Mesenchymal Stem Cells: Methods and Protocols. Springer, ISBN: 978-1-60327-169-1.

Sinclair, U., 1905. The Jungle. Doubleday, Page & Co.

Specht, E., Welch, D.R., Rees-Clayton, E.M., Lagally, C.D., 2018. Opportunities for applying biomedical production and manufacturing methods to the development of the clean meat industry. Biomed. Eng. J. 132, 161–168.

Starr, R.R., 2015. Too little, too late: ineffective regulation of dietary supplements in the United States. Am. J. Public Health 105 (3), 478–485.

Swann, J.P., 2006. How chemists pushed for consumer protection: the Food and Drugs Act of 1906. Chem. Herit. 24 (2), 6–11. https://www.fda.gov/media/110307/download.

Waltz, E., 2021. Lab-Made Chicken Reaches Select Diners in Singapore. Scientific American, Nature/Biotechnology. https://www.scientificamerican.com/article/lab-made-chicken-reaches-select-diners-in-singapore/.

CHAPTER 10

History of GRAS

Kelly A. Magurany

NSF International, Ann Arbor, MI, United States

Introduction

The following chapter provides a history of the GRAS (Generally Recognized as Safe) regulatory framework for ingredients added to human food as regulated by the US Food and Drug Administration (US FDA). Although it is recognized that ingredients added to animal feed may also be designated as GRAS within Title 21 of the Code of Federal Regulations (CFR) Part 582, the scope of this chapter is limited to the application of GRAS in human food. Further, substances that have been deemed not to be GRAS either through Federal Register (FR) notices or by regulation are excluded from the scope of this chapter. These include color additives and ingredients derived from new plant varieties especially those that are genetically modified plants (per 57 FR 22984, May 29, 1992). Finally, GRASE, or Generally Recognized as Safe and Effective, was introduced into the US FDA regulations for over-the-counter drugs (OTC); however, this regulatory topic is out of the scope of food ingredient regulations and therefore is also not covered in this text.

An overview of the timeline of the history of GRAS regulations in human food and notifications of GRAS substances to the US FDA is provided in Fig. 1.

Promulgation of GRAS status

Legislation for the protection of the public to potentially unsafe food additives was enacted in 1906 as the first Federal food law, the Pure Food and Drug Act, and administered by the Bureau of Chemistry of the Department of Agriculture. The primary purpose was stated to be "…for preventing the manufacture, sale or transportation of adulterated or poisonous or deleterious foods, drugs, medicine, and liquors, and for regulating traffic therein"

History of Food and Nutrition Toxicology
https://doi.org/10.1016/B978-0-12-821261-5.00005-2

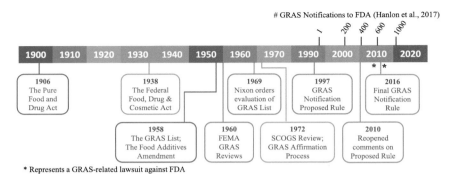

Fig. 1 Key milestones for GRAS regulations and GRAS notifications. (Modified from US FDA, 2018. FDA's Approach to the GRAS Provision: A History of Processes. FDA.)

(Siu et al., 1977). Inspiration for Congress to enact the legislation was alleged to be partly in response to Upton Sinclair's *The Jungle*, which described significant food safety abuses in the Chicago meatpacking industry and partly as a result of public outcry to economic adulteration of foods that commonly occurred at that time (e.g., adding sawdust to bread, colorants to spent tea, or formaldehyde to milk) (Burdock and Carabin, 2004). Extension of the law was enacted in 1938 when the Pure Food and Drug Act became the Federal Food, Drug, and Cosmetic Act; however, premarket approval for the use of additives in foods, by what is now the US FDA, was not required until the institution of the Food Additives Amendment of 1958, which prohibited the use of food additives that have not been adequately tested to establish their safety (H.R. 13254, 1958). An unsafe food additive as defined in Sec. 409 of the Amendment and now 21 USC 348 of the act was defined based on the approved status of a food additive. Specifically, "A food additive shall…be deemed unsafe… unless…(2) there is in effect, and it and its use or intended use are in conformity with, a regulation issued under this section…." The petition process to the secretary for regulation prescribing the conditions of safe use is described in part (b) of 21 USC 348 and was further codified as 21 CFR Part 121.51–121.52 and is currently codified in the Federal Regulations as 21 CFR Part 171: Food Additive Petitions.

GRAS, or Generally Recognized as Safe, refers to those substances that have been determined to be safe for addition to food either through a long history of safe use (prior to January 1, 1958) or based on the general availability and scientific consensus within the peer-reviewed literature that there would be no concern for the use of the ingredient in foods based on the proposed conditions of use (US FDA, 2018b). The GRAS terminology was first used as part of the 1958 Food Additives Amendment and was intended to alleviate the need for premarket approval of food ingredients that were broadly recognized to be safe (US FDA, 2018b). Specifically, the 1958 Amendment defined a food additive as "…any substance the intended use of which results or may reasonably be expected to result, directly or indirectly, in its becoming a component or otherwise affecting the characteristics of any food…if such substance is not generally recognized…to be safe under the conditions of its intended use…" (21 USC 321(s)).

Eligibility for classification of a substance as GRAS was incorporated into the regulation as 21 CFR Part 121.3 (36 FR 12093, June 25, 1971) and is now codified in 21 CFR Part 170.30 and requires that general recognition of safety be "…based only on the views of experts qualified by scientific training and experience to evaluate the safety of substances directly or indirectly added to food…[and]…requires common knowledge throughout the scientific community…that there is reasonable certainty that the substance is not harmful under the conditions of its intended use…" ("reasonable certainty of no harm" is also known as the standard of safety). Two paradigms to establish GRAS are now described in 21 CFR Part 170.30 by way of an amendment to clarify GRAS procedures on December 7, 1976 (41 FR 53600) and include GRAS based on common use in food prior to January 1, 1958, or by scientific procedures. Common use in food is further described in 21 CFR Part 170.30(d) as "…A food ingredient of natural biological origin that has been widely consumed for its nutrient properties in the United States prior to January 1, 1958, without known detrimental effects, which is subject only to conventional processing as practiced prior to January 1, 1958, and for which no known safety hazard exists…" [use outside the United States may also be considered. See 21 CFR Part 170.30(c)(2)]. For these substances, it is acknowledged in this part that it is not practicable to list all such substances and specific inclusion of such GRAS substances in the regulations is not necessary. GRAS established based on scientific procedures is applicable to those substances not used in food prior to January 1, 1958, and such an assessment is required per 21 CFR Part 170.30(b) to "…require the same quantity and quality of scientific evidence as is required to obtain approval as a food additive…."

The GRAS list

Although at the time of the 1958 Amendment it was considered impracticable to identify all possible GRAS substances, a list of food ingredients deemed to be commonly used in food was identified. Substances added directly to food, and those added indirectly to food as components of food contact materials, such as cotton fabrics or paper and paperboard, were included. A proposed rule for the "GRAS List" was published in the Federal Register on December 9, 1958, as 21 CFR Subpart B—Exemption of Certain Food Additives from the Requirement of tolerances, 121.100—Substances that are generally recognized as safe (23 FR 9511, 1958) and finalized on November 20, 1959, as 21 CFR 121.101(d) (24 FR 9368, 1959). The list is currently codified as 21 CFR Part 182. The original "GRAS List" is provided in Tables 1 and 2 and includes substances listed without inclusion of a tolerance, or maximum allowable use level (Table 1), and those listed with the inclusion of a tolerance (Table 2) (note: other categories of substances including spices, seasonings, and flavorings were later added to the GRAS list in subsequent rulemakings (25 FR 404, January 19, 1960; and 26 FR 3991, May 9, 1961)). In addition, some of those substances that were allowed in food before September 6, 1958, through directives or formal opinions from the FDA (e.g., letters of no objection that were issued upon request by an individual manufacturer) were considered "prior-sanctioned" substances and were added to the code and are now recognized as 21 CFR Part 181 (US FDA, 2018b). "Opinion letters" issued by the US FDA prior to January 1, 1958, were officially revoked on April 9, 1970, through the Federal Register (35 FR 5810, 1970), which was later codified as 21 CFR Part 170.6. However, these opinion letters could have been replaced "by qualified and current opinions" (21 CFR Part 170.6(e)) if the recipient of such a letter were to submit the original letter and request to the US FDA prior to July 23, 1970. Thus some prior-sanctioned substances remain unlisted in the CFR. At the time in which the GRAS and prior-sanctioned substances were added to the Federal Register, no effort was made to collect and evaluate the available scientific literature, as at the time, they were considered common food ingredients (SCOGS, 1982).

Self-affirmations of GRAS

Although not explicitly stated in the Food Additives Amendment of 1958, the GRAS "exemption" from premarket approval by the US FDA allowed for any party to establish the GRAS status of an ingredient added to food without notification to US FDA, assuming the principles of GRAS were followed. In other words, general recognition of safety for the intended use of an ingredient may be established, provided the conclusion of GRAS was based on scientific consensus of experts qualified by scientific training

Table 1 1958 GRAS list, compounds with no tolerance specified (24 FR 9368, 1959).

Chemical preservatives	Emulsifying agents (con't)	Nutrients (con't)
Ascorbic acid	Mono- and diglycerides from the glycerolysis of edible fats or oils	Niacin
Ascorbyl palmitate		Niacinamide
Calcium ascorbate	Monosodium phosphate	D-pantothenyl alcohol
Calcium propionate	derivatives of mono-	Potassium chloride
Erythorbic acid	and diglycerides from the glycerolysis of edible fats or oils	Pyridoxine hydrochloride
Potassium sorbate	Propylene glycol	Riboflavin
Propionic acid	**Miscellaneous**	Riboflavin-5-phosphate
Sodium ascorbate	Acetic acid	Sodium pantothenate
Sodium propionate	Aluminum sodium sulfate	Sodium phosphate (mono-, di-, tribasic)
Sodium sorbate	Aluminum sulfate	
Sorbic acid	Butane	Thiamine hydrochloride
Tocopherols	Calcium phosphate, tribasic	Thiamine mononitrate
Buffer and neutralizing agents	Caramel	a-Tocopherol acetate
Acetic acid	Carbon dioxide	Vitamin A
Aluminum ammonium sulfate	Carnauba wax	Vitamin A acetate
Aluminum sodium sulfate	Citric acid	Vitamin A palmitate
Aluminum potassium sulfate	Glycerin	Vitamin B12
Ammonium bicarbonate	Glycerol monostearate	Vitamin D2
Ammonium carbonate	Helium	Vitamin D3
Ammonium hydroxide	Magnesium carbonate	**Sequestrants**
Ammonium phosphate (mono- and dibasic-)	Magnesium hydroxide	Calcium acetate
	Monoammonium glutamate	Calcium chloride
Calcium carbonate	Nitrogen	Calcium citrate
Calcium chloride	Papain	Calcium diacetate
Calcium citrate	Phosphoric acid	Calcium gluconate
Calcium gluconate	Propane	Calcium hexametaphosphate
Calcium hydroxide	Propylene glycol	Calcium phytate
Calcium lactate	Triacetin (glyceryl triacetate)	Citric acid
Calcium oxide	Tricalcium phosphate	Dipotassium phosphate
Calcium phosphate	Sodium carbonate	Disodium phosphate

Continued

Table 1 1958 GRAS list, compounds with no tolerance specified (24 FR 9368, 1959)—cont'd

Citric acid	Sodium phosphate	Monocalcium acid
Lactic acid	Sodium	phosphate
	tripolyphosphate	
Magnesium carbonate	**Nonnutritive**	Monoisopropyl citrate
	sweeteners	
Magnesium oxide	Calcium cyclohexyl	Potassium citrate
Potassium acid tartrate	sulfamate	Sodium acid phosphate
Potassium bicarbonate	Calcium saccharin	Sodium citrate
Potassium carbonate	Saccharin	Sodium diacetate
Potassium citrate;	Sodium cyclohexyl	Sodium gluconate
Potassium hydroxide	sulfamate	
	Sodium saccharin	Sodium
		hexametaphosphate
Sodium acetate	**Nutrients**	Sodium metaphosphate
Sodium acid	Ascorbic acid	Sodium phosphate
pyrophosphate		(mono-, di-, tribasic)
Sodium aluminum	Calcium carbonate	
phosphate		
Sodium bicarbonate	Calcium oxide	Sodium potassium tartrate
Sodium carbonate	Calcium pantothenate	Sodium pyrophosphate
Sodium citrate	Calcium phosphate	Sodium tartrate
Sodium hydroxide	(mono-, di-, tribasic)	Sodium
		tetrapyrophosphate
Sodium phosphate	Calcium sulfate	Sodium tripolyphosphate
(mono-, di-, tri-)		
Sodium potassium	Carotene	Tartaric acid
tartrate		
Sodium sesquicarbonate	Ferric phosphate	**Stabilizers**
Sulfuric acid	Ferric pyrophosphate	Agar-agar
Tartaric acid	Ferric sodium	Carob bean gum (locust
	pyrophosphate	bean gum)
Emulsifying agents	Ferrous sulfate	Carrageenin
Diacetyl tartaric acid	Iron, reduced	Guar gum
esters of mono- and	1-Lysine	
diglycerides from the	monohydrochloride	
glycerolysis of edible fats		
or oils		

Table 2 1958 GRAS list compounds with specified use and/or tolerance.

Chemical	Tolerance	Uses
Anticaking agents		
Aluminum calcium silicate	2%	In table salt
Calcium silicate	5%	In baking powder
Calcium silicate	2%	In table salt
Magnesium silicate	2%	
Tricalcium silicate	2%	
Chemical preservatives		
Benzoic acid	0.10%	—
Butylated hydroxyanisole	Total content of antioxidants not to exceed 0.02%	Of fat or oil content, including essential (volatile) oil content, of food
Butylated hydroxytoluene		
Caprylic acid	—	In cheese wraps
Dilauryl thiodipropionate	Total content of antioxidants not to exceed 0.02%	Of fat or oil content, including essential (volatile) oil content, of food
Gum guaiac	0.10% (equivalent antioxidant activity)	In edible fats or oils
Nordihydroguaiaretic acid	Total content of antioxidants not to exceed 0.02%	Of fat or oil content, including essential (volatile) oil content, of food
Potassium bisulfite	—	Not in meats or foods recognized as a source of vitamin B_1
Potassium metabisulfite	—	
Propyl gallate	Total content of antioxidants not to exceed 0.02%	Of fat or oil content, including essential (volatile) oil content, of food
Sodium benzoate	0.10%	—
Sodium bisulfite	—	Not in meats or foods recognized as a source of vitamin B_1
Sodium metabisulfite	—	
Sodium sulfite	—	
Sulfur dioxide	—	
Thiodipropionic acid	Total content of antioxidants not to exceed 0.02%	Of fat or oil content, including essential (volatile) oil content, of food

Continued

Table 2 1958 GRAS list compounds with specified use and/or tolerance—cont'd

Chemical	Tolerance	Uses
Emulsifying agents		
Cholic acid	0.01%	Dried egg whites
Deoxycholic acid	0.01%	
Glycocholic acid	0.01%	
Ox bile extract USP (solids)	0.01%	
Taurocholic acid (or its sodium salt)	0.01%	
Miscellaneous		
Caffeine	0.02%	In cola type beverages
Ethyl formate	0.0015%	As a fumigant for cashew nuts
Magnesium stearate	–	As migratory substances from packaging materials when used as a stabilizer
Sorbitol	7.0%	In foods for special dietary use
Triethyl citrate	0.25%	Egg whites
Nutrients		
Copper gluconate	0.005%	–
Cuprous iodide	0.01%	In table salt as a source of
Potassium iodide	0.01%	dietary iodine
Sequestrants[a]		
Isopropyl citrate	0.02%	In salt
Sodium thiosulfate	0.1%	
Stearyl citrate	0.15%	

[a] No attempt has been made to designate those chemicals that function as both sequestrants and chemical preservatives.
Modified from 24 FR 9368, 1959. 24 Federal register 9368: rules and regulations: chapter I—food and drug administration, Department of Health, Education, and Welfare. Subchapter B—Food and Food Products. Part 121—Food Additives. Subpart B—Exemption of Certain Food Additives from the Requirement of Tolerances. Substances Generally Recognized as Safe.

and experience to evaluate the safety of substances directly or indirectly added to food, either by confirming the "common use" of the substance in food prior to January 1, 1958, or through scientific procedures (21 CFR Part 170.30(a)). GRAS conclusions supported by the industry became known as "self-affirmations" of GRAS. Expectations for self-affirmations of

GRAS were consistent with those of GRAS affirmations submitted to the US FDA and included:

(1) "…General recognition of safety requires common knowledge throughout the scientific community knowledgeable about the safety of substances directly or indirectly added to food that there is reasonable certainty that the substance is not harmful under the conditions of its intended use…" (i.e., there is general consensus among qualified experts that a substance is safe for the intended use) (21 CFR 170.30(a) as amended by the 1997 GRAS proposed rule, 53 FR 18938).

(2) "General recognition of safety should require the same quantity and quality of scientific evidence as is required to obtain approval of a food additive (21 CFR 170.30(b))."

(3) "General recognition of safety through scientific procedures shall be based upon the application of generally available and accepted scientific data, information, or methods, which ordinarily are published, as well as the application of scientific principles, and may be corroborated by the application of unpublished scientific data, information, or methods (21 CFR 170.30(c)." (This is in contrast to a food additive, which does not require that data be generally available and accepted, otherwise known as the "common knowledge element." This "common knowledge element" thus sets a higher bar for GRAS as the scientific evidence should be published in a peer-reviewed scientific journal, i.e., generally available and accepted. Although the scientific evidence supporting the safety of a food additive should be of the same quantity and quality, the "common knowledge element" is not required (62 FR 18938, 1997).)

(4) "…General recognition of safety through experience based on common use in food prior to January 1, 1958, shall be based solely on food use of the substance prior to January 1, 1958, and shall ordinarily be based upon generally available data and information. An ingredient not in common use in food prior to January 1, 1958, may achieve general recognition of safety only through scientific procedures… (21 CFR 170.30(c))." (Common use in food may be established based on consumption in the United States or internationally based on an amendment to the regulation in May of 1988 (53 FR 16544, 1988) that is now codified as 21 CFR 170.30(c)(2).)

(5) GRAS is based on the intended use of the ingredient. If a use is proposed, other than the use that was evaluated in the conclusion on GRAS, that use is not GRAS unless a conclusion of GRAS for that intended use has been established (21 CFR 170.30(i)).

(6) "…New information may at any time require reconsideration of the GRAS status of a food ingredient… (21 CFR 170.30(l))."

(7) Any substances designated as GRAS shall be used within the principles of good manufacturing practices (21 CFR 182.1(b)), i.e.,

    (1) "The quantity of a substance added to food does not exceed the amount reasonably required to accomplish its intended physical, nutritional, or other technical effect in food; and

    (2) The quantity of a substance that becomes a component of food as a result of its use in the manufacturing, processing, or packaging of food, and which is not intended to accomplish any physical or other technical effect in the food itself, shall be reduced to the extent reasonably possible.

    (3) The substance is of appropriate food grade and is prepared and handled as a food ingredient."

US FDA has reiterated the position that "persons have the right to make independent GRAS determinations" within many forums and often with updates to GRAS regulations through the Federal Register (53 FR 16544, 1988; 62 FR 18938, 1997; 81 FR 54960, 2016), with the logic that "… it is on the basis of the GRAS exception of the 'food additive' definition that many ingredients derived from natural sources (such as salt, pepper, vinegar, vegetable oil, and thousands of spices and natural flavors), as well as a host of chemical additives (including some sweeteners, preservatives, and artificial flavors), are able to be lawfully marketed today without having been formally reviewed by FDA and without being the subject of a food additive regulation. The judgment of Congress was that subjecting every intentional additive to FDA premarket review was not necessary to protect public health and would impose an insurmountable burden on FDA and the food industry (57 FR 22984, 1992)."

Self-affirmation of GRAS by the flavor and extracts manufacturers association (FEMA)

With the advent of the Food Additives Amendment of 1958, the burden of proof for the safety of ingredients added to food was largely shifted to industry. Those ingredients that were currently added to food that were not either GRAS for their intended use or regulated within an effective food additive regulation were at risk of enforcement action by US FDA (although a grace period was allowed by Congress) (Hallagan and Hall, 1995). Thus efforts to establish regulatory compliance for these ingredients were a priority for industry. One effort that has demonstrated best practice, both in the GRAS approach and the effective partnership with the US FDA, was that of the Flavor and Extracts Manufacturers Association (FEMA). FEMA is a consortium of US flavor additive manufacturers that was established in 1909 (FEMA, 2022). The goal of FEMA was to establish a program for the evaluation of flavor ingredients (that included natural and artificial flavors as now defined in 21 CFR Part 101.22) that was consistent with the four key aspects of GRAS: (1) general recognition of safety by qualified experts, (2) demonstration of qualified experts through training and experience, (3) safety established based on scientific procedures or common use in food prior to January 1, 1958, and (4) GRAS contingent upon the conditions of intended use.

Several early milestones were integral for establishing the FEMA GRAS program. To begin, in 1959, FEMA evaluated the depth and breadth of flavor use within commerce by conducting an industry survey. Secondly, they worked to establish a panel of experts, independent of industry, that was successfully instituted in 1960 (Cohen et al., 2018; Hallagan and Hall, 1995, 2009). Experts for the panel were identified based on technical training in toxicology, pharmacology, metabolism, biochemistry, analytical chemistry, veterinary medicine, pathology, and statistics, and preference was given to those with specific experience evaluating the safety of flavor ingredients.[a] Lastly, the process for the scientific assessment of flavor ingredients needed to be implemented, where a key component of success was to establish general recognition of safety. To accomplish this, the FEMA Expert Panel developed GRAS lists of flavor ingredients and Scientific Literature Reviews (SLRs) that provided the basis of the panel's conclusions of GRAS that were published upon the completion of an assessment and only after US FDA review. The SLRs were originally developed through a contract with US FDA and available through the National Technical Information Service (NTIS). Since 1965, the identity and maximum use levels of FEMA GRAS flavors have also been published in the journal, *Food Technology*. In more recent years, safety assessments of the FEMA GRAS Panel for structurally related groups of single chemical flavors and natural flavor complexes have been published in the peer-reviewed literature (Hallagan and Hall, 2009).

[a]FDA policy and regulations do not define what credentials are required to consider someone to be an expert and based on several court cases examining the GRAS status of ingredients, the final determination has been left to the courts (Hallagan and Hall, 1995); however, in November 2017, US FDA provided a draft guidance document for the convening of a GRAS panel that describes the recommended expertise (US FDA, 2017a).

With the advent of the internet, FEMA GRAS publications may now be found on the FEMA website at femaflavor.org (FEMA, 2022). Through these procedures, FEMA established transparency for the GRAS evaluations and general recognition through publication in the peer-reviewed literature. After 60 years of practice and operating under the authority of the US FDA 1958 Food Additives Amendment, the FEMA GRAS program has been recognized for its expertise, independence, and transparency in the conduct of GRAS evaluations for flavor ingredients (FEMA, 2022; GAO, 2010).

From a technical perspective, the FEMA GRAS program has evolved substantially over the years in the conduct of the assessments, leveraging the latest advances in scientific evaluation and risk assessment. From the start, the components of the GRAS evaluation included: (1) the identity and purity of a substance, (2) its chemical and pharmacological relationship to analogous substances, (3) its presence and level as a naturally occurring substance in food, and (4) any relevant metabolic or toxicological data (Oser and Ford, 1977). However, in the early assessments, establishment of GRAS based on common use in food prior to January 1, 1958, was a major factor in the conclusion of GRAS status (Cohen et al., 2018; Hall and Oser, 1965). At the time, "common use" was established through an industry survey of flavor manufacturers that were part of FEMA, the National Association of Chewing Gum Manufacturers, and several independent manufacturers of candy products. To date, FEMA conducts poundage surveys of flavor ingredients in foods approximately every 5 years.

Regarding the nature of a flavor ingredient, it was acknowledged that these ingredients are often complex mixtures and that evaluation of individual components of a flavor mixture that may be in food at very low levels (parts per million to parts per trillion) was not practical (Hallagan and Hall, 1995). It was also acknowledged that any one flavor component, e.g., benzaldehyde, may be contributed from multiple flavor ingredients and that these ingredients may be used at varying concentrations depending on the food type. For example, clove oil may be used as a minor flavor note in a food product at trace parts per million levels (ppm) but may be used as the primary flavor note in a candy at 1000 ppm and thus exposure in the total diet, including beverages, baked goods, candy, chewing gum, and desserts, was considered a key component of the safety assessment (Hall and Oser, 1965). Based on the evaluation of maximum use levels, it was found that on average, flavor ingredients are not typically used at more than five times the average use level in any food type (Hall and Oser, 1965). For the assessment of safety and in addition to the available toxicologic and pharmacologic data, per capita intake (PCI) levels were calculated for the intended food uses and consumption ratios were calculated to compare added and naturally occurring concentrations in the food (Hallagan and Hall, 1995).

Overall, early assessments were primarily based on the long history of safe use in foods, the intended use as a flavor considering maximum use levels in different food types, and based on the principle of self-limitation. This principle submits that flavor ingredients used at high concentrations would be unpalatable and therefore there is a high likelihood that flavor ingredients would be used at very low levels in foods (Cohen et al., 2018). Based on recent information, concentrations of individual flavoring ingredients added to food are, almost without exception, <0.1%, or 1000 ppm, with the majority at <0.001%, or 10 ppm (Smith et al., 2005a). In addition, it was assumed per 21 CFR Part 121.101 (now 21 CFR Part 182.1) that the flavor ingredient was used under the principles of Good Manufacturing Practice, i.e., "…the quantity of a substance added to food does not exceed the amount reasonably required to accomplish its intended physical, nutritional, or other technical effect in food…" and that "…the substance is of appropriate food grade and is prepared and handled as a food ingredient." Importantly, based on the principle of self-limitation and GMP, the maximum use levels identified by the FEMA GRAS Panel were to be considered typical use levels and in no way were to be regarded as tolerance levels in food. Further, the GRAS status of the flavor ingredient applied only to the condition of use included in the assessment with a reevaluation required for expanded use conditions. In the 1965 publication, the FEMA Expert Panel's GRAS list consisted of more than 1100 flavor ingredients including 265 natural flavoring compounds that are now listed in 21 CFR Part 172.510 and 21 CFR Part 182.20 (Cohen et al., 2018; Hall and Oser, 1965). By 1995, of the 1783 GRAS substances that had been reviewed, more than 1400 had been found to be naturally occurring in foods (Hallagan and Hall, 1995).

The scientific procedures of the FEMA GRAS Panel have been dynamic, progressing with advances in science. As changes have been made, publications reviewing the FEMA approach have been communicated (Gerarde, 1973; Oser and Ford, 1977; Woods and Doull, 1991). In addition, to ensure that historical assessments were maintained with current science, FEMA periodically reevaluated the GRAS status of flavor ingredients; this exercise became known as affirmation of GRAS. The first reevaluation was completed in 1985 (including a review of >1200 flavor ingredients) and a second in 1993 (completed in 2005) and included review of >2000 flavor ingredients. The latest reevaluation inspired the implementation of a 5-year review period that would incorporate any new data into the SLRs that were identified during that period (Hallagan and Hall, 2009). Currently, a 10-year rotating safety review is in place to evaluate structurally similar chemical groups of flavoring ingredients (Smith et al., 2005a). Up until 2009 and as a result of the reevaluation, eight flavors have had their GRAS status revoked, including alkanet root extract, brominated vegetable oil, calamus, calamus oil, musk ambrette, 3-nonanon-1-ol, 2-methyl-5-vinylpyrazine, and o-vinylanisole. A ninth flavor, cinnamyl anthranilate, was voluntarily abandoned by industry and later banned by US FDA (Hallagan and Hall, 2009). Several hundred flavor ingredients were not affirmed as GRAS due to data insufficiencies, and many assessments have been updated with new data and reaffirmed as GRAS (Hallagan and Hall, 1995).

To date, the FEMA GRAS Panel has established the GRAS status of more than 2800 flavoring ingredients that are used by industry with more than 1000 single chemical defined flavor substances evaluated since 1995 (Cohen et al., 2018; FEMA, 2022). Single chemical flavor ingredients, identified as discrete compounds, are evaluated consistent with the procedures outlined by Smith et al. (2005a), which is largely consistent with the evaluation of food additives established by the European Food Safety Authority (EFSA, 2021) and the Joint FAO/WHO Expert Committee on Food Additives (JECFA, 2020). These substances may be isolated from natural sources or synthetically derived. Almost without exception, the chemical nature of synthetically derived flavors, which are not found in nature, is structurally related to naturally occurring compounds. In addition, more than 250 natural flavoring complexes (NFCs) have been reevaluated according to the most current scientific procedures published by Smith (2004), Smith et al. (2005b), and Cohen et al. (2018). NFCs are defined as mixtures of chemicals obtained from botanical sources through physical separation methods that may include fractional distillation, topping (removal of volatile parts), solvent extraction, supercritical extraction, thin-film evaporation, and molecular distillation (Smith, 2004). A summary of the procedures for single chemical flavor ingredients and natural flavor complexes may be found in Fig. 2. In all cases, to reach a GRAS decision, there must be (1) an understanding of the known or anticipated biochemical fate of the substance and its potential to produce toxicity, and (2) the panel must come to consensus that there is a reasonable certainty of no harm, i.e., the substances are safe, at the level of use of the substances in the context of its toxic potential. For further details on the procedures, readers are referred to Smith (2004), Smith et al. (2005a, b), and Cohen et al. (2018) publications.

Data inputs

1) Description of the starting material and isolation method, including as applicable
   a. All recognized natural/botanical and geographical sources
   b. All commercially used plant parts and degrees of maturity
   c. All commercially used isolation methods and the variability inherent in the isolation method
2) Complete analytical characterization, including statistical summary
3) Specifications that support identity and purity for food use
4) Data that supports technical efficacy for the intended use
5) All available safety data on the NFC and its constituents
   a. Chemical structure and mode of action on biological systems
   b. Metabolic and pharmacologic characteristics
   c. Toxicity testing including that for general toxicology, carcinogenicity, genotoxicity screening, and developmental and reproductive toxicology, immunotoxicity, and neurotoxicity
6) Data to support total exposure including
   a. History of use
   b. Intake of the natural levels of the flavor in foods
   c. Intake of the added levels of the flavor for the subject food use

Procedures

Part A. Congeneric Groups

1. Identify Congeneric Groups[1] and Cramer Class[2] for all known constituents
2. Confirm no *in vivo* genotoxicity risk for constituents. If not possible, stop or generate data.
3. Calculate the mean % and *per capita* intake (PCI x 10 method)[3]
4. Confirm total intake < TTC for Cramer Class[2] for each group. If not,
5. Evaluate toxicity data; confirm ADI[4] > intake. If not, stop. If data gaps, generate data. If intake > ADI, NFC is not GRAS.

Procedures (con't)

Part B. Unknown constituents (NFCs only)

1. Calculated the mean % and per capita intake (PCI x 10 method)[3]
2. Calculate the Consumption Ratio[5]. If intake is significantly greater than natural levels in food, stop. NFC is not GRAS.
3. Confirm no risk of TTC excluded class[6]. If risk, stop. NFC is not GRAS.
4. Confirm no *in vivo* genotoxicity risk. If risk, intake must be < 0.15 µg/person/day or negative genotoxicity for NFC to establish GRAS. If not, stop or generate data.
5. Confirm intake < TTC for Cramer Class III[2]. If not,
6. Evaluate toxicity data; confirm adequate MOS[7] for intake. If not, stop. If data gaps, generate data. If inadequate MOS, NFC is not GRAS.

Part C. Other Considerations

1. Confirm no other concerns for safe use exist (e.g. use by infants or children, higher toxicity metabolites). If concerns, stop. If data gaps, generate data. If unreasonable risk, NFC is not GRAS. If no other concerns, NFC is GRAS.

---

[1] Congeneric groups are groups of structurally-related compounds expected to have similar toxicologic properties (see Table below).

[2] Cramer classes (I, II and III) have been established that define a threshold of toxicological concern (TTC), based on safety data for structurally similar compounds, below which there would be no concern for toxicity (calculated from the 5% of the distribution of NOELs of the dataset for each class and using a safety factor of 100x). Compounds lacking data may be assigned to a Cramer class based on a decision tree that evaluates its structure. The TTC's for each class are I- 1800 µg/kg-day, II- 540 µg/kg-day and III- 90 µg/kg-day (Cramer et al., 1976; Kroes et al., 2004, 2000; Munro et al., 1996)

[3] The PCI x 10 method provides a µg/person/day intake level estimation based on the following equation, where 0.8 is an adjustment factor to account for the volume of potentially unreported flavor usage (Cohen et al., 2018):

$$\text{Flavor usage (kg/yr)} \times 10^9 \text{ µg/kg} \quad \times 10 = \text{µg/person/day}$$
$$\text{US population} \times 0.8 \times 365 \text{ days}$$

[4] ADI = Acceptable Daily Intake

[5] The consumption ratio for a flavor ingredient is: $\dfrac{\text{consumption in food}}{\text{consumption of added flavor}}$

[6] Excluded chemical classes from TTC include aflatoxin-like-, azoxy- and N-nitroso-compounds; heavy metals; proteins; 2,3,7,8-dibenzo-p-dioxin and it's analogues; polyhalogenated dibenzo-p-dioxins,- dibenzofurans and-biphenyls; steroids; nanomaterials; and radioactive materials (Kroes et al., 2004).

[7] Margin of Safety

Fig. 2 FEMA GRAS procedures for single chemical and natural flavor complexes (NFCs). (Modified from Smith, R.L., Cohen, S.M., Doull, J., Feron, V.J., Goodman, J.I., Marnett, L.J., Munro, I.C., Portoghese, P.S., Waddell, W.J., Wagner, B.M., Adams, T.B., 2005. Criteria for the safety evaluation of flavoring substances. Food Chem. Toxicol. 43, 1141–1177. https://doi.org/10.1016/j.fct.2004.11.012 and Cohen, S.M., Eisenbrand, G., Fukushima, S., Gooderham, N.J., Guengerich, F.P., Hecht, S.S., Rietjens, I.M.C.M., Davidsen, J.M., Harman, C.L., Taylor, S.V., 2018. Updated procedure for the safety evaluation of natural flavor complexes used as ingredients in food. Food Chem. Toxicol. 113, 171–178. https://doi.org/10.1016/j.fct.2018.01.021.) *(Continued)*

Congeneric groups

1. Saturated aliphatic, acyclic, linear primary alcohols, aldehydes, carboxylic acids and related esters
2. Saturated aliphatic, acyclic, branched-chain primary alcohols, aldehydes, carboxylic acids and related esters
3. Aliphatic linear and branched-chain alpha, beta-unsaturated aldehydes and related alcohols acids and esters
4. Aliphatic allyl esters
5. Unsaturated linear and branched-chain aliphatic, non-conjugated aldehydes, related primary alcohols, carboxylic acids and esters
6. Aliphatic primary alcohols, aldehydes, carboxylic acids, acetals and esters containing additional oxygenated functional groups
7. Saturated alicyclic primary alcohols, aldehydes, acids and related esters
8. Saturated and unsaturated aliphatic acyclic secondary alcohols, ketones and related esters
9. Aliphatic acyclic and alicyclic alpha-diketones and related alpha-hydroxyketones
10. Alicyclic ketones, secondary alcohols and related esters
11. Pulegone and structurally and metabolically related substances
12. Aliphatic and aromatic tertiary alcohols and related esters
13. Aliphatic, alicyclic, alicyclic-fused and aromatic-fused ring lactones
14. Benzyl derivatives
15. Hydroxy- and alkoxy-substituted benzyl derivatives

16. Cinnamyl alcohol, cinnamaldehyde, cinnamic acid and related esters
17. Phenyl-substituted primary alcohols, aldehydes, carboxylic acids and related esters
18. Phenyl-substituted secondary alcohols, ketones and related esters
19. Aliphatic and aromatic hydrocarbons
20. Phenol derivatives
21. Hydroxyallylbenzenes and hydroxypropenyl-benzene derivatives
22. Phenethyl alcohol, phenylacetaldehyde and related acetals and esters
23. Aliphatic and aromatic ethers
24. Furfuryl alcohol, furfural and related substances
25. Furan derivatives
26. Aliphatic and aromatic sulfides and thiols
27. Sulfur-substituted furan derivatives
28. Sulfur-containing heterocyclic and heteroaromatic derivatives
29. Aliphatic acyclic diols, triols and related substances
30. Aliphatic and aromatic amines and related amides
31. Nitrogen containing heterocyclic and heteroaromatic substances
32. Pyrazine derivatives
33. Anthranilate derivatives
34. Amino acids
35. Maltol derivatives
36. Epoxide derivatives

Fig. 2, cont'd

The select committee on GRAS substances
History and scope of work

In review of the regulation on food additives, the White House Conference on Food, Nutrition and Health suggested to the current administration that the GRAS substances listed in the regulation be critically evaluated for their safe use. This recommendation was also inspired by the removal by the US FDA of various cyclamate salts from the GRAS list as nonnutritive sweeteners due to concerns regarding bladder tumors in rats (34 FR 17063, October 21, 1969). On October 30, 1969, President Richard M. Nixon directed the US FDA (Bureau of Foods, now the Center for Food Safety and Nutrition) to evaluate the current list of GRAS substances by summarizing the available scientific literature and providing a recommendation on any restrictions for use in food that may be necessary (US FDA, 2018b). US FDA announced through the Federal Register the intent to conduct a comprehensive study of substances presumed to be GRAS (35 FR 18623, December 8, 1970). Components of this effort included extensive literature and consumer consumption surveys; a generous supply of information and data from governmental, industrial, and academic sources; and some biological testing that was contracted by the US FDA. The resulting data were provided to a Select Committee that was organized in June 1972 by the Life Sciences Research Office (LSRO), a contractor of the US FDA, that was established in 1962 by the Federation of American Societies for Experimental Biology (FASEB). The Select Committee was tasked with conducting the GRAS substance safety evaluations, that included review of the available data and further research (as needed), by individual committee members and LSRO contractors (SCOGS, 1982; Siu et al., 1977). This evaluation became known as the SCOGS review or the review by the Select Committee on GRAS Substances.

The Select Committee was made up of independent experts and scientists from the LSRO and several additional scientists contracted by the LSRO that were qualified by training and experience to join the Select Committee. The resulting committee included 11 total members (Senti, 1983). The final members of the Select Committee were as follows: J.F. Borzelleca, PhD (pharmacology); G.W. Irving, Jr., PhD (biochemistry), Chairman; B.N. La Ou, Jr., MD, PhD (pharmacology); J.R. McCoy, VMD (pathology); G.L. Plaa, PhD (pharmacology); R.G.H. Siu, PhD (organic chemistry); J.L. Wood, PhD (biochemistry) that served for the duration of the committee. Members that served limited periods included A.M.

Altschul, PhD (biochemistry), 1972–73; H.G. Day, ScD (chemistry), 1973–82; S.J. Foman, MD (pediatrics), 1974–82; S.A. Miller, PhD (biochemistry), 1972–78; M.B. Shimkin, MD (oncology), 1974–82; M.E. Swendseid, PhD (nutrition), 1979–82 (SCOGS, 1982).

The scope of work initially committed by the Select Committee included the comprehensive safety evaluation of 235 GRAS substances codified within 21 CFR Part 121.1 (now 21 CFR Part 182), excluding flavors, spices, and essential oils. However, with additional submissions of self-affirmed GRAS and prior-sanctioned substances, the final scope of the work by the Select Committee was over 450 substances including direct food additives and additives used in the manufacture of packaging materials (Fisher, 1982; SCOGS, 1982; Senti, 1983; Siu et al., 1977; US FDA, 2018b).

SCOGS conclusions

At the completion of the reviews, SCOGS had published 141 comprehensive reports and several supplemental reports from 1972 to 1982 on 468 GRAS or prior-sanctioned substances that included 422 substances that were evaluated for direct addition to food and 46 substances that were evaluated as components of packaging materials (Fisher, 1982; SCOGS, 1982; Senti, 1983). Notice of draft reports from the Select Committee was issued through the Federal Register and interested parties were welcomed to present any comments to the Select Committee for consideration. Where hearings were requested, the hearing dates and names and affiliations of witnesses were also published in the Federal Register by the US FDA (SCOGS, 1982). Finalized reports from the Select Committee were approved by the director of the LSRO, then were reviewed and approved by the LSRO Advisory Committee that included representatives from the FASEB societies and were finally approved by the executive director of FASEB that ultimately delivered the reports to US FDA (US FDA, 2018b). The overall operational procedures leading to the affirmation of GRAS are provided in Fig. 3.

The conclusions of the Select Committee were standardized with the intention to force a decision within predetermined guidelines so that qualified conclusions and exceptions could not be made and so that interpretation of the conclusion by independent bodies, including the US FDA, would be less difficult. This approach worked in most cases; however, some more complicated evaluations were necessary that included weighing the risks and benefits of certain additive applications. As such, conclusions were not assigned to all substances (SCOGS, 1982). The five conclusions that were assigned were as follows (US FDA, 2018c):

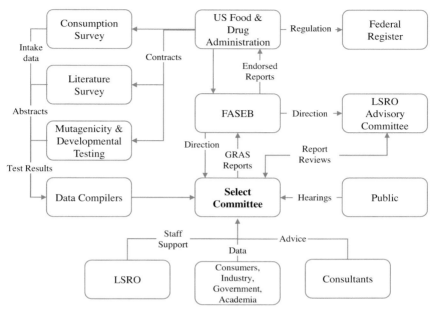

Fig. 3 Operational overview of the SCOGS evaluation process. (Modified from Siu, R.G., Borzelleca, J.F., Carr, C.J., Day, H.G., Fomon, S.J., Irving, G.W., La Du, B.N., McCoy, J.R., Miller, S.A., Plaa, G.L., Shimkin, M.B., Wood, J.L., 1977. Evaluation of health aspects of GRAS food ingredients: lessons learned and questions unanswered. Fed. Proc. 36, 2519–2562.)

1. "There is no evidence in the available information on [substance] that demonstrates, or suggests reasonable grounds to suspect, a hazard to the public when they are used at levels that are now current or might reasonably be expected in the future.

2. There is no evidence in the available information on [substance] that demonstrates a hazard to the public when it is used at levels that are now current and in the manner now practiced. However, it is not possible to determine, without additional data, whether a significant increase in consumption would constitute a dietary hazard.

3. While no evidence in the available information on [substance] demonstrates a hazard to the public when it is used at levels that are now current and in the manner now practiced, uncertainties exist requiring that additional studies be conducted.

4. The evidence on [substance] is insufficient to determine that the adverse effects reported are not deleterious to the public health should it be used at former levels and in the manner formerly practiced.

5. In view of the almost complete lack of biological studies, the Select Committee has insufficient data upon which to evaluate the safety of [substance] as a [intended use]."

The breakdown of the number of substances for each conclusion is reported by Fisher (1982) and included 339 substances concluded as #1, 69 substances concluded as #2, 21 substances concluded as #3, 5 substances concluded as #4, and 34 substances concluded as #5. Any opinions associated with the Select Committee conclusions may be requested through the National Technical Information Service (NTIS, 2017) using the NTIS Accession number that is provided in the US FDA SCOGS database (US FDA, 2018c). A total number of 115 SCOGS reports for over 370 substances is reported in the database. An explanation for the discrepancy between the number of reports and substances described by Fisher (1982) and the US FDA SCOGS database was investigated, and a listing of those substances included in the original SCOGS report, but not in the current US FDA SCOGS database is summarized in Table 3. Some of the chemicals listed in the original SCOGS report (SCOGS, 1982) were consolidated into other chemical classes in the current database or the SCOGS report was simply not available in the US FDA database; although some of the substance that are not reported in the database, e.g., wheat gluten and corn gluten, are listed in 21 CFR as GRAS.

Substances that were determined to be GRAS after the Select Committee review were affirmed as GRAS by the US FDA through notice of proposed rulemaking in the Federal Register and subsequent updates to 21 CFR Parts 184 and 186 (US FDA, 2018c). The US FDA affirmed GRAS status through the affirmation process that was developed in 1972 through rulemaking in the Federal Register (37 FR 6207, 1972; 37 FR 25705, 1972) and subsequently outlined in 21 CFR Part 170.35(a) and (b). For those substances that were self-affirmed as GRAS and not included in the original US FDA GRAS List nor submitted for review by the Select Committee were invited by the US FDA for submission through the GRAS affirmation petition process outlined in 21 CFR Part 170.35(c). Successful petitions from these submissions are also listed in 21 CFR Parts 184 and 186.

SCOGS policy and safety recommendations

Having spent a decade evaluating GRAS substances within the safety framework of the US FDA legislation, and subsequent to publishing the conclusions of GRAS evaluations, the Select Committee made several recommendations on the next steps associated with the GRAS approach. The

Table 3 Substances reviewed by the select committee not in US FDA database.

Ingredient	Conclusion	SCOGS report #	PB No.	Listing on US FDA database?
Acetooleins	1	30	254536	Listed as glycerin and glycerides
Acetostearins	1	30	254536	
Activated carbon	1-Majority / 5-Minority	11–6	82160375	Not available
Beef fat	1	11–15	82108671	Not available
Benzoyl peroxide	1	11–2	81127854	Not available
Borax (packaging)	1	11–4	81121410	Not available
Boric acid (packaging)	1	11–4	81121410	Not available
Cloves	1	19	238792	Consolidated with clove oil and similar
isoButane	1	112	80112022	Not available; helium gas is listed for this PB#
n-Butane	1	112	80112022	
Butterfat, enzyme modified	1	11–15	82108671	Not available
Calcium sulfate	1	33	262652	Listed as sulfuric acid
Chicken fat, enzyme modified	1	11–15	82108671	Not available
Citrus bioflavonoids (orange, grapefruit, tangerine)	5	11–3	82192931	Not available
Collagen	1	11–8	81229221	Not available
Corn gluten	1	11–2	82155482	Not available
Cornmint oil	5	11–9	82160391	Not available
Diacteyl tartaric acid esters of diglycerides	1	30	254536	Listed as glycerin and glycerides
Diacteyl tartaric acid esters of monoglycerides	1	30	254536	
Diglycerides of edible fats or oils or edible fat-forming fatty acids	1	30	254536	

Continued

Table 3 Substances reviewed by the select committee not in US FDA database—cont'd

Ingredient	Conclusion	SCOGS report #	PB No.	Listing on US FDA database?
Eugenol	1	19	238792	Consolidated with clove oil and similar
European dill seed oil	1	22	238906	Not available
Ferrocyanide salts for fining of wine	1	11–10	82155474	Not available
Ferrous oxide (packaging)	1	35	80176676	Listed as ferric oxide
Glucono delta-lactone	1	11–11	82108663	Not available
Glyceryl lactooleate	1	30	254536	Listed as glycerin and glycerides
Glyceryl lactopalmitate	1	30	254536	
Hesperidin complex	5	11–3	82192931	Not available
Hesperidin, purified	5	11–3	82192931	Not available
Lemon bioflavonoid complex	5	11–3	82192931	Not available
Mace	3	18	266878	Listed as nutmeg and mace
Mace oil				
Mace oleoresin				
Malt extract	1	11–13	81121402	Not available
Maltodextrins				
Malt syrup				
Methyl polysilicones	1	11–14	81229239	Not available
Milk fat, enzyme modified	1	11–15	82106871	Not available
Monoglyceride citrate	1	30	254536	Listed as glycerin and glycerides
Monoglycerides of edible fats and oils or edible fat-forming fatty acids	1	30	254536	
Monophosphate derivatives of diglycerides	1	30	254536	
Monosodium phosphate derivatives of monoglycerides	1	30	254536	
Naringin	5	11–3	82192931	Not available

Nitrogen	1	112	80112022	Not available; helium gas is listed for this PB#
Nitrous oxide	1	112	80112022	Not available; helium gas is listed for this PB#
Oat gum	5	11–23	82192930	Not available
Oiticica oil	5	11–16	81239409	Not available
Okra gum	5	11–23	82192930	Not available
Oxystearins	3	30	254536	Listed as glycerin and glycerides
Peptones (beef tissue, casein, defatted fatty tissue, gelatin, soy meal, soy protein concentration, soy protein isolate)	1	11–17	82155466	Not available
Potassium bisulfite	2	15	265508	Listed as potassium metabisulfite
Potassium sulfate	1	33	262652	Listed as sulfuric acid
Propane	1	112	80112022	Not available; helium gas is listed for this PB#
Psyllium seed husk gum	1	11–23	82192930	Not available
Pyroligneous acid	5	11–7	82160359	Not available
Quince seed gum	5	11–23	82192930	Not available
Regenerated cellulose	1	25	274667	Listed as cellulose
Shellac	5	11–19	82160383	Not available
Shellac wax	5	11–19	82160383	Not available
Smoke flavoring, aqueous condensates	3	11–7	82160359	Not available
Smoke flavoring, aqueous extracts	3	11–7	82160359	Not available
Smoke flavoring, aqueous emulsifier extract of vegetable oil extract	5	11–7	82160359	Not available
Smoke yeast flavoring	5	11–7	82160359	Not available
Sodium salts of aminotris (methylene-phosphonic) acid (packaging)	5	11–1	82107087	Not available

Continued

Table 3 Substances reviewed by the select committee not in US FDA database—cont'd

Ingredient	Conclusion	SCOGS report #	PB No.	Listing on US FDA database?
Sodium sulfate	1	33	262652	Listed as sulfuric acid
Sodium zinc metasilicate	5	11–20	82160367	Not available
Stearyl alcohol	1	11–22	81118424	Not available
Sulfoacetate derivatives of diglycerides	1	30	254536	Listed as glycerin and glycerides
Sulfoacetate derivatives of monoglycerides	1	30	254536	
Triacetin	1	30	254536	
Wheat gluten	1	11–12	82155482	Not available
Zein	1	11–12	82155482	Not available

recommendations considered GRAS policy and technical perspectives as it relates to the conduct of the safety evaluations (Senti, 1983; US FDA, 2018c).

From a policy perspective, the Select Committee suggested that the GRAS List be phased out and that a single system for the evaluation of food ingredients be used. The basis for this conclusion was that the GRAS approach, although pragmatic for its purpose at the time, did not have a scientific basis by which to maintain GRAS substances and food additives independent of each other. They also suggested that these terms may cause confusion and that all but a few substances (e.g., sucrose, corn starch, and gelatin) should be designated as GRAS food additives going forward. As many of the GRAS substances that were evaluated would meet the criteria for clearance as food additives, significant limitations in taking this step were not identified. However, the Select Committee considered the implications of the Delaney Clause on the movement away from the use of the GRAS approach. The Delaney Clause is a provision added within the 1958 Food Additives Amendment that prohibits the regulation of a food additive deemed to be unsafe, where "…it is found to induce cancer when ingested by man or animal, or if it is found, after tests which are appropriate for the evaluation of the safety of food additives, to induce cancer in man or animal…" (21 USC 348(c)(3)(a)). By definition, a GRAS substance is exempt from regulation as a food additive and therefore the Delaney Clause does not apply (21 USC 321(s)). The Select Committee, therefore, recommended that the Delaney Clause be modified to allow for scientific interpretation of safety data by qualified experts and to eliminate prescriptive legislation of safety that is scientifically counterproductive to the assurance of food safety. The Delaney Clause is implied by the Select Committee to be an example of "…political judgments [that] have been invoked, not for the purposes of overall risk/benefit determination, but as a substitute for specific scientific assessment of health risk." (For further information on the state of the science associated with carcinogenicity risk assessment and evidence that suggests in some cases that tumors observed in animals may not be relevant to human cancer risk, the reader is directed to a 2021 Toxicology Forum workshop summarized by Felter et al., 2022.)

From a technical perspective, the Select Committee identified six key areas for the supporting data of a GRAS evaluation needing special attention (SCOGS, 1982) including:

(1) Substance identification: The committee recommended that complete characterization and specification data be provided and that specifications include toxicologically relevant substances such as heavy

metals and cyclic hydrocarbons. Without an appropriate specification, there is no assurance that the food ingredient is the same as that represented in the toxicological evidence. Deficiencies were noted for some substances especially complex natural products such as gums, waxes, and algae, and mixtures obtained through fermentation. It was recommended that the source materials and production steps, range of physical characteristics, and chemical components be provided for the end product to further support any available characterization data.

(2) Consumer exposure data: Rough estimates of consumer exposure were generally available, but significant improvements in the safety evaluation may be made with more detailed information. Suggested improvements included obtaining the total amount of a food substance added to food and the per capita disappearance data in use, consumption data for at-risk subpopulations known to consume an ingredient, the extent of exposure to ingredient reaction products in food, and the migration information on additives used in packaging materials.

(3) Efficacy of food substances: although efficacy data were and are a requirement of food additive petitions per 21 CFR 170.3, many of the GRAS substances reviewed by the Select Committee did not have available efficacy data. It was suggested that efficacy data be required for GRAS substances.

(4) Human data: The committee recommended that controlled evaluation in human subjects of substances added to human food should be conducted and in a tiered manner with the initial support of animal testing.

(5) Behavioral tests: It was recommended that behavioral endpoints be further developed in animal testing to account for this less well-developed area of toxicology, but one of particular interest for human safety.

(6) Hypersensitivity: Due to the risks of anaphylactic reactions to ingredients in foods and the general paucity of methodology to adequately investigate this endpoint, it was recommended that anaphylaxis induction tests in animals be extended and additional techniques for evaluating hypersensitivity endpoints be explored.

GRAS proposed rule

Although the GRAS affirmation procedure outlined in 21 CFR Part 170.35 had served its purpose for the reevaluation of GRAS substances from 1974 to 1990, industry GRAS affirmation requests submitted after 1990 were taking extended time periods to complete. More than 12 submissions were identified as taking more than 72 months: an untenable timeline for the US FDA and a deterrent to industry to petition the US FDA on GRAS (US FDA, 2018a). The extensive timeline was, in part, because a GRAS affirmation petition required the lengthy process of rulemaking, including: (1) publishing a notice of the filing in the Federal Register, followed by (2) a comment period for the petitioned request. Then, (3) a comprehensive review of the data and the comments received as part of the filing notice would be conducted by the US FDA to establish that the petitioned use is GRAS; and (4) a detailed explanation developed by the US FDA for the basis of GRAS was required. Finally, (5) this explanation had to be published in the Federal Register (62 FR 18938, 1997).

To use US FDA resources more efficiently and to inspire industry to notify US FDA of their self-affirmations of GRAS, a GRAS notification procedure was proposed to replace the GRAS affirmation process (62 FR 18938, 1997; US FDA, 2018a). Under the notification procedure, the notifying party would conduct the GRAS assessment and submit the notice of the GRAS conclusion to the US FDA. The US FDA would then review the notice (within 90 days) to determine whether they agree that there is sufficient basis for GRAS and that no other data that the US FDA is aware of may raise any issue that the ingredient may not be GRAS for the notified intended use. However, US FDA would not "…conduct a detailed evaluation of the data that the notifier relies on to support a determination that a use of a substance is GRAS or to affirm that a substance is GRAS for its intended use…" (62 FR 18938, 1997). The US FDA would respond to the notifications in one of three ways: (1) "FDA has no questions"; (2) "The notice does not provide a basis for a conclusion of GRAS"; and (3) "At the notifier's request, FDA ceased to evaluate the notice."

The US FDA invited parties to submit notifications prior to the finalization of the proposed rule in what was referred to as an "interim period" that was intended to identify any modifications that were needed to the notification process. This interim period lasted until 2010 when the GRAS comments to the proposed rule were reopened (75 FR 81536, 2010) and continued until the rule was finalized in 2016 (81 FR 54960, 2016). During that time, more than 600 GRAS notifications were submitted to the US FDA with an average response time of ~200 days (Hanlon et al., 2017). More than 80% of the US FDA responses resulted in "no questions," ~17% were withdrawn, and only ~3% were concluded to have "no basis" for a conclusion of GRAS (Hanlon et al., 2017).

In the notice of proposed rulemaking for GRAS, the US FDA identified a series of benefits to both the public and industry in the implementation of the GRAS notification program (62 FR 18938, 1997). These included:

(1) The notification procedure would eliminate the extensive rulemaking process allowing the US FDA to direct its resources to issues of GRAS deemed to be a priority to the protection of public health.

(2) The procedure was more straightforward for industry and would be an incentive to notify the US FDA of their GRAS determinations.

(3) With an increase in industry GRAS notifications, the US FDA would have a better understanding of the occurrence of GRAS substances in the food supply and subsequently a more accurate picture of the cumulative dietary exposure to these substances.

(4) Public health would be better served if the US FDA were able to devote more time to developing industry guidance documents on key food safety issues.

(5) Resources would be more readily available to review food and color additive petitions.

However, the US FDA also reiterated that a manufacturer may legally market a GRAS substance added to food without informing the agency.

As a 90-day timeframe for a response to a GRAS notification was proposed by the US FDA, standardization and consistency in submissions to the agency were considered critical.

As such, the proposed rule included clarity around the expected components to be included in a GRAS notification. These are summarized as follows in Table 4. The inventory for GRAS Notices filed to the US FDA, since 1998, is publicly available and may be found at www.fda.gov/food/generally-recognized-safe-gras/gras-notice-inventory. Included within the inventory are the name and address of the notifier, the GRAS ingredient, the intended conditions of use, the GRAS Notice file no., date of submission, and links to supporting documents including the US FDA response letter and the GRAS notification document as submitted.

US FDA guidance documents to support safety evaluations

As the regulatory framework for the safety of food ingredients does not provide detailed technical guidance to conduct comprehensive safety evaluations to the US FDA expectations, the US FDA has published numerous guidance documents to provide their interpretation of the most appropriate approach to develop and interpret data to support a food ingredient safety

Table 4 Components of a GRAS notification per the 1997 proposed rule.

Component	Description
GRAS exemption claim	This is to be a letter with a statement that the substance is exempt from premarket approval by the US FDA as the intended use of the substance had been determined to be GRAS. The letter would include the notifier name and address, the common or usual name of the substance, the conditions of use including the food types, levels of use and purpose, the intended target population for consumption, the basis for the GRAS determination (common use or scientific procedures), a statement that the data that provide the basis for GRAS are available upon request by the agency, and the letter should be dated and signed by the notifier
Identity and specifications	Detailed information about the substance identity should be provided and would include, as applicable: the Chemical Abstracts Service (CAS) registry no., Enzyme Commission (EC) number, empirical formula, structural formula, quantitative composition, method of manufacture (excluding trade secret information), characteristic properties, any potential human toxicants, and the food grade specification
Self-limiting levels of use	Where applicable, the level of a substance that would render the food unpalatable, unappealing, or otherwise unfit for consumption should be provided
Scientific procedures data	The data to support a conclusion of GRAS based on scientific procedures may be variable but, in general, includes the identity, characteristic properties, methods of manufacture, toxicological studies, and information on dietary exposure
Technical evidence of safety (scientific procedures)	This is a detailed summary of the basis for the determination of GRAS and should include a comprehensive discussion with references to the generally available and accepted scientific data, information, methods, or principles that the notifier relies on to establish safety. This should include the probable level of consumption in the diet and the effects of cumulative exposure considering other known uses, and a summary of any data that may be inconsistent with the conclusion of GRAS. Also to be included in the summary should be a statement regarding the basis for concluding expert consensus that the substance is GRAS for the intended use and that the data present a reasonable certainty of no harm. This may be established through supporting data, i.e., the evidence suggests there are no safety concerns that experts would need to resolve. It may also be based on the opinion of safe use from a specially convened expert panel or an authoritative body, such as the National Academy of Sciences

Continued

Table 4 Components of a GRAS notification per the 1997 proposed rule—cont'd

Component	Description
Common use data	These data should provide evidence for a substantial history of consumption for a significant number of consumers. Technical data that would support GRAS based on scientific procedures may also be relevant and included, as applicable
Technical evidence of safety (common use)	This is a detailed summary of the basis for the determination of GRAS and should include a comprehensive discussion with references to the generally available and accepted data supporting common use in food. In addition, the summary should include technical data, and any data and a discussion of that data that may be inconsistent with a conclusion on GRAS. Further, a discussion on whether the use in food was widespread enough such that any adverse effects would have been observed and recorded, and finally, a summary regarding the basis of expert consensus that the substance is GRAS for the intended use and presents a reasonable certainty of no harm

evaluation. As the technical component of a GRAS evaluation is consistent with the quantity and quality of a food additive petition, these guidance documents are relevant for both regulatory paradigms and others, such as color additives, that are not included in the scope of this chapter. "Toxicological Principles for the Safety Assessment of Food Ingredients," now known as the "Redbook 2000, or Redbook I," was originally published in 1982 (US FDA, 2019). It was intended to provide guidance to notifiers regarding the need for toxicological studies; how to design, conduct, and report toxicology studies; how to conduct statistical analysis of data; how to review histological data; and direction on the submission of these data to the US FDA. A draft revision to the Redbook was published by US FDA in 1993 as notified through the Federal Register (58 FR 16536, 1993) and became known as "Redbook II" (US FDA, 2019). In 2006, the US FDA issued an additional guidance document titled, "Guidance for Industry: Summary Table of Recommended Toxicological Testing for Additives Used in Food" that provided a summary of the minimum toxicological testing recommendations based on the cumulative concentration of the substance in the diet (from all uses) and the concern level for that substance. The concern level is identified as A, B, or C and is based on the toxicological potential of the substance predicted from its chemical structure (US FDA, 2006a).

An equally important component of a food ingredient safety evaluation is the estimation of dietary intake. Two key components are included: (1) the estimated dietary intake from the notified use of the GRAS substance and (2) the estimated data intake from all dietary uses or the cumulative dietary intake. To support this evaluation, in 2006, the US FDA published a guidance document titled, "Guidance for Industry: Estimating Dietary Intake of Substances in Food" (US FDA, 2006b). This guidance document provides detailed information on the scope of the dietary intake that should be considered (e.g., impurities in addition to the GRAS substance), sources of food consumption data, and methods for estimation of probable intake. An additional guidance document that also provides some information on intake, but primarily focuses on chemical identity, purity, and related data, was also published and is titled, "Guidance for Industry: Recommendations for Submission of Chemical and Technological Data for Direct Food Additive Petitions" (US FDA, 2009). Although the 2009 guidance document was written in the context of direct food additive petitions, much of the information also applies to GRAS.

Guidance documents specific to the GRAS regulatory framework are also available including a document recently published titled, "Guidance for Industry: Regulatory Framework for Substances Intended for Use in Human Food or Animal Food on the Basis of the Generally Recognized as Safe (GRAS) Provision of the Federal Food, Drug, and Cosmetic Act" that provides direction on how to navigate the GRAS framework (US FDA, 2017b). A frequently asked questions guidance on GRAS is also available that provides answers to common questions on the regulatory process and other regulatory considerations regarding GRAS (US FDA, 2016).

One way to establish consensus for the designation of an ingredient as GRAS for its intended use is for the notifier to convene a GRAS panel of experts that are qualified by training and experience to evaluate the safety of food ingredients. The conduct of a GRAS panel sponsored by industry has been a topic of debate, where the panel is to remain independent, nonbias, without conflicts of interest, such that a scientifically defensible conclusion of GRAS may be established. Recognizing this issue, the US FDA published a draft guidance document in November 2017 that provides their thinking on the best practice approach for convening a GRAS panel (US FDA, 2017a). This guidance provides advice on how to prevent bias, how to create a balance of expertise as relevant for the food ingredient, how to organize and manage the deliberation of the panel, and how to reduce conflicts of interest and appearance issues.

This summary provides a limited scope of the available guidance documents issued by the US FDA. However, the reader is directed to the US FDA website that lists all available guidance documents relevant to the food topic that may be found here: https://www.fda.gov/food/guidance-regulation-food-and-dietary-supplements.

Challenges to GRAS

In practice, the GRAS exemption from premarket approval of a food ingredient is a regulatory paradigm that is unique to the United States with no other known international parallel. Not unexpectedly, the GRAS exemption has been met with harsh criticism as notification to the US FDA of a new GRAS ingredient or the expanded use of an existing GRAS ingredient in food is recommended but not required. Although self-affirmations of GRAS are expected to be conducted with the same scientific rigor as any GRAS notification made to the US FDA, critics contest that there are significant risks of bias in a safety assessment of an ingredient sponsored and potentially even prepared by industry. Allegations of the "fox guarding the chicken coop" and self-affirmations referred to as "Generally Recognized as Secret" have been reported (Hallagan and Hall, 2009; Neltner et al., 2014; Wenner, 2008). In addition, part of the GRAS process includes the estimation of the cumulative dietary exposure of an ingredient to be sure that levels in food from all possible use applications do not exceed a safe level. Assessment of cumulative exposure is difficult where there is not visibility to those ingredients that have been designated as GRAS based on self-affirmation (Faustman et al., 2021). Finally, the GRAS notification process was proposed in the Federal Register in 1997 (62 FR 18938, 1997) and the comment period for the proposed rule for GRAS notification was re-opened in 2010 (75 FR 81536, 2010), which raised significant concern that the process was not promulgated and therefore incomplete, yet industry had been operating within the proposed rule since 1997. As the result of a lawsuit filed in 2014 against the US FDA by the Center for Food Safety, the GRAS Notification Proposed Rule was finalized in 2016. Significant lawsuits associated with GRAS against the US FDA are summarized in Table 5.

In 2010, the US Government Accountability Office (GAO) issued a report to Congress that the US FDA should strengthen its oversight of food ingredients determined to be generally recognized as safe (GAO, 2010). In the report, the GAO, based on a rigorous review of the GRAS program, alleged that the US FDA does not have full oversight of all GRAS

Table 5 Significant lawsuits filed against the US FDA regarding GRAS.

Date	Defendant	Allegation
2/20/2014	Center for Food Safety (n.d.)	It is unlawful for FDA to exempt ingredients added to food under a proposed rule. Alleged examples of the failure of the GRAS proposed rule include volatile of mustard (its primary constituent allyl isothiocyanate was later identified as a potential human carcinogen), Olestra (caused anal leakage, severe diarrhea, and other GI distress), and Quorn (caused severe allergic reaction). *Court decision*: US FDA entered into a consent decree with the Center for Food Safety that called for the US FDA to submit a final rule for the GRAS notification process by August 31, 2016
5/22/2017	Center for Food Safety et al. (n.d.)	The GRAS final rule (81 FR 54960, 2016) allows potentially unsafe food additives to be used in the food supply. Self-affirmations of GRAS remain entirely secret from the FDA and the public, abdicating FDA's responsibility to protect the food supply and eliminating the opportunity to conduct an accurate assessment of the cumulative effect of an ingredient in food. The GRAS exemption does not prohibit the self-certification of a carcinogen as GRAS. *Court decision*: On September 30, 2021, the Southern District Court of New York denied the motion of a summary judgment by the Center for Food Safety et al. and supported the legality of the GRAS Framework

determinations and thus does not have full oversight of the safety of the food supply where GRAS determinations have not been notified to the US FDA. In addition, it was recognized, at the time, that sufficient guidance had not been provided to industry in how to appropriately document GRAS conclusions, and no monitoring of industry self-affirmations of GRAS by the US FDA was identified by the GAO. Further, they recognized the credibility issue presented by operating under a proposed rule that was published in 1997. The GAO also alleged that US FDA has not enacted a systematic reevaluation of substances determined to be GRAS since the SCOGS review was completed in the early 1980s, although reference to the regulation, 21 CFR Part 170.30(l), requires a reassessment of new data to maintain

GRAS status. Lastly, they recognized the potential for nanomaterials to be in the food supply as GRAS with a lack of US FDA oversight. This report likely prompted the reopening of the GRAS proposed rule for comment in December 2010.

Faustman et al. (2021) reported on the status of the 2010 recommendations, summarizing the six primary recommendations of the GAO report as follows:

1. To develop a strategy to require companies to provide FDA with basic information about GRAS substances, e.g., identity and intended uses, which would be publicly accessible
2. To develop a strategy to minimize the potential for conflicts of interest in companies' GRAS determinations
3. To develop a strategy to monitor the appropriateness of companies' GRAS determinations through random audits or some other means, including issuing guidance on how to document GRAS determinations
4. To develop a strategy to finalize the rule that governs the voluntary notification program
5. To develop a strategy to conduct reconsiderations of the safety of GRAS substances in a more systematic manner
6. To develop a strategy to help ensure the safety of engineered nanomaterials that companies market as GRAS substances without the agency's knowledge.

In review of the status of these primary recommendations from the GAO, Faustman et al. (2021) reported that recommendations 3, 4, and 6 have been adequately addressed and draft guidance for best practices in convening a GRAS panel, which would address recommendation 2, was published in 2017. Recommendations 1 and 5 remain unaddressed to date.

Presumably inspired by the GAO report, nongovernmental organizations including the Pew Charitable Trusts and the Natural Resources Defense Council (NRDC) began to conduct their own investigations of the self-affirmations of GRAS sponsored by industry (Hallagan et al., 2020). Neltner et al. (2014) investigated the likely occurrence of substances self-affirmed as GRAS without disclosure to the US FDA. The investigation included a review of publicly available literature claiming GRAS status to identify candidate chemicals and a follow-up to individual manufacturers requesting additional information that would support the GRAS basis. In total, 56 companies were included and an estimated 275 chemicals having GRAS status by self-affirmation were identified. Many of the manufacturers did not respond to requests for additional information and therefore these numbers may not present an accurate picture of the scope of current industry self-affirmations with some reports that the actual number is closer to 1000. The Pew Charitable Trusts also conducted an assessment of the GRAS program within a multistakeholder approach that included industry, the public interest community, and government. Detailed reports of this assessment were provided in the published literature and summarized in a 2013 article (The Pew Charitable Trusts, 2013). They reported that with more than 10,000 additives estimated to be used in foods, observing health effects from any one additive would be extremely difficult unless the nature of the health effect was immediate and severe. Further, they suggest that the US FDA would have to prove harm before the substance could be restricted in the food supply. In addition, they suggest that the law does not currently give the US FDA the authority to obtain the information necessary to identify chemicals of concern and they lack visibility to the additives in the supply chain in order to effectively fulfill their mission to protect public health by ensuring all food additives are safe.

Despite the challenges, the GRAS process, including self-affirmations of GRAS, remains well supported by the US FDA. This support is based on the clear guidance provided by the US FDA through the GRAS proposed and final rules for the conduct of the GRAS assessments, the recommendation to engage a panel of experts to confirm consensus for safe use, and the additional guidance documents provided by the US FDA that further describe data requirements. There is also a recognition that the former absence of the GRAS program was a significant barrier to innovation in industry with food additive petitions to the US FDA taking upwards of 6 years to complete. In addition, expending precious FDA resources to evaluate the safety of ingredients well recognized to be safe is not considered value added, given the breadth of ingredients and contaminants raising food safety concerns of which US FDA resources are often focused. Although self-affirmations of GRAS remain a legal basis by which to establish safe use of a food ingredient, the US FDA continues to encourage manufacturers to notify them of conclusions on GRAS status.

GRAS final rule

The final GRAS notification rule was published in the Federal Register on August 17, 2016 (81 FR 54960, 2016) and codified within 21 CFR Parts 170.203–170.285. The rule eliminated the GRAS affirmation process

(21 CFR Part 170.35) and formally implemented the GRAS notification program at the US FDA effective October 17, 2016. In the text of the rule, the US FDA clarified the criteria for eligibility for a substance to be classified as GRAS and established new administrative procedures for notification. Components of a GRAS notification were clearly divided into seven unique sections. The following summarizes each section's requirements and expectations in alignment with the guidance provided within the final GRAS Rule and codified within 21 CFR as cited.

Component of a GRAS notification per the GRAS final rule: Part I—Signed statements and certification (21 CFR §170.225)

- name and address of the organization;
- name, signature, and position of the person(s), attorney(s), or agent(s) signing the GRAS notice;
- name of the notified substance (using an appropriately descriptive term, not the trade or proprietary name), the intended conditions of use (include food(s), level(s), purpose), and any information related to the subpopulation to be exposed, where applicable;
- statutory basis for the GRAS conclusion (scientific procedures in accordance with 21 CFR §170.30(a) and (b) or common use in food in accordance with 21 CFR §170.30(a) and (c)); and
- required statements:
  - informational statement on submission of a GRAS notice consistent with subpart E, that is to your knowledge to be complete, representative, and balanced (including unfavorable information);
  - view that the notified substance is not subject to premarket approval requirements of the FD&C Act based on the conclusion of GRAS;
  - view on whether data or information in Parts 2–7 are exempt from disclosure under FOIA (Confidential business information), and whether this information shall be shared with FSIS, where applicable; and
  - agreement that FDA has authority to access data and information during customary business hours, upon request.

Note: This section should not include information that is considered trade secret or confidential business information.

Part II—Identity, method of manufacture, specifications, and physical and technical effect (21 CFR §170.230)

- substance identity—use an appropriately descriptive term for the GRAS substance, not common name:

  – provide supporting data that identifies the substance and any known toxicants that may be present; and
  – biological origin: include genus, species, subspecies (variety or strain or both), source (plant or animal part).
  – include food grade specifications;
- provide the method of manufacture in sufficient detail to determine safety; and
- provide supportive data regarding the intended physical or technical effect in the food and the levels at which the effect is produced.

Part III—Dietary exposure (21 CFR §170.235)
- identify the amount of the GRAS substance that consumers are expected to ingest as part of the total diet:
  – exposure from intended use
  – exposure from all sources in the diet; and
  – provide the source of the food consumption data that is used.
- identify any substance that is expected to be formed in or on food due to use of the GRAS substance;
- identify any contaminant that is expected to be present naturally or due to the manufacture of the GRAS substance; and
- provide any assumptions that were used to estimate dietary exposure.

Part IV—Self-limiting levels of use (21 CFR §170.240)
- provide data or other information to support self-limited use, where the GRAS substance is limited in use by technical practicality or organoleptic properties; and
- if the use of the substance is not self-limited, provide a statement in this part to this effect.

Part V—Common use in food before 1958 (21 CFR §170.245)
- include the basis and supporting data and information for common use in food prior to 1958.

Part VI—GRAS narrative (21 CFR §170.250)
- provide a basis that the GRAS substance is safe under the intended conditions of use:
  – consider the subject use and all dietary sources; and
  – consider any chemically or physically related substance in the diet.
- provide a summary of the generally available data and other data cited from Part 7 of the notification;
- provide an interpretation of the data (including any unfavorable data) that explains why a conclusion of GRAS for the notified substance relative to the estimated exposure was determined;

- provide an explanation as to how a basis for GRAS was achieved without access to nonpublic safety-related data and information shall be included; and
- per a favorable conclusion, state that the substance is generally recognized, among qualified experts, to be safe under the conditions of its intended use:
- identify any data that is exempt from disclosure under FOIA.

Part VII—Supporting data and information

- list of all data and information that was used and referenced in Parts 5 and 6 of the GRAS notification; and
- specify in the list which data are generally available and which are not generally available.

Future directions of GRAS status

The regulatory framework for GRAS, although unique and perhaps not without issues, is a paradigm that is unlikely to be repealed in the near future. It continues to be supported by the US FDA and remains a lawful method for evaluating the safety of food ingredients in the United States based on the favorable outcomes of recent lawsuits challenging its legality (Center for Food Safety et al., n.d.). In addition, the US FDA continues to advise industry to notify them of their GRAS determinations. As many self-affirmations of GRAS remain industry trade secret, efforts to improve the US FDA oversight of self-affirmations of GRAS and the methods to establish the GRAS status of a substance in food are expected to continue. One recent initiative is the Toxic Free Foods Act of 2021, a partisan bill sponsored by Representative Rosa DeLauro (D-CT-03). This bill would require the US FDA to publish a revision to the GRAS final rule requiring an ingredient manufacturer to notify the US FDA of a GRAS determination. It would also require that each GRAS determination and the supporting information be made public. The bill would place additional restrictions on what substances are eligible for consideration as GRAS.

In September 2014, the food industry initiated an effort to develop an auditable standard for the conduct of a GRAS determination. This effort was sponsored by the Grocery Manufacturers Association, now the Consumer Brands Association, and led by NSF International, a standards development body that operates as an independent, global, not-for-profit organization with a long, rich history of protecting public health. At the time, the initiative was to develop a science-based framework that defines the content and conduct of GRAS determinations of food ingredients that will meet the regulatory requirements under sections 201(s) and 409 of the Food, Drug, and Cosmetic Act, and implementing regulations in 21 CFR 170.3 and 21 CFR 170.30 and in accordance with the GMA GRAS Code of Practice. The GRAS publicly available specification (PAS) was meant as a tool, especially for those self-determinations of GRAS not notified to the US FDA, to ensure that consistent, robust, and sound GRAS assessments and conclusions are conducted across the industry to provide further confidence that food is safe for consumers (further background on the impetus of this standard may be found in Hartung (2018)). Importantly, the GRAS PAS was not intended to supplant or supersede the FDA's GRAS regulations or Notification Program, but as a tool intended to complement the FDA's regulations and guidance documents. The intention of the collaboration was to form a consensus body in accordance with NSF International standards development procedures which requires a balanced committee of experts across academia, industry, consumer and other advocacy groups, regulators, and other interested organizations to develop the GRAS PAS standard. The GRAS PAS remains in development as of January 2022.

References

23 FR 9511, 1958. 23 Federal Register 9511: Proposed Rule Making: Food Additives.

24 FR 9368, 1959. 24 Federal register 9368: rules and regulations: chapter I— food and drug administration. In: Subchapter B— Food and Food Products. PART 121— Food Additives. Subpart B— Exemption of Certain Food Additives from the Requirement of Tolerances. Substances Generally Recognized as Safe. Department of Health, Education, and Welfare.

35 FR 5810, 1970. 35 Federal Register 5810: Rules and Regulations; Subpart A—Definitions and Procedural and Interpretative Regulations Food Additive Status Opinion Letters; Statement of Policy.

37 FR 25705, 1972. 37 Federal Register 25705: Rules and Regulations Food Additives; GRAS and Food Additive Status Procedures.

37 FR 6207, 1972. 37 Federal Register 6207: Proposed Rule Making GRAS and Food Additive Status; Procedures for Affirmation and Determination.

53 FR 16544, 1988. 53 Federal Register 16544: Rules and Regulations. Eligibility for Classification of Food Substances as Generally Recognized as Safe. Final Rule.

57 FR 22984, 1992. 57 Federal Register 22984: Notices. Statement of Policy: Foods Derived From New Plant Varieties.

58 FR 16536, 1993. 58 Federal Register 16536: Draft Revised "Toxicological Principles for the Safety Assessment of Direct Food Additives and Color Additives Used in Food"; Availability. https://www.govinfo.gov/content/pkg/FR-1993-03-29/pdf/FR-1993-03-29.pdf.

62 FR 18938, 1997. 62 Federal Register 18938: Proposed Rules: Substances Generally Recognized as Safe.

75 FR 81536, 2010. 75 Federal Register 81536. Proposed Rules: Substances Generally Recognized as Safe; Reopening of the Comment Period.

81 FR 54960, 2016. 81 Federal Register 54960. Rules and Regulations. Substances Generally Recognized as Safe. Final Rule.

Burdock, G.A., Carabin, I.G., 2004. Generally recognized as safe (GRAS): history and description. Toxicol. Lett. 150, 3–18. https://doi.org/10.1016/j.toxlet.2003.07.004.

Center for Food Safety, n.d. Center For Food Safety v US FDA. Case No. 1:14-cv-267. Filed February 20, 2014.

Center for Food Safety, Earthjustice, Stella, C.R., Tomaselli, P.M., Gartner, E.C., Lehner, P., n.d. Center for Food Safety, Breast Cancer Prevention Partners, Center for Science in the Public Interest, Environmental Defense Fund, and Environmental Working Group v. US FDA. Case No. 1:17-cv-03833. Filed May 22, 2017.

Cohen, S.M., Eisenbrand, G., Fukushima, S., Gooderham, N.J., Guengerich, F.P., Hecht, S.S., Rietjens, I.M.C.M., Davidsen, J.M., Harman, C.L., Taylor, S.V., 2018. Updated procedure for the safety evaluation of natural flavor complexes used as ingredients in food. Food Chem. Toxicol. 113, 171–178. https://doi.org/10.1016/j.fct.2018.01.021.

EFSA, 2021. Food Additives. EFSA. [WWW Document]. URL https://www.efsa.europa.eu/en/topics/topic/food-additives. (Accessed 29 January 2022).

Faustman, C., Aaron, D., Negowetti, N., Leib, E.B., 2021. Ten years post-GAO assessment, FDA remains uninformed of potentially harmful GRAS substances in foods. Crit. Rev. Food Sci. Nutr. 61, 1260–1268. https://doi.org/10.1080/10408398.2020.1756217.

Felter, S.P., Bhat, V.S., Botham, P.A., Bussard, D.A., Casey, W., Hayes, A.W., Hilton, G.M., Magurany, K.A., Sauer, U.G., Ohanian, E.V., 2022. Assessing chemical carcinogenicity: hazard identification, classification, and risk assessment. Insight from a Toxicology Forum state-of-the-science workshop. Crit. Rev. Toxicol., 1–42. https://doi.org/10.1080/10408444.2021.2003295.

FEMA, 2022. About FEMA GRAS Program. FEMA. [WWW Document]. URL https://www.femaflavor.org/gras. (Accessed 22 January 2022).

Fisher, K.D., 1982. A successful peer review program for regulatory decisions. Regul. Toxicol. Pharmacol. 2, 331–334. https://doi.org/10.1016/0273-2300(82)90006-X.

GAO, U.S.G.A, 2010. Food Safety: FDA Should Strengthen Its Oversight of Food Ingredients Determined to Be Generally Recognized as Safe (GRAS). [WWW Document]. URL https://www.gao.gov/products/gao-10-246. (Accessed 7 January 2022).

Gerarde, H.W., 1973. Survey update: determining safety for flavor chemicals. Food Prod. Dev. 7, 82–85.

H.R. 13254, 1958. Food Additives Amendment of 1958. Public Law 85–929. 72 Stat. 1784.

Hall, R.L., Oser, B.L., 1965. The safety of flavoring substances. In: Gunther, F.A. (Ed.), Residue Reviews/Rückstands-Berichte. Springer New York, New York, NY, pp. 1–17, https://doi.org/10.1007/978-1-4615-8440-7_1.

Hallagan, J.B., Hall, R.L., 1995. FEMA GRAS—a GRAS assessment program for flavor ingredients. Flavor and Extract Manufacturers Association. Regul. Toxicol. Pharmacol. 21, 422–430. https://doi.org/10.1006/rtph.1995.1057.

Hallagan, J.B., Hall, R.L., 2009. Under the conditions of intended use—new developments in the FEMA GRAS program and the safety assessment of flavor ingredients. Food Chem. Toxicol. 47, 267–278. https://doi.org/10.1016/j.fct.2008.11.011.

Hallagan, J.B., Hall, R.L., Drake, J., 2020. The GRAS provision—the FEMA GRAS program and the safety and regulation of flavors in the United States. Food Chem. Toxicol. 138, 111236. https://doi.org/10.1016/j.fct.2020.111236.

Hanlon, P.R., Frestedt, J., Magurany, K., 2017. GRAS from the ground up: review of the Interim Pilot Program for GRAS notification. Food Chem. Toxicol. 105, 140–150. https://doi.org/10.1016/j.fct.2017.03.064.

Hartung, T., 2018. Rebooting the generally recognized as safe (GRAS) approach for food additive safety in the US. ALTEX, 3–25. https://doi.org/10.14573/altex.1712181.

JECFA, 2020. Principles and Methods for the Risk Assessment of Chemicals in Food. [WWW Document]. URL https://www.who.int/publications-detail-redirect/9789241572408. (Accessed 29 January 2022).

Neltner, T., NRDC, Maffini, M., 2014. Generally Recognized as Secret: Chemicals Added to Food in the United States 14.

NTIS, 2017. NTIS | Home. [WWW Document]. URL https://www.ntis.gov/. (Accessed 13 January 2022).

Oser, B.L., Ford, R.A., 1977. Recent progress in the consideration of flavoring ingredients under the food additives amendment 10. GRAS substances. Food Technol., 65–74.

SCOGS, 1982. Insights on Food Safety Evaluation. FDA Report No. FDA/BF-83/1S. National Technical Information Service.

Senti, F.R., 1983. Insights on food safety evaluation: a synopsis. Regul. Toxicol. Pharmacol. 3, 133–138. https://doi.org/10.1016/0273-2300(83)90037-5.

Siu, R.G., Borzelleca, J.F., Carr, C.J., Day, H.G., Fomon, S.J., Irving, G.W., La Du, B.N., McCoy, J.R., Miller, S.A., Plaa, G.L., Shimkin, M.B., Wood, J.L., 1977. Evaluation of health aspects of GRAS food ingredients: lessons learned and questions unanswered. Fed. Proc. 36, 2519–2562.

Smith, R., 2004. Safety evaluation of natural flavour complexes. Toxicol. Lett. 149, 197–207. https://doi.org/10.1016/j.toxlet.2003.12.031.

Smith, R.L., Cohen, S.M., Doull, J., Feron, V.J., Goodman, J.I., Marnett, L.J., Munro, I.C., Portoghese, P.S., Waddell, W.J., Wagner, B.M., Adams, T.B., 2005a. Criteria for the safety evaluation of flavoring substances. Food Chem. Toxicol. 43, 1141–1177. https://doi.org/10.1016/j.fct.2004.11.012.

Smith, R.L., Cohen, S.M., Doull, J., Feron, V.J., Goodman, J.I., Marnett, L.J., Portoghese, P.S., Waddell, W.J., Wagner, B.M., Hall, R.L., Higley, N.A., Lucas-Gavin, C., Adams, T.B., 2005b. A procedure for the safety evaluation of natural flavor complexes used as ingredients in food: essential oils. Food Chem. Toxicol. 43, 345–363. https://doi.org/10.1016/j.fct.2004.11.007.

The Pew Charitable Trusts, 2013. Fixing the Oversight of Chemicals Added to Our Food. [WWW Document]. URL http://pew.org/2yJXHbu. (Accessed 7 January 2022).

US FDA, 2006a. Guidance for Industry: Summary Table of Recommended Toxicological Testing for Additives Used in Food. US Food Drug Adm. [WWW Document]. URL https://www.fda.gov/regulatory-information/search-fda-guidance-documents/guidance-industry-summary-table-recommended-toxicological-testing-additives-used-food. (Accessed 7 January 2022).

US FDA, 2006b. Guidance for Industry: Estimating Dietary Intake of Substances in Food. US Food Drug Adm. [WWW Document]. URL https://www.fda.gov/regulatory-information/search-fda-guidance-documents/guidance-industry-estimating-dietary-intake-substances-food. (Accessed 7 January 2022).

US FDA, 2009. Guidance for Industry: Recommendations for Submission of Chemical and Technological Data for Direct Food Additive Petitions. US Food Drug Adm. [WWW Document]. URL https://www.fda.gov/regulatory-information/search-fda-guidance-documents/guidance-industry-recommendations-submission-chemical-and-technological-data-direct-food-additive. (Accessed 7 January 2022).

US FDA, 2016. Guidance for Industry: Frequently Asked Questions about GRAS for Substances Intended for Use in Human or Animal Food. US Food Drug Adm. [WWW Document]. URL https://www.fda.gov/regulatory-information/search-fda-guidance-documents/guidance-industry-frequently-asked-questions-about-gras-substances-intended-use-human-or-animal-food. (Accessed 31 January 2022).

US FDA, 2017a. Best Practices for Convening a GRAS Panel: Guidance for Industry Draft Guidance Guidance for Industry 30.

US FDA, 2017b. Guidance for Industry: Regulatory Framework for Substances Intended for Use in Human Food or Animal Food on the Basis of the Generally Recognized as Safe (GRAS) Provision of the Federal Food, Drug, and Cosmetic Act.

US FDA, 2018a. FDA's Approach to the GRAS Provision: A History of Processes. FDA.

US FDA, 2018b. History of the GRAS List and SCOGS Reviews. FDA.

US FDA, 2018c. GRAS Substances (SCOGS) Database. FDA. [WWW Document]. URL https://www.fda.gov/food/generally-recognized-safe-gras/gras-substances-scogs-database. (Accessed 7 January 2022).

US FDA, 2019. Redbook 2000: I Introduction. US Food Drug Adm. [WWW Document]. URL https://www.fda.gov/regulatory-information/search-fda-guidance-documents/redbook-2000-i-introduction. (Accessed 31 January 2022).

Wenner, M., 2008. Magnifying taste. Sci. Am. 299, 96–99. https://doi.org/10.1038/scientificamerican0808-96.

Woods, L.A., Doull, J., 1991. GRAS evaluation of flavoring substances by the expert panel of FEMA. Regul. Toxicol. Pharmacol. 14, 48–58. https://doi.org/10.1016/0273-2300(91)90051-V.

CHAPTER 11

Food safety compliance and legislation history

D. Detwiler
Northeastern University, Boston, MA, United States

A common mistake in looking at the history of an event or, in this case, a set of policies, is to examine the recent history and not go back to look at the early years of a topic, such as food toxicology. In this case, we know more about attitudes, ideas, and even governance around the toxicology of food from what can be found outside the science of this field.

A brief look at the early history of food safety compliance and legislation in Britain

Common in many parts of the world today, drinking tea became trendy in London and spread throughout England by the late 17th century. Through the 18th century, the British replaced beer and ale with tea and coffee as their national drinks. These became viewed as part of an elevated diet for the social and wealthy. As they became hugely expensive and heavily taxed, consumers battled a new problem—growing fraud in tea and coffee.

As a result, Great Britain's Parliament took action to curb these crimes and passed the **Adulteration of Coffee Act of 1718** (5 Geo. 1 c. 11)— "An Act against clandestine running of uncustomed Goods, and for the more effectual preventing of Frauds relating to the Customs" making it illegal to debase coffee (Mews et al., 1896). This early act imposed a rather hefty penalty for any use of "water, grease, butter, or such like material whereby the same is made unwholesome and greatly increased in weight" that would impact "the prejudice of His Majesty's Revenue, the health of his subjects, and to the loss of all fair and honest dealers" (Lely, 1894). Here, one can find evidence from over 300 years ago that the British Parliament had a keen awareness of not only the different ways and opportunities prior to consumption that a food item could be adulterated, but also the existence of the means to detect a range of evidence of potential toxicants or banned

History of Food and Nutrition Toxicology
https://doi.org/10.1016/B978-0-12-821261-5.00002-7

substances in the drink. Also important is that they not only acknowledge in this act the impact on public health but also the possible economic impact.

In 1724 Great Britain's Parliament amended the Act with **"An Act for More Effectual Preventing Frauds and Abuses in the Public Revenues"** (11 Geo. 1, c. 30). Whereas the earlier act focused on the wholesomeness of the product, it did not address situations where a characteristic other than wholesomeness was at issue. The new act included words such as "counterfeit," "adulterate," "alter," and "fabricate." This new act also prohibited actions to increase the weight of the product or to manufacture with certain food additives and dyes or with any drug or drugs (Lely, 1894).

Whereas this new amendment increased the penalty amount, it also included much greater depth of clarity in terms of what qualifies as adulterating the commodity. Six years later, this act was again amended to focus on additional commodities with the **Act to Prevent Frauds in the Revenue of Excise, With Respect to Starch, Coffee, Tea, and Chocolates (1730)** (4 Geo. 2, c, 14). This time, the description of the illegal acts included much more clarity:

> … *if any person or persons who shall be a dealer in or seller of tea, shall dye, fabricated, or manufacture any sloe leaves, liquorish leaves, or the leaves of tea that have been used, or the leaves of any other tree, shrub or plant in imitation of tea, or shall mix, color, stain or dye such leaves or tea with terra japonica, sugar, molasses, clay, logwood, or with any other ingredients or materials whatsoever…*
>
> **(Lely, 1894.)**

Here, one can find a wider awareness of the range of ways in which such adulteration is accomplished, a range of when and where such acts are carried out, a range of materials used as adulterants, and a range of means with which to impact victims.

Britain again saw more clarification regarding fraud and tea with the **1776 Adulteration of Tea Act** (17 Geo. 3. c. 29.). This act provided for "…the more effectual Prevention of the manufacturing of Ash, Elder, Sloe, and other leaves, in imitation of Tea, and to prevent Frauds in the Revenue of Excise in respect to Tea" (Lely, 1894).

Starting in the mid-1800s, attention on adulteration now focused on food in general. Frederick Filby, in his 1934 book *History of Food Adulteration and Analysis*, credits the work of the German chemist Frederick Accum for having "finally brought the storm over adulteration in 1820…. From that time onward, adulteration has come more and more before public attention" (Filby, 1934). Thus the push for the authenticity of food is an effort with roots that date back to the early 19th century. Accum began his crusade for national adulteration legislation with the publishing of his groundbreaking 1820 writing—"A Treatise on Adulteration of Food and Culinary Poisons: Exhibiting the Fraudulent Sophistications of Bread, Beer, Wine, Spirituous Liquors, Tea, Oil, Pickles, and Other Articles Employed in Domestic Economy. And Methods of Detecting Them." In this, Accum exposed and criticized the food processing industry for "normal" practices, especially the use of chemical additives (Accum, 1820). This work also marked the beginning of public awareness of the need for food safety oversight. Of particular note is the artwork that appeared in Accum's Treatise, with the familiar use of a skull to indicate death and the words "There is *Death* in the Pot" (see Fig. 1).

Some 30 years after the publishing of Accum's Treatise, *The Lancet*, a British medical journal, published a series of devastating reports in the 1850s on food adulteration, relying on commissioned analyses of food samples (Wilson, 2005). Dr. Arthur Hassall, a British physician and chemist, exposed many unsavory practices. For instance, he showed how pickled vegetables were dyed with lead- and copper-based colors. Profit drove adulteration of common items, such as milk (watered), flour (alum added), and beer (lead acetate added) (Clayton, 1908). In their summary of investigations into these incidents, the British Parliament's House of Commons Committee on Adulteration of Food mostly gave up on the belief that "the forces of competition and the knowledge of the consumer were sufficient to guarantee the sale of unadulterated foodstuffs of adequate quality" (House of Commons, 1872).

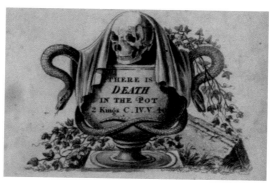

Fig. 1 Artwork from cover of Accum's (1820) work. Note the message and symbolism. *(Retrieved from The Public Domain Review https://publicdomainreview.org/collection/a-treatise-on-adulteration-of-food-and-culinary-poisons-1820.)*

Hassall used *The Lancet* as a platform to "name and shame" individual shops for the fraudulent products they sold. His work led directly to the passage of the **1860 Food Adulteration of Food and Drink Act** and later British legislation against these practices (Coley, 2005). The 1860 act has long been viewed as a failure. Though it involved, for the first time, the appointment of public analysts, very few were appointed, thus the regulation was not generally acted upon.

To reverse this, Parliament passed the **Adulteration of Food and Drink and Drugs Act of 1872** that mandated the appointment of public analysts. This new act designated the sale of mixtures, such as additives along with main ingredients, as illegal unless clearly declared at the point of sale. Also, as evident by the act's name, the act covered drugs for the first time. This act described how adulteration causes a "great hurt" to Her Majesty's subjects and endangers their lives (Lely, 1894).

The Sale of Food and Drugs Act of 1875 made a positive impact on improving food quality, continued the progress of preventing widespread adulteration, and made new efforts to define and regulate food purity. A key element of the act's effectiveness was its emphasis on strict liability. Another act that year, **The Public Health Act of 1875**, granted powers for food inspection and seizure. The **Sale of Food and Drugs Act of 1875** further defined the term "food," required consumer-driven standards, and set strict liability for food-related offenses (Lely, 1894).

While the **1879 Sale of Food and Drugs Amendment Act** introduced changes to solve conflicts in court interpretations and decisions from courts in England and Scotland (Howman, 1901), **The Sale of Food and Drugs Act of 1899** is notable in how it clarified that the definition of food would now include "any article which ordinarily enters into or is used in the composition or preparation of human food." As a result, this act placed significant focus on food quality and nutrition.

The British **Food and Drugs Act of 1938** combined food, drugs, and public health legislation relating to food. Specific wording included that the act "prohibited the addition of substances to foods so as to render the food injurious to health." For the first time, truth in food labels gained legislation, as the act authorized policymakers to make regulations governing the labeling of food and set forth penalties for false or misleading labels and advertisements. Further, the United Kingdom now designated food poisoning as a reportable communicable disease across the country.

The legislation directed to protect consumers from adulteration of specific foods and commodities was broadened to a more general approach to all foods and even drugs. These developments in the policy reflect changes

Table 1 Timeline of British Food Law 1718–1938.

1718	Adulteration of Coffee Act
1724	An Act for More Effectual Preventing Frauds and Abuses in the Public Revenues
1730	Act to Prevent Frauds in the Revenue of Excise, With Respect to Starch, Coffee, Tea, and Chocolates
1776	Adulteration of Tea Act
1860	Food Adulteration of Food and Drink Act
1872	Adulteration of Food and Drink and Drugs Act
1875	Public Health Act
1875	Sale of Food and Drugs Act
1879	Sale of Food and Drugs Amendment Act
1899	Sale of Food and Drugs Act
1938	The British Food and Drugs Act

in behavior—offender, industry, retail, consumer, and legal/political. The many revisions can also be interpreted as a potential weakness—detrimental to food crimes' response (Table 1).

What this series of British acts reveals is not only the growth of adulteration in food but also the advancement of technology to detect such acts against consumers. Each time a new adulterant or method was added, the acts read as a reflection of science's ability to detect substances entered into or is used in the composition or preparation of human food.

Similar momentum on the toxicology of food can be found in the United States around the end of the 19th century.

During the US Civil War, President Lincoln signed an act on May 15, 1862, establishing the US Department of Agriculture (USDA) with a focus mostly on research and discovery. This newly established USDA financed agricultural exploration in foreign lands and hired botanists trained to search for new plants and varieties that would launch new agriculture in the United States. At this time, however, Congress had not granted the USDA authority to regulate and inspect meat.

Some two decades after the USDA was established, the Commissioner of Agriculture appointed Harvey W. Wiley, MD as its chief chemist in 1883 (Harvey Washington Wiley, 2020). Wiley soon focused his attention and government funding toward the investigation of food adulteration (Harvey Washington Wiley, 2018). Within 4 years, Wiley published, at the direction of the Commissioner of Agriculture, a series of Technical Bulletins on Foods and Food Adulterants (U.S. Department of Agriculture, 1887). By the end of the decade, the USDA issued Bulletin 25: "A Popular Treatise on the Extent and Character of Food Adulterations," clearly advocating for national legislation on food adulteration (Wedderburn, 1890). In a number of unsuccessful attempts between 1897 and 1901, Wiley worked with various organizations to propose various versions of pure-food legislation to Congress (Harvey Washington Wiley, 2018).

As Wiley began his work, a sea of evidence for the need for improved food toxicology and supporting regulations was presented to the court of public opinion.

On the front page of the March 12, 1884, issue of *Puck* magazine (a popular political magazine at the time), Frederick Opper, regarded as one of the nation's pioneers of newspaper comic strips, drew readers' attention to

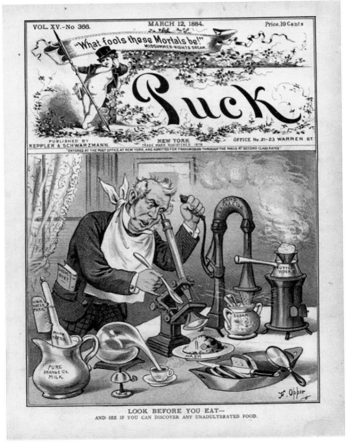

From Opper, F. (1884, March 12). "Look before you eat." *Puck.* Retrieved from: https://www.visitthecapitol.gov/exhibitions/artifact/look-you-eat-chromolithograph-frederick-burr-opper-puck-march-12-1884.

adulterated foods with his color image "Look before you eat: And see if you can discover any unadulterated food" (Opper, 1884). Testing his breakfast food and coffee, our main character holds a chemistry book in his pocket while using the technology of that day to look deep into his food. He extracts sand from his sugar, measures the water in his milk, sees hair in his butter, and finds a button in his hash. Note that the title of the chromolithograph states "see if you can discover any unadulterated food" implying that consumers—even with all the knowledge and technology—would have a hard time finding food that is pure and wholesome.

While readers of *Puck* magazine in 1884 may have had their first exposure to the issue of adulterated food, readers of a Socialist political newspaper called *Appeal to Reason* gained much more than an eyeful from an image 20 years later. In 1904 investigative journalist Upton Sinclair spent 7 weeks working undercover in Chicago's meatpacking plants. A year later, he wrote a series of articles in *Appeal to Reason* where he exposed how unsanitary working conditions were in the plants and how the meat industry was putting consumers at risk for disease. Sinclair soon published his exposé in the form of his 1906 novel *The Jungle*, allowing the world their first significant notice of the unseen dangers on their dinner plates. Even though Sinclair's intended message was support for socialism, readers paid a great deal of attention to the two chapters in which he described in detail the conditions under which meat was prepared.

Readers' concerns soon became a political issue and escalated into a full-blown "meat scandal" in President Theodore Roosevelt's administration. Though initially referred to by Roosevelt as a "Muckraker" for his role as an investigative journalist who exposed a social/corporate ill, Sinclair would later engage directly with the president over the food conditions in Chicago. In one of many letters between Sinclair and President Roosevelt, the author described how the industry in Chicago took steps, after he published his novel, to prevent others from taking a look at what took place inside the processing facilities or, as Sinclair wrote: "The lid is on in Packingtown" (Sinclair, 1906). In response, President Roosevelt sent his own team of commissioners who ultimately proved that the conditions reported by Sinclair were authentic.

On May 23, 1906, coinciding with the release of Upton Sinclair's *The Jungle*, *Puck* magazine would again include an image focusing on impure food with their centerfold illustration "Watch the Professor: A Monstrous and Amazing Feat of Magic" by Udo J. Keppler. This image shows a magician on a stage, with a skeleton for a face, wearing a tuxedo, and a sash labeled "Beef Trust." He shoves animals labeled as "Diseased Livestock" into a long white tube labeled "Packingtown" to magically produce multiple packages of "Pure Meat Products." Behind the "Professor" on stage stands what looks to be a small man in uniform with a ribbon naming him as "The Prof's Assistant," also wearing a cap labeled "Inspector."

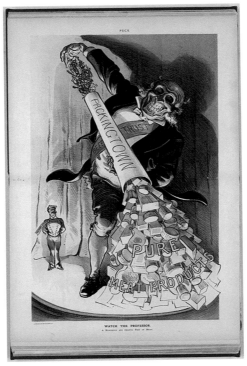

From Keppler, Udo J. (1906, May 23). "Watch the Professor: A Monstrous and Amazing Feat of Magic" Illus. In: *Puck*, v. 59, no. 1525 (1906, May 23). Washington, DC, Library of Congress, Prints and Photographs Division, FSA—OWI Collection. ppmsca 26062 //hdl. loc.gov/loc.pnp/ppmsca.26062. (Accessed 4 August 2021).

The impact of Sinclair's novel on readers can be seen in an excerpt from *The London Times* Literary Supplement review of the book in 1906, where the reviewer connected Sinclair's material to its real-world context and validated the truth exposed through the novel's content. The review reinforced *The Jungle* as a factual warning and accurately predicted the concerns Americans would continue to face today.

This book is published as a novel, and it might claim to be reviewed, therefore, under the head of fiction. But the very first thing to be said about it is that, if it is a novel, a work of imagination and invention, the conduct of an author who invented and published in a form easily accessible to all readers, young or old, male or female, such disgusting, inflammatory matter as this would deserve the severest censure. Unhappily we have good reason for believing it to be all fact, not fiction. The action of the President, who send commissioners to inquire into the truth or falsehood of Mr. Sinclair's statements, and the known tenour [SP] of the commissioners' reply remove all doubt, and give the book very great importance. By its truths or its untruths the story stands or falls, and it is with nothing less than horror that we learn it to be true. Unhappily we have good reason for believing it to be all fact, not fiction.… it is with nothing less than horror that we learn it to be true. The things described by Mr. Sinclair happened yesterday, are happening today, and will happen tomorrow and the next day, until some Hercules comes to cleanse the filthy stable.

From The London Times. (1906, June 1). "The Jungle." Literary Supplement. Microfilm collection, Western Washington University.

Despite the efforts of major meat companies to counter the findings and arguments against the industry, including the Franco-American Food Company's nearly whole page "Open Letter to President Roosevelt and the American Nation" in the *New York Times*, in which they described themselves as the "Packers of Honestly and Cleanly Made" products (The Franco-American Food Company, 1906), the American public was already convinced of the deplorable conditions in the meatpacking industry and were not persuaded by food industry attempts to improve public relations. Consumers across the nation, as well as merchants in many other countries who lost sales due to the "scandal" with bad meat from Chicago, supported strong food safety legislation. This, along with the findings of Roosevelt's investigative commission, no doubt gave strength to the president's decision to sign into law two key pieces of food safety legislation:

1. **The Federal Meat Inspection Act of 1906 (FMIA)** established authority for federal meat inspection.
2. **The Pure Food and Drug Act of 1906** banned the manufacture, sale, or transportation of adulterated or misbranded or poisonous or deleterious foods, drugs, medicines, and liquors and established what would later become the US Food and Drug Administration (FDA).

The Pure Food and Drug Act was later described by R.W. Dunlap, the acting Secretary of Agriculture, in 1925 as "one of the most beneficent pieces of legislation ever passed by Congress" (Dunlap, 1925). Change did not happen overnight, however, as the distribution of food to international markets would continue to plague consumers and retailers (see Fig. 2). A series of postcards attacking the American meatpacking industry—specifically in Chicago—circulated in South Africa in 1907. Robert Bacon, the (then) acting Secretary of State, wrote a letter to the US ambassador to the United Kingdom discussing these postcards and including a set of the postcards as a response to the complaint raised by Armour and Company for "working great harm to their business" (Bacon, 1907).

Not only do these postcards reflect the artist's attempt to bring food toxicology to a more visible level—in terms of the visible adulteration as well as the postcards' circulation—but the letter demonstrated the lengths to which the food industry would go to use political avenues to stop the growth of consumer awareness of the lack of standards in terms of food safety and the need for more broad policy regarding food safety regulations.

The Food, Drug, and Cosmetic Act of 1938, a subsequent law, repealed some of the 1906 FMIA while empowering the FDA to require

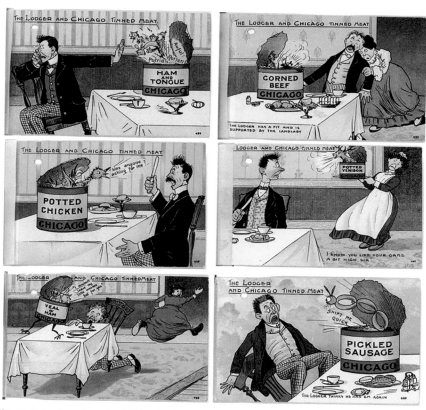

Fig. 2 Set of postcards, 1907. *(Enclosed in Bacon, R. (1907, September 9). "Letter from Acting Secretary of State Robert Bacon to U.S. Ambassador to the United Kingdom Whitelaw Reid Discussing Postcards Regarding the Chicago Meatpacking Industry." General Records of the Department of State, Record Group 59. National Archives Identifier: 2657925. Retrieved from https://catalog.archives.gov/id/2657925.)*

food (other than that regulated by the USDA) to conform to three kinds of food standards:

(1) Standards (definitions) of identity,

(2) Standards of quality, and

(3) Standards regulating the fill of containers.

No provisions were established by this time, however, for federal inspection by the FDA related to food defense or authenticity, let alone food safety.

From public and government awareness of failures in our food system came new regulations and greater levels of regulatory control. These did not come without criticisms and opposition from some within the food industry. Experts, including Harvey Wiley, the USDA chief chemist 1883–1912, criticized the often-relaxed implementation of new food safety regulations.

In 1925 Wiley wrote a letter to President Calvin Coolidge in which he addressed "a 'shocking' neglect on the part of the United States Government to enforce the Food and Drugs Act, for which I labored incessantly [*sic*] for twenty-five years" (Wiley, 1925). He did not technically send the letter to the president, as he published the letter in *Good Housekeeping* magazine, then the director of the Bureau of Foods, Sanitation, and Health for the magazine. Wiley criticized the government for having often turned a blind eye on specific cases that appeared to violate the law, and he discussed how "failures to administer the law" by those superior to him were so "shocking" that he ultimately retired voluntarily. Wiley noted in his letter that "the proper enforcement of the Food and Drugs Act is intimately related to the public health," but offered his assessment in that "the health and efficiency of our citizens are continually threatened" (Wiley, 1925). Though Wiley's criticisms may have been justified, food safety had come a long way since the turn of the century.

Taking a summary review, England's **1860 Adulteration Act** and America's **1906 Pure Food and Drug Act** are two of the earliest pieces of legislation to provide generalized regulation of food and drugs on a national scale. In both the European and American events, political landscapes conducive to reform in food toxicology related to protecting consumers and becoming modern regulatory states came about through the hard work of individuals who campaigned for legislation to prevent adulteration. Legislative changes came about after the hard work of investigative journalists who were enthusiastic to bring the evils of adulteration to the forefront of the public mind and the ignited demands from consumers.

Over the next several decades, new sciences; new food production technologies; and new consumer trends, demands, and behaviors would collide to erode the level of food safety and reverse some of the progress that had been made. Frozen foods and improved means of transportation allowed for raw ingredients and prepared foods to last longer and travel farther. At the same time, mid-century Americans were gradually beginning consuming more meals outside the home and, along with Americans' passion for driving, fast food restaurants eventually grew in numbers and popularity, even securing their place as part of the "American culture."

In the mid-1980s, new threats emerged as followers of Bhagwan Shree Rajneesh, a mystic, guru, and spiritual teacher in India, carried out "the first and largest bioterrorism attack in the U.S., of Food Poisoning/Bioterrorism on American soil" (Powell, 2018). The "1984 Rajneeshee Incident" resulted in 751 recorded illnesses, 45 hospitalizations, (no deaths) of citizens in The Dalles, Oregon, from *Salmonella enterica* Typhimurium (Detwiler, 2016).

A lengthy investigation by the Oregon Health Department and various other local and federal authorities found that the perpetrators spread liquids tainted with the *Salmonella* pathogen on surfaces in many public places, including a county courthouse. Perpetrators introduced the pathogen into the drinking water, salad bars, and even salad dressings at nearly a dozen restaurants in The Dalles, Oregon. Their purpose was later determined to be as insidious as the act itself—to incapacitate voters to influence the outcome of a local 1984 election in their favor, placing cult members, known as Rajneeshees, into office. This unprecedented act of terrorism would eventually force policymakers to focus on food defense in the form of "defining the illegality of ill-intended use, production, dissemination, or storage of biological agents" (Ryan and Glarum, 2008).

Food toxicology as an element of food safety took on an increased priority after the 1993 "Jack in the Box" *Escherichia coli* outbreak. Health officials reported over 700 people becoming ill, nearly 150 hospitalizations, and four deaths of young children as a result of contaminated hamburger patties being undercooked by grill operators in this restaurant chain. According to Bill Marler, regarded as the nation's leading foodborne illness attorney, this outbreak was the catalyst for "unprecedented food safety changes in US government regulations, the meat industry, and consumer practices in the 1990s. No other event had radically changed the meat industry since Upton Sinclair's book: *The Jungle*" (Marler, 2020). For some, the changes were too few and did not come soon enough. For some in the food industry, these changes transformed everything they knew about foodborne pathogens.

On September 28, 1994, Michael R. Taylor, then the USDA's food safety inspection service administrator, stunned the audience in a speech before the AMI when he said:

> To clarify an important legal point, we [the USDA] consider raw ground beef that is contaminated with E. coli O157:H7 to be adulterated within the meaning of the Federal Meat Inspection Act. We are prepared to use the Act's enforcement tools, as necessary, to exclude adulterated product from commerce. We plan to conduct targeted sampling and testing of raw ground beef at plants and in the marketplace for possible contamination. We know that the ultimate solution to the [E. coli] O157:H7 problem lies not in comprehensive end-product testing but rather in the development and implementation of science-based preventive controls, with product testing to verify process control.

(Taylor, 1994.)

In other words, the USDA was declaring *E. coli* O157:H7 an illegal adulterant in meat and poultry under the USDA's regulatory authority and initiating a "zero tolerance" policy for the pathogen, implying potential legal ramifications for meat manufacturers. With this, the USDA had to rethink its Pathogen Reduction plan to include a new focus on science, especially related to inspection and testing. The toxicological advances available to this effort had not been fully supported until this time and the USDA inspection efforts centered chiefly around organoleptic (what is available through the human senses—see, smell, touch) inspection.

Food toxicology as an element of national defense became a priority after the 1984 Rajneeshee bioterror attack and after the attacks on September 11, 2001. Not even a year had passed since the 9/11 attack on New York's World Trade Center buildings and on the Pentagon when the World Health Assembly, the decision-making body of the World Health Organization (WHO), adopted a 2002 resolution expressing serious concern about threats against civilian populations by the deliberate use of agents disseminated via food.

Within a year, WHO published "Terrorist Threats to Food: Guidance for Establishing and Strengthening Prevention and Response Systems"—a food safety/food terrorism document for national government policymakers (WHO, 2003). Focusing on food, food ingredients, and water (in the forms of food ingredients and bottled water), the document classifies food safety as an essential element of modern, global public health security. It goes on to define "food terrorism" as.

an act or threat of deliberate contamination of food for human consumption with biological, chemical, and physical agents or radionuclear materials for the purpose of causing injury or death to civilian populations and/or disrupting social, economic or political stability.

In outlining the potential effects of food terrorism, the WHO utilized data from "unintended" foodborne disease outbreaks to describe the toll of potential disease and death. The document looks at how a single incident of "unintentional contamination" of just one kind of food can infect hundreds of thousands of people with a "serious debilitating disease," then goes on to extrapolate the effects of some more deliberate and dangerous attack on our food supply.

The impact on trade and the economy is discussed as a "primary motive" for food terrorism. Recalls in American markets of foreign fruits resulted in the bankruptcy of international growers and shippers after consumers around the globe shunned such products. The WHO document details specific events in recent history when individual US recalls of domestic ground beef contaminated with *E. coli* O157:H7 and lunch meats contaminated with *Listeria* numbered in the tens of millions of pounds of affected product each.

The USDA's Food Safety Inspection Service (FSIS) lists on its webpage a great amount of information online for each recall issued in the United States. The number of entries for individual recalls is staggering. Not only are the examples listed by the WHO the tip of the iceberg in terms of the numbers of recalls and the quantity of food products adulterated, but a look at data from the Bureau of Labor Statistics shines more light on the scope of this economic impact. When analyzing Consumer Price Index average price data specific for the products and the year of the recalls, one learns that the approximate dollar value loss of just the two beef recalls listed in the WHO document come in at $44 million and $61 million, respectively.

Again, the WHO points to the significant financial impact on the market and related stakeholders. Beyond the loss of profit and the closing of businesses and the financial toll on individual countries, however, the WHO uses lessons learned from outbreaks and recalls over the last 20 years to emphasize that foodborne diseases have the potential of causing the disruption of global trade and economic stability and may even impact political stability.

While the WHO published "Terrorist Threats to Food" to provide member governments with guidance on preventing the deliberate contamination of food, some of this document's main points hold significant meaning for unintentional food problems. The understanding of those in the industry of every facet of the food chain, from farm to table, is critical in identifying and preventing failures and violations of the system.

The United States House of Representatives introduced the Public Health Security and Bioterrorism Preparedness Response bill as H.R. 3448 on December 11, 2001. It passed the House the next day almost unanimously, then passed the Senate unanimously on December 20, 2001, as **The Public Health Security and Bioterrorism Preparedness Response Act of 2002**—an act "to improve the ability of the United States to prevent, prepare for, and respond to bioterrorism and other public health emergencies." Surrounded by leaders from the Department of Health and Human Services, and the USDA, President George W. Bush signed the act into law as Public Law 107–188 on June 12, 2002.

The act established procedures for preparation for bioterrorism and public health emergencies, as well as the National Disaster Medical System, comprised of teams of health professionals. Further, the rules under this act include security risk assessment of individuals who have access to the select agents and toxins, with the purpose being to restrict access from any person who meets the criteria of a "restricted person" as defined in the **USA Patriot Act of 2001** (PL 107–56—October 26, 2001). The act was signed into law by President George W. Bush the previous year.

A subpart of the Public Health Security and Bioterrorism Preparedness Response of 2002, the **Agricultural Bioterrorism Protection Act of 2002** (80 FR 10627, 7 CFR 331, 9 CFR 121), provides for the regulation of certain biological agents and toxins that have the potential to pose a severe threat to human, animal, and plant health, or animal and plant products.

Under this act, 67 select agents and toxins as per 7 CFR Part 331, 9 CFR Part 121, and 42 CFR Part 73 are categorized into three areas (Select Agents and Toxins List, 2017).

- First, those subject to regulation by HHS—specifically the Centers for Disease Control and Prevention (CDC), such as SARS, Ricin, Ebola, and South American Hemorrhagic Fever viruses.
- Second are those subject to regulation by the USDA—specifically the Animal and Plant Health Inspection Service (APHIS), such as Avian influenza virus, swine fever virus, and USDA plant protection and quarantine agents and toxins.
- Finally—those that overlap and are subject to regulation by both agencies, such as various Bacillus and Brucella agents and Venezuelan equine encephalitis virus.

New concerns and new technologies will continue to place food toxicology as a major tool, both reactive and proactive, in regulatory compliance and in providing for the health and safety of consumers.

Over the past two decades, in addition to food safety and food defense, food toxicology has grown as a concern in the United States and on a global scale in terms of food authenticity, with the rise in fraud and related crimes within a wide range of commodities. Major international events, such as the 2008 melamine scandal in China (when adulterated milk and infant formula caused over 300,000 illnesses, some 54,000 infant hospitalizations, and the deaths of six babies (Huang, 2014)) as well as the 2013 horsemeat scandal in Europe (where horse DNA was found in processed beef products), prompted new laws and new agencies to investigate and prevent.

Part of the reality that needs to be considered is that the legal or political definition of an event (food safety, defense, authenticity, etc.) comes well after consumers are harmed and public health has been threatened.

Food toxicology must advance in isolation of corporate and legal influences. The true value of food toxicology comes in its ability to provide industry insight, regulatory frameworks, and consumer safety.

References

Accum, F., 1820. A Treatise on Adulteration of Food and Culinary Poisons. Longman, Hurst, Rees, Orme, and Brown, London. Republished electronically on The Public Domain Review. Retrieved from https://publicdomainreview.org/collections/a-treatise-on-adulteration-of-food-and-culinary-poisons-1820/.

Bacon, R., 1907, September 9. "Letter from Acting Secretary of State Robert Bacon to U.S. Ambassador to the United Kingdom Whitelaw Reid Discussing Postcards Regarding the Chicago Meatpacking Industry." General Records of the Department of State, Record Group 59. National Archives Identifier: 2657925. Retrieved from https://catalog.archives.gov/id/2657925.

CDC, 2017. Select agents and toxins list. In: Federal Select Agent Program. CDC, USDA. Retrieved from https://www.selectagents.gov/SelectAgentsandToxinsList.html.

Clayton, E.G., 1908. Arthur Hill Hassall: Physician and Sanitary Reformer. A Short History of his Work in Public Hygiene, and of the Movement Against The Adulteration of Food and Drugs. Bailliere, Tindall, and Cox, London. Retrieved from https://archive.org/details/arthurhillhassa00claygoog/page/n9.

Coley, N., 2005, March 1. The fight against food adulteration. Educ. Chem. 52 (2). Royal Society of Chemistry. Retrieved from https://eic.rsc.org/feature/the-fight-against-food-adulteration/2020253.article.

Detwiler, D., 2016. Death should not be on the menu. EC Nutr. 5 (3), 1148–1149. Retrieved from https://www.ecronicon.com/ecnu/pdf/ECNU-05-0000158.pdf.

Dunlap, R.W., 1925, June 13. Letter of USDA Acting Secretary R.W. Dunlap to President Calvin Coolidge. Archival Copy. Retrieved from https://6sd6hj41ya-flywheel.netdna-ssl.com/images/pdfs/109_Dunlapletter.pdf.

Filby, F.A., 1934. A History of Food Adulteration and Analysis. Allen & Unwin, London.

Harvey Washington Wiley, 2018, January 10. Science History Institute. Retrieved from https://www.sciencehistory.org/historical-profile/harvey-washington-wiley.

Harvey Washington Wiley, 2020, February 24. FDA. https://www.fda.gov/about-fda/fda-leadership-1907-today/harvey-wiley#person-bio.

House of Commons, 1872, March 6. Report from the Select Committee on Adulteration of Food etc. 1856, 379, viii, 1, p iv; Parl Deb HC vol 209. (HC 1872). The Stationery Office, London.

Howman, M., 1901. The Sale of Food and Drugs Acts, 1875 to 1899 with Notes: Decided Cases in England and Scotland, and Appendix Containing Forms, Etc. William Green & Sons, Edinburgh.

Huang, Y., 2014, July 16. The 2008 Milk Scandal Revisited. Forbes Magazine. Retrieved from http://www.forbes.com/sites/yanzhonghuang/2014/07/16/the-2008-milk-scandal-revisited/#41a6bb204428.

Lely, J.M., 1894. Statutes of Practical Utility: Arranged in Alphabetical and Chronological Order with Notes and Indexes: Being the 5th Edition of Chittys Statutes. vol. IV Sweet & Maxwell, London.

Marler, B., 2020. In: Detwiler, D. (Ed.), FOOD SAFETY: Past, Present, and Predictions. Elsevier Academic Press, Cambridge, MA, ISBN: 9780128182192.

Mews, J., Gordon, W.E., Spencer, A.J. (Eds.), 1896. The Law Journal Reports for the Year 1896. vol. 65. Stevens and Sons, London, p. 19.

Opper, F., 1884, March 12. Look Before You Eat. Puck. Retrieved from https://www.visitthecapitol.gov/exhibitions/artifact/look-you-eat-chromolithograph-frederick-burr-opper-puck-march-12-1884.

Powell, D., 2018, December 2. Your Vomit and Diarrhea is Our Bread and Butter: Portland's outbreak museum. Barf Blog. Retrieved from https://www.barfblog.com/tags/bill-keene/.

Ryan, J., Glarum, J., 2008. Biosecurity and Bioterrorism: Containing and Preventing Biological Threats. Elsevier, Burlington, MA.

Sinclair, U., 1906, March 10. Letter from Upton Sinclair to President Theodore Roosevelt. 03/10/1906 (National Archives Identifier: 301981); Letters Received, 1893–1906; Records of the Office of the Secretary of Agriculture, 1839–1981; Record Group 16, National Archives. Retrieved from https://www.archives.gov/historical-docs/todays-doc/?dod-date=310.

Taylor, M., 1994. Change and opportunity: harvesting innovation to improve the safety of food. In: Speech Before the American Meat Institute Annual Convention, San Francisco, CA. Available from: https://www.foodsafetynews.com/AMI%20Speech%20September%201994.pdf.

The Franco-American Food Company, 1906, June 8. An Open Letter to President Roosevelt and the American Nation. The New York Times. Microfilm collection, Western Washington University.

U.S. Department of Agriculture, 1887. Technical Bulletin 19330—Number 13: Foods and Food Adulterants. Retrieved from https://archive.org/details/foodsfoodadulter13unit/page/n10.

Wedderburn, A., 1890. U.S. Department of Agriculture Technical Bulletin 25: "A Popular Treatise on the Extent and Character of Food Adulterations". Retrieved from https://archive.org/details/populartreatiseo25wedd/page/n2.

Wiley, H., 1925, September. Letter to President Coolidge: Enforcement of the Food Law. Good Housekeeping Magazine. Archived copy. Retrieved from https://6sd6hj41ya-flywheel.netdna-ssl.com/images/pdfs/53_Letters%20to%20President.pdf.

Wilson, B., 2005, February 27. Food Scares are One of the Great British Traditions. The Telegraph. Retrieved from https://www.telegraph.co.uk/news/uknews/1484479/Food-scares-are-one-of-the-great-British-traditions.html.

World Health Organization, 2003. Terrorist Threats to Food: Guidance for Establishing and Strengthening Prevention and Response Systems. Retrieved from https://apps.who.int/iris/handle/10665/42619.

Further reading

Detwiler, D., 2020. Food Safety: Past, Present, and Predictions. Elsevier AP.

Keppler, U.J., 1906, May 23. "Watch the Professor: A Monstrous and Amazing Feat of Magic" Illus. in: Puck, v. 59, no. 1525. Library of Congress, Prints and Photographs Division, FSA—OWI Collection, Washington, DC. ppmsca 26062 hdl.loc.gov/loc.pnp/ppmsca.26062. (Accessed 4 August 2021).

The London Times, 1906, June 1. The Jungle. Literary Supplement. Microfilm collection, Western Washington University.

CHAPTER 12

Food safety assessment and methodologies for GMOs and new or novel foods

Richard E. Goodman

Department of Food Science, Food Allergy Research and Resource Program, University of Nebraska-Lincoln, Lincoln, NE, United States

Introduction

Food production, food protection, and food consumption have taken many turns in the history of each society. In most countries, food choices have been dictated by those plants and animals available for consumption in specific geographical locations and by the cultural practices such as fermentation that reduces risks from many microbes. There have been limited guidelines on food preparation, cooking, and spices from historical uses over many decades to centuries. In recent history, many societies have developed broader food preferences and practices. Some changes bring potential new risks and questions for consumers, developers, and regulators. Certainly, the safe consumption of foods commonly consumed within a society forms a basis for acceptable foods in each culture. But the world changes. I was born in Washington State in the United States. I first consumed Paneer Tikka Masala which includes bovine milk proteins but no meat, in New Delhi, India, in 2002. Five years later I purchased a frozen package of Paneer Tikka Masala in Lincoln, Nebraska. It was manufactured in India and was labeled appropriately for US regulations as containing milk to protect milk–allergic consumers. Some food changes are due to choices of selection influenced by consumer preferences; some are due to the ease and economics of food production, transportation, and storage; and some are due to the influence of advertisements and social media.

Regulations exist for packaged foods in most countries to help control the levels of significant contaminants and of major allergen sources and glutens involved in celiac disease (CeD) that are in human food. The safety of foods prepared in restaurants, buffets, and private homes is less restricted and ends up being the responsibility of the consumer to ask the right questions and to be cautious if they have food allergies or have CeD. Food safety systems are not perfect, but current guidelines for packaged foods and commodity crops do afford protection for most at-risk consumers including those with specific allergies or celiac disease and those with some metabolic restrictions such as diabetes. It is important to consider at-risk consumers when evaluating food safety as there are many potential risks and the health status of the consumers can vary over time.

Food safety regulations in the United States

The US government's primary food safety agency is the Food and Drug Administration for most foods and the US Department of Agriculture for meat and some egg products. According to the archive of the Food and Drug Administration (https://www.fda.gov/about-fda/about-website/fdagov-archive), food chemical analysis was begun in 1848, which was performed by the Department of Agriculture and transferred to the Food and Drug Administration in 1862. In 1930 the Pure Food and Drugs Act was passed making it illegal to adulterate or misbrand food and drugs that were sold across state lines. The agency has evolved over time and with legal changes directed by Congress. Currently, the Center for Food Safety and Applied Nutrition (CFSAN) of the FDA has the overall responsibility of evaluating the safety of genetically engineered organisms intended for food use and new food types. The US Environmental Protection Agency (EPA) has responsibility for the safety of GM crops that have insecticidal, bactericidal, or virus-resistant traits following the guidelines of the FDA. Other divisions are responsible for biologics, devices, drugs, veterinary medicine, toxins, and regulatory issues. Regulations for food and drugs are published in the Code of Federal Regulations (CFR) Title 21, defining the Food and Drug Administration as being responsible for regulatory activities ensuring food safety. Since risks vary to some extent for individual consumers due to genetics and environmental factors, the assessment of risks must be comprehensive and often individualized to subpopulations. Specific chapters in the book *Nutritional Toxicology* (Kotsonis and Mackey, 2002) present information about nutrition and risk factors in foods including key components, risks of allergy, celiac disease, and toxicity. New food crop regulations differ to some extent between the United States and Europe. Regulations are specific to the legal entities of a country, but with increasing global food trade there are efforts to harmonize, if not standardize evaluations across countries.

The introduction of genetically engineered (or genetically modified) food crops was a stimulus for a change that emerged in the early 1990s (FDA, 1992; Nordlee et al., 1996; Harlander, 2002). Focused international evaluation guidelines were written for evaluating potential risks of genetically modified or genetically engineered foods. The FDA in the United States published recommendations in the Federal Register providing guidance based on overall food safety including the history of safe use, nutrition, potential risks of allergy and toxicity, and potential unexpected effects similar to natural plant breeding (FDA, 1992). The policy was to use existing US regulations to evaluate potential risks. For international guidance, independent scientific experts of food allergy met under the joint consultations of the Food and Agriculture Organization and the World Health Organization of the United Nations in 1991. Updates were published in 1996, 2000, and 2001, reporting potential food safety evaluations for food derived from plants produced by biotechnology focusing primarily on the substantial equivalence of already accepted food crop varieties through FAO/WHO Consultations, the Organization for Economic Co-operation and Development (OECD). The CODEX Alimentarius Commission of the United Nations was designed to produce collaborations of the Food and Agricultural Organization (FAO) and the World Health Organization (WHO), both bodies within the United Nations. From 2003 the CODEX Alimentarius Commission accepted separate guidelines for the safety assessment of plants, animals, and microbes that were altered using biotechnology (CODEX, 2009). Individual countries have either adopted the CODEX guidelines, adopted similar procedures, or rely on other countries for food ingredients and foods that cross international boundaries.

Evaluating the safety and utility of genetically engineered food crops following CODEX guidelines

Description of the principles and practices in CODEX for foods derived from modern biotechnology is divided into a General Principles document that provides an overall introduction with a history of safe use of the source organism as a primary consideration (CAC/GL 44-2003). Specific guidelines were defined by the CODEX Alimentarius Commission for modifications of plants, microbes, and animals in additional documents (CAC/GL 45-2003, CAC/GL 46-2003, and CAC/GL68-2008). For all three classes of food sources, characterization of the organism and associated risks are integral to the assessment for food safety. The developer has the overall responsibility for producing the information and data, but it is reviewed critically by regulatory authorities including the FDA and EPA in the United States.

A general nutrient profile is required for each GMO, often with multiple geographically grown samples to measure proteins, amino acids, lipids, carbohydrates, vitamins, and minerals. These must be described and compared to a non-GM organism of a similar type to judge "substantial equivalence." That does not mean identical but within the range of current similar varieties that are being used for food and feed now.

A description of any added DNA is required along with function, regulatory elements, and position of inserts relative to the endogenous DNA of the modified organism. The developer must describe the expected intended changes and demonstrate the stability of the DNA and its characteristics over three or more reproductive cycles to ensure DNA stability. The number of DNA inserts must be described and the DNA sequence at the ends of the insert(s) reported along with expected protein or RNA products. Unintended effects must be predicted and described, for instance, any proteins predicted from open reading frames at the insertion site or DNA junctions in the insert.

Comparisons of all new proteins and potential proteins at DNA junctions in a transgenic organism should be made to proteins known to cause allergy, toxicity, or celiac disease. Glutens and gluten-like proteins are expected from natural genes in modified wheat, barley, or rye species, which can be evaluated based on DNA and amino acid sequence comparisons. If a new plant food was developed from a species or genes of the Pooideae grass family, sequences of predicted or known proteins should be compared to those of known celiac disease-causing (CeD) proteins using a database such as the Celiac Database in AllergenOnline.org that became publicly available in 2012 within the www.AllergenOnline.org website.

The CODEX guidelines were developed by scientific consultations in limited public meetings of member country representatives and those of specific nongovernmental entities (NGOs). The CODEX drafts were published and discussed following a specific procedure of the CODEX before member country votes were cast, over a period of months to years. For GMOs, draft guidelines were finalized at a meeting in Vancouver, British Columbia (Canada), September 9–13, 2001. The overall guideline and documents for plants and microbes were accepted by the votes of the CODEX member countries in 2003. For animals, the document was finalized in 2008. The CODEX documents are guidelines and individual countries can accept or ignore the recommendations. The United States has accepted the CODEX guidelines. The European Food Safety Authority (EFSA) and the European Commission (EC) have adopted more stringent guidelines with some additional tests that could delay GM acceptance and approval, as well as increased costs. It is not clear that the extra tests have improved safety. An organism is considered a GMO under CODEX if specific DNA has been taken from one source and transformed into another organism by either physical means (gene gun, chemical insertion) or by recombinant organism by infection with a recombinant Agrobacterium or similar vector. There have been disputes in various countries about the status of gene-editing techniques such as the use of CRISPR-Cas9. The United States decided that unless a detectable foreign gene is inserted, the organism would not be considered a GMO. The EC has decided that gene-edited organisms are still GMOs (Existing guidance appropriate for assessment of genome editing in plants | EFSA (europa.eu).

Procedures for evaluating potential hazards and risks

Publications describe procedures for evaluating potential hazards and risks from GM crops based on the safety of the organism being modified and the genes and proteins introduced. For whole new food sources such as an alga, insect species, or a new fungus, the process is more complicated but may be done in a similar fashion.

The evolutionary relationship of the gene donor and gene recipient organisms and known risks and hazards associated with them are important. Scientific literature searches performed for peer-reviewed publications using NCBI PubMed, NCBI Taxonomy, Web of Science, and some more public resources such as Wikipedia can often provide useful information. Individual country procedures for judging safety are guided by the rules of the country. In the United States, the basic rule was established in 1958 under the FDA approach to GRAS (Generally Recognized as Safe) Provisions under food additives. There have been updates in the process with the most recent in 1997 under the Code of Federal Regulations. The EU has a similar definition with a food safety history date limit of 1997 as the cutoff of the history of safe use.

Food allergy is an important hazard as is toxicity. Both should focus on known hazards and risks from commonly consumed foods. The major biotechnology companies, academic scientists, and regulatory scientists have collaborated on defining tests and processes for safety evaluation including procedures for bioinformatics and stability of proteins during digestion. Comparisons of sequences of new proteins to known allergens have been used to evaluate current GM crops (Hileman et al., 2002; Goodman et al., 2008; Siruguri et al., 2015; Jin et al., 2017; Delaney et al., 2018). Some have proposed focusing on the E score of FASTA or BLASTP rather than the percent identity of matches (Silvanovich et al., 2009). However E scores vary markedly due to the length of the proteins and size of the database so it seems some important matches might be missed and many other irrelevant matches emphasized. The procedure originally looked for identity matches of 8 contiguous amino acids to known allergens. But that has moved to finding identity matches of >35% identity over 80 amino acids and to full-length identity matches with FASTA or BLASTP in the CODEX guideline. Different allergen databases could be used for these comparisons, but importantly the number of allergens used in the comparisons has moved from a few hundred in 1996 to more than 2200 proteins in 2021 in databases including www.AllergenOnline.org. The bioinformatics at www.AllergenOnline.org has three options for sequence comparisons. One is a full-length FASTA and a match of >50% identity is likely to be cross-reactive for IgE-mediated allergens and likely to require serum IgE testing to confirm possible risks. The sliding 80-amino acid match by FASTA allows matches of <80 amino acids as there is a calculated adjustment to correct the percent identity to being equivalent to an 80-amino acid alignment by multiplying by the actual number of amino acids in the alignment and dividing by 80. Thus a match of 72 amino acids of the peanut allergen Ara h 2 which is 100% identical to Ara h 2 would be scored as 90% identical over 80 amino acids. Some databases would not flag that as a protein with risk, but that segment has at least two IgE epitopes (Goodman, 2021). And although it is not a useful comparison, the eight-amino acid match can be performed in the AllergenOnline.org database. The important point is that higher identity matches are more likely to indicate possible risks of allergy or cross-reactivity. As demonstrated by Abdelmoteleb et al. (2021), matches greater than 35% identity to proteins in AllergenOnline.org are common from proteomes predicted by whole genome sequences. The much higher identity matches of protein that are evolutionarily conserved across broad taxonomic categories including humans and many foods that are commonly eaten indicate a need to readjust the criterion of >35% identity over 80 amino acids based on the protein type. Many share >50% identity and common exposure without recorded allergies being reported for those sources indicates no need to perform serum IgE binding tests.

Serum IgE tests are needed when the source of a new gene or food is known to be a common cause of allergies and especially if there is a high sequence identity match to an allergen. Serum samples must be from willing volunteers with specific allergies relevant to the protein or food source, or at least self-described as having allergies and with symptoms that match short time of exposure, multiple events with the same food. Specific IgE tests with ImmunoCAPs are useful for confirmation. Tests should include natural and reduced, denatured forms of the protein if possible using individual human samples and controls. IgE detection should be performed with validated monoclonal antihuman IgE. For samples testing positive by direct binding, inhibition assays should be performed with proteins from the sequence matched source (Goodman et al., 2013; Panda et al., 2013). Basophil activation or histamine release provides useful information to demonstrate clinically important recognition of two or more IgE epitopes by IgE from a serum sample for overall risk assessment (Eiwegger et al., 2019).

IgE binding to proteins is a prerequisite to immediate reactions to allergens. However, binding to IgE performed in laboratory samples and using laboratory methods of immunoblots, ELISA, or RAST inhibition studies using purified proteins in ratios beyond the abundance in foods can be misleading. Diagnosis of food and airway allergy by clinicians is often based on clinical history, skin prick tests positivity (SPT), and laboratory test results including ImmunoCAP tests using Thermo Fisher reagents (van Hage et al., 2017). The binding of IgE to proteins can be tested for biological activity using food challenges, skin prick tests, or basophil reactivity to demonstrate that at least two IgE epitopes are present on a protein and the relevance of IgE from individual subjects (Santos et al., 2021).

Importantly the range of tests described does not need to be performed for every GM product or every novel food. The priority should be the history of safe use. The likelihood of risk of allergy and cross-reactivity should be based first on the sequence comparisons and if needed, based on serum IgE binding. If there is IgE binding, then measurement of bioactivity using basophil tests, skin prick tests, or antigen challenges are the final steps for demonstrating potential risks of allergy.

The stability of the introduced proteins to digestion by pepsin at an acidic pH was judged useful as a number of food allergens are stable in pepsin in a simple test tube assay (Astwood et al., 1996; Thomas et al., 2004; Ofori-Anti et al., 2008). The assay is a simple fixed conditions test tube assay with readouts of stainable proteins in an SDS-PAGE gel. It has been criticized in some peer-reviewed journals as a number of allergens are digested in a short time, while some dietary proteins are very stable in pepsin but without evidence of allergy. The assays often are not performed uniformly and the determinations are generally subjective (Fu et al., 2002; Bogh and Madsen, 2016). Judging the time of digestion has been contentious because the characterization of some tested proteins do not appear to correlate stability with allergenicity (Herman et al., 2007; Ofori-Anti et al., 2008). Other researchers try to mimic human physiological digestion by adding saliva, stomach, intestinal fluid, and more with extended times and detection of peptides but those have not correlated for allergy (Verhoeckx et al., 2019). The assay is a simple test tube assay with a fixed amount of protein, fixed pH, and purified pepsin from swine. An important consideration is the definition of allergens and the frequent lack of information about the dose of the protein in the foods where they are present. Some scientists have added intestinal fluid digestion following digestion in pepsin, yet the relevance of intestinal digestion for food allergy is not clear as immune system sampling of intestinal lumen contents occurs immediately after leaving the stomach. Peyer's patches are present throughout the small and large intestines. In addition, some of the food proteins that are stable have other properties such as stimulation of T helper 1 cells, rather than T helper 2 cells. Furthermore, not all Th2 cells stimulate B cells to make IgE antibodies, some stimulate IgG production by B cells and more information is accumulating regarding immunosuppressive T cells and B cells. Results of stability in pepsin are interesting but should be judged with a measure of the abundance of the protein in food fractions of food, yet it is clear that some commonly consumed proteins are abundant and stable in pepsin.

The combined results of these assessments are needed to judge risks and/or safety. It is important to remember that the results of each step need to be judged in the context of risks, whether high or low, for allergy. Source, bioinformatics, serum IgE test if needed, stability in pepsin, and abundance are other parameters to be considered (Fig. 1).

Example of evaluation of MON810 insect-resistant maize

Monsanto Company developed maize (corn) plants resistant to the European corn borer (*Ostrinia nubilalis*) and other lepidopteran insect pests due to the expression of low levels of Cry1Ab from *Bacillus thuringiensis*, a microbe that was used effectively as a microbial organic pesticide

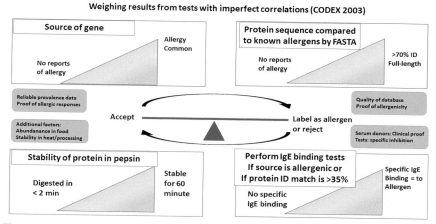

Fig. 1 Interpretation of the CODEX 2003 guideline processes requires scaled judgment as there are significant gradients of the potency of allergen sources, of sequence identity across protein types for risks of cross-reactivity, for grading specific IgE binding and stability of the proteins to digestion. (From Goodman, R.E., Vieths, S., Sampson, H.A., Hill, D., Ebisawa, M., Taylor, S.L., van Ree, R., 2008. Allergenicity assessment of genetically modified crops—what makes sense? Nat. Biotechnol. 26(1), 73–81.)

in the 1960s. The Bt bacteria have approximately 5000 genes and potential proteins. Original YieldGard corn was developed using biolistic DNA insertion of the *cry1Ab* gene along with DNA regulatory elements and the kanamycin-resistant antibiotic gene *nptii* from a different bacterium. It was tested for food and feed safety and regulatory approval in the United States in 1996 for food, feed, and cultivation. Canada approved all three uses (food, feed, and cultivation) in 1997 and Argentina in 1998. The source of the gene, the DNA sequence of the transformation molecules, and characterization of the DNA insert and proteins produced in the plant were studied and compared to known allergens, toxins, and antinutrients before approvals. The studies demonstrated the characteristics of the GM plants, stability of the DNA over multiple generations, and the nutritional properties of the maize were compared to genetically similar non–GMO maize (Petrick et al., 2020). Separate studies were conducted at Monsanto to consider potential allergenicity, toxicity, and overall food safety according to the Food and Drug Administration (FDA) in the Federal Register in 1992 (Sanders et al., 1998). Characterization of the genetic changes were studies demonstrating that the DNA insert was at a single site and that the protein expressed was as expected (Petrick et al., 2020). A toxicity assessment was performed according to the Environmental Protection Agency (EPA) as described in 1998 (EPA, U.S. Reregistration eligibility, 1998). The safety of Bt proteins was considered by McClintock et al. (1995) and the Cry 1 proteins were judged to be nontoxic for mammals. Broiler chicken studies were performed comparing corn grain from YieldGard (Mon810) and crossed YieldGard and Roundup Ready (GA21) maize with nontransgenic control and commercial maize feed chickens (Taylor et al., 2003). The composition of the grain from the MON810 maize was similar within statistical parameters to nontransgenic maize as similar studies have shown for many GM events (Herman and Price, 2013). The process of testing and evaluating food and feed materials from GM crops is complex, taking from 8 to 12 years to complete, including the submission of studies to multiple countries before the commercial sale of the seeds to farmers. The history of safe use of the source of the introduced gene and protein must include literature searches for possible allergenicity and toxicity. Published scientific evidence of consumption or human exposure is important. The most important tests for safety are bioinformatics comparisons of the amino acid sequence of newly expressed proteins from inserted DNA to allergens in an established allergen database (www.AllergenOnline.org) as well as public protein databases (NCBI protein at www.ncbi.nlm.nih.gov/protein; or UniProt at www.uniprot.org/uniprot/) for identification of allergens or potentially IgE cross-reactive proteins (Goodman et al., 2016).

A similar bioinformatics search should be performed for matches to toxins, which is difficult as there are no general toxicity databases though there are specific databases on spider and wasp venoms. The European Food Safety Authority has developed a rather elaborate recommendation document for toxicity assessment (Palazzolo et al., 2020). However, the original charge for the grant to Palazzolo et al. was for toxin assessment and the authors did not accomplish that. Instead, they described the complexity of judging risks of toxicity that have been faced by those developing GM crops and submitting safety evaluations to regulators. The bioinformatics to toxins can be accomplished by searches of proteins in the NCBI Protein database with keyword limits of "toxicity" and "toxins," though that is more difficult with changes to the database in 2019 that included removing keyword limits.

Large biotech companies seek approvals from the United States, Canada, Australia/New Zealand, Japan, and recently from South Korea and China before commercial sales anywhere. They also attempt to gain approvals from the European Union, although mostly for food and feed use as few European countries will grow GM crops. Japan also does not allow the cultivation of GM crops but does allow sales for food and feed. Argentina, Brazil, and a few other countries in South America have approved some GM crops as outlined in the ISAAA GM crop website (https://www.isaaa.org/gmapprovaldatabase/).

Herbicide-tolerant crops

Several herbicide-tolerant (HT) crops have been developed. Each is tolerant to moderate doses of specific chemical herbicides. HT maize, cotton, and sugar beets have been produced by transformation with a bacterial enzyme, CP4 EPSPS, that is not bound by or inhibited by glyphosate, a small organic chemical that is an analog of the amino acid glycine. Glyphosate is a broad-spectrum small molecular weight organophosphate compound that inhibits the natural enzyme 5-enolpyruvylshikimate-3-phosphate synthase in most plants. The action blocks the production of aromatic amino acids and some other aromatic metabolites. It can be used as a postemergent herbicide in plants containing this gene. Glyphosate is one of the most used herbicides because of the HT traits in a number of GMO crops and low-impact environmental consequences in terms of safety for insects, mammals, and birds, compared to some other herbicides. Many studies have been performed over years using animal models to estimate potential toxicity including genotoxicity and have not found substantial risks compared to many other agricultural chemicals (Wikipedia: Glyphosate—Wikipedia, accessed December 6, 2021). However, a few scientists have performed studies and reported a correlation of exposure to some cases of non-Hodgkin's lymphoma in 2015. And IARC (International Agency for Research and Cancer) has classified glyphosate as a probable human carcinogen in 2015. However, many scientific panels and regulators have not been able to replicate claims of cancer or long-term toxicity of glyphosate, although various surfactants used in farm formulations of glyphosate may have some risks but they too have been evaluated for safety by regulatory agencies in both the United States and Europe. HT GMOs that have been made for tolerance to other chemical herbicides (2,4-D, dicamba, glufosinate, and Isoxaflutole) have been approved for specific crops (www.ISAAA.org/gmapprovaldatabase). All the approved GM crops that are used commercially in the United States have been through a testing and evaluation process that is consistent with the CODEX guidelines. The HT products allow more efficient farming of many important food and feed crops which holds down production costs. Farm practices must of course follow techniques that control chemical pesticide exposure including protecting ground and surface waters.

Many other GM crops including maize, soybeans, cotton, canola, sugar beets, papaya, beans, cowpea, squash, rice, wheat, sugarcane, eggplant, tomato, and potatoes have been approved. Each inserted gene, protein, and the transformed crop has been evaluated for approval to grow for food and feed and commercial plant production. Some of the GM events do not express a new protein; rather, they express RNA to inhibit viral replication (papaya ringspot virus resistance, potato yellows, and leaf roll-resistant potatoes) or to alter the expression of endogenous genes. Some GM crops include multiple genes. Some GM crops are reproductively crossed with plants having multiple events to produce more stable insect resistance or to combine herbicide tolerance with insect resistance. Are extra evaluations needed for food safety if the two parental lines are judged safe?

Viral, fungal, and bacterial plant pest control

Many important food and feed crops are attacked by viral, fungal, and bacterial organisms that cause considerable crop losses and impact food quality. Some GM crops have been created that help control these infections and losses. Potatoes in the United States are impacted by at least two important viruses and by a fungal-like organism, *Phytophthora infestans,* and by Colorado potato beetles. Monsanto Company made multiple versions of GM Russet Burbank including a triple stack with two antiviral genes, one against potato leaf roll virus and one against potato yellow virus as well as a Cry 3 A gene that stops the Colorado potato beetle. However, market pressures from major food companies halted the expanding commercial development with campaigns against GMOs. Potatoes resistant to *Phytophthora infestans* that cause the Irish Potato famine have been constructed by researchers at the J.R. Simplot Company (Habig et al., 2018) and in an African potato line (Ghislain et al., 2019), both by insertion of three RB genes from related wild potato species. Field test data and safety evaluations of these events appear good, without noticeable adverse environmental or plant effects.

Papaya trees and fruit in Hawaii were heavily infected with papaya ringspot virus in the 1990s. Dennis Gonsalves constructed a transformation cassette with part of the DNA sequence from the virus to transform trees in Hawaii (Gonsalves, 1998). Two lines were produced, and one became the dominant breeding line, Rainbow Papaya line 55-1. Planting the GM variety in Hawaii saved the industry and was effective at reducing the overall viral presence there. The mechanism of resistance is due to RNAi (RNA interference) that stops production in the cells of the infected plants. This papaya was approved for use in the United States and Japan. Related viruses are endemic in SE Asia, Bangladesh, China, India, and Pakistan. In 2006 Chinese scientists developed a resistant Huanong No. 1 GM line that was found to be resistant to the ringspot virus, but in 2018 the strain was no longer resistant to wild-type virus in South China (Wu et al., 2018). Other research in South Asia showed there are diverse viruses infecting papaya in countries like Bangladesh and Pakistan (Hamim et al., 2019; Saleem et al., 2021).

Bacterial wilt disease is common in bananas in East Africa. Leena Tripathi and colleagues transferred genes from two commonly consumed peppers into banana explants and grew plants that were demonstrated to be resistant to the bacteria. The GM bananas have not been commercialized yet, but their safety appears acceptable (Jin et al., 2017). Citrus greening disease, also called Huanglongbing, infects citrus trees in most areas of the world now (Singerman and Rogers, 2020). It is caused by a bacterium *Candidatus Liberibacter africanus* that is spread among trees by sucking insects that are becoming resistant to chemical pesticides (Wang et al., 2017). A problem for trees, in general, is the process of growing new varieties of trees since a new infection can overcome resistance, as the bacteria get into the phloem of the tree through the saliva of sucking insects and grows there, causing damage to the nutrient transport system. There may be an option if a viral "vaccine" can be developed for citrus greening disease by transferring expression cassettes to phloem with RNAi constructs or with genes for plant defensin proteins that can be dispersed in the tree killing the bacteria (NAS, 2018). Research on those options is ongoing.

Nutritionally enhanced GM events

Golden Rice provides an important example of a nutritionally enhanced food crop. The concept is to have beta-carotene produced at moderate to high levels in a variety of white rice consumed in many Asian countries including the Philippines, Bangladesh, and India, and some countries in Africa, where yellow and green vegetables that have high levels of beta-carotene are not commonly consumed and animal products that have vitamin A as an important nutrient are also not commonly consumed.

The developers included academics from Zurich and scientists from Syngenta. Development happened in stages as the first constructs included one gene from a bacterium and another from the daffodil flower that demonstrated accumulation of beta-carotene and a second using a different phytoene synthase (Burkhardt et al., 1997; Beyer et al., 2002). Second generation events used different genes to produce beta-carotene. One study of DNA transformation events showed promising results (Paine et al., 2005). Additional transformations were performed in the Japonica rice cultivar Kaybonnet and one, GR2E, was finally chosen as having the best single DNA insertion and performance (Swamy et al., 2019). These transformations included three genes, pmi (phosphomannose isomerase) as a marker gene, crti phytoene desaturase from *Pantoea ananatis,* and phytoene synthase Zmpsy1 from *Zea mays* (maize or corn). One event (GR2R) transformed with the final cassette was inserted into an intron of an important rice root promoter gene but it did not perform well in the field (https://www.irri.org/golden-rice). The final GR2E event was a single insert and performed well as demonstrated in published studies (Swamy et al., 2019, 2021; Biswas, et al., 2021). Regulatory authorities in the United States (2018), Canada (2018), Australia and New Zealand (2017), and the Philippines (2019) approved this variety following detailed scientific reviews. The reviews evaluated the GM rice used in food and feed. The Philippines is the only country so far to consider the cultivation of GR2E event, but others including Bangladesh may follow (https://www.isaaa.org/gmapprovaldatabase/event/default.asp?EventID=528&Event=GR2E).

A study to demonstrate the nutritional properties of Golden Rice to improve the vitamin A status of consumers who are deficient in vitamin A and prone to vision problems and low immunity against malaria and other tropical diseases was conducted in Huanan, China. The study was well designed except the parents of children fed in the study were not informed that the rice was from a GM event (Tang et al., 2009). Some parents thought the material had not been evaluated properly for safety and the published report was retracted. It was partly funded by grants from the US Dept. of Agriculture (Retraction, 2015; original publication Tang et al., 2012). The results of the nutrition study were not questioned and showed a diet of GR was as efficient as purified vitamin A fed in a capsule, and more efficient than spinach in raising the vitamin A levels in the vitamin A-deficient children aged 6–8 years by 21 days. The retraction demonstrates the need to have all ethical and other information for studies performed correctly to support or reject the science of any specific GMO. The lesson is to follow all rules for ethical compliance and protection of study subjects. No one was hurt by the study, but the parents were upset, and the retraction hurt the public image for Golden Rice and GMOs in general.

General food availability enhanced by GMOs

Some question the need for GMOs in the food supply and the answers differ between crops, countries, and traits of the GMO. Golden Rice fulfilled a nutritional need for enhancing beta-carotene in the diets of populations in countries where white rice is the major food energy source. In this case, the question is not rice availability but nutritional availability, i.e., vitamin A. In other cases, GMOs can help preserve food that provides protein or other nutritional components. The Rainbow and Sunup papayas were transformed to inhibit ringspot virus in Hawaii by protecting the crops from the virus that destroys the papayas in a short time. Papaya is a good source of vitamins and fiber. The resistant varieties successfully preserved the crops and the industry in Hawaii.

Other crops such as Cassava (*Manihot esculenta*) contain limited nutrients beyond starch for energy. Depending on the variety of cassava and preparation conditions with breeding programs, higher levels of carotene will increase vitamin A in consumers (Peprah et al., 2020). Cassava is a staple crop in Africa, Southeast Asia, and South America. A GM cassava, resistant to the brown streak virus, was approved in June 2021 for use in Kenya. It is an RNAi construct, so it does not express a novel protein, but the nutrients, DNA stability, and growth conditions were evaluated to ensure that it is suitable for food production under the growing conditions in these regions. Other possible GM cassava under development includes increased ferritin protein for enhanced iron and improved carotene expression.

Disease-resistant GM crops with reduced risks to bananas and potatoes from bacterial diseases are available but not yet approved for widespread cultivation or for food sales. These are not high protein crops, but they provide nutrients, including calories, and are staple foods for a significant population in Africa.

The case for insect-resistant crops such as moth- and storage beetle-resistant cowpea is important for sub-Saharan Africa. These products reduce chemical pesticide needs and help by preserving harvested cowpeas during storage. The Bt cowpea has been approved in Nigeria to stop the pod borer (*Maruca vitrata*) and another GMO with alpha-amylase inhibitor cowpea to stop the storage beetle (Luthi et al., 2013) should be reviewed by regulators soon. Both are potentially very useful for smallholder farmers and the general population.

Gene editing of conventional crops and animals

Gene editing using TALENs or CRISPR-Cas9 is maturing as a method to alter endogenous gene expression to improve nutritional products or phenotypic characteristics including alterations in mosquito reproduction capacity and reduction in plants for disease susceptibility. Some countries including the United States do not regard gene-edited crops to be GMO unless there is a clearly defined DNA insertion. The crops still require nutritional profiling to ensure they are a reasonable food crop. However, in the European Union, gene-edited crops are considered to GMOs and presumably, the EFSA and the European Commission will require the same broad safety and nutritional evaluation that is required for all GMOs.

Developers are looking to gene editing to improve crop performance or improve nutritional values. They are also considering for knocking out potentially harmful genes such as those encoding glutens that cause celiac disease or specific allergens (Jouanin et al., 2018; Assou et al., 2021). Other developers are attempting to improve agricultural productivity by reducing the need to cull male chicks in poultry production and risks in the farm for mechanically removing the horns from bovines. The gene editing does little more than make genetic changes that can happen by gene mutations.

New foods and novel foods

Each country can define a new food based on historical use and sometimes based on the year of introduction within their country based on clear documentation. In Europe, foods that were introduced before 1997 are not considered novel (Regulation EU, 2015). In the United States, food safety is regulated under the Code of Federal Regulations, title 21. In the US regulations, foods in common use in the American diet by 1958 are considered generally recognized as safe (GRAS). New foods are considered food additives unless they fall under the definition of GRAS (generally recognized as safe until 21, CFR 170.30). New ingredients after that date can be accepted as GRAS if they go through a science-based self-evaluation process that is strengthened by FDA review. The evaluation must consider safety and nutritional components. The process has become more formalized in the 1970s and 1980s as described in 21 CFR 170.35. An FDA determination responds to requests for review with a letter indicating there are questions to be answered or no questions remain. The US Food, Drug and Cosmetic Act (FD&C), section 201(f) indicates that food be produced, packaged, stored, and transported under sanitary conditions. It must also be properly labeled (Section 403). There are guidelines for the FDA to respond in restricted time that have gotten shorter since 2005 which are also posted on the US Food & Drug Administration website (www.fda.gov/food/generally-recognized-safe-gras/). The GRAS process was updated in 2016 (Federal Register vol 81, No. 159, August 17, 2016/Rules and Regulations).

Examples of whole new foods requiring safety evaluation

Food availability and safety challenges in a variety of countries today include the presence of mycotoxins in grain crops. The European Union and some other countries have tight standards for limiting levels of specific fumonisin levels while some maize producing countries in Africa do not have acceptable limits for domestic human consumption (WHO, Fumonisins, 2018: https://www.who.int/foodsafety/FSDigest_Fumonisins_EN.pdf). Due to grain mixing differences and differences in the use of grain for animal feed, ethanol production, and human foods, domestic human consumption in some countries includes levels of some mycotoxins above the accepted safe limits set by the WHO (Pinotti et al., 2016). Control of grain quality is evaluated at shipping points since farm-level measurements are not practical. The normal food production system means that some agricultural production countries end up accepting much higher levels of some mycotoxins which may put the local consumers at risk due to high levels in the foods than grains shipped to tightly controlled venues in Europe.

Introduction of algae, fungi, and insects as food sources

Consider a new food source, such as an alga that can be grown in ponds or closed laboratory like production facilities (Bleakley and Hayes, 2017). The history of safe human consumption is an important consideration, even for closely related species. *Chlorella* sp. and *Spirulina* sp. have been consumed as food primarily in Asia and in health food products in the United States (Fig. 2). Other algal species such as *Chlamydomonas reinhardtii* are being developed now and expect to be marketed as alternative food sources (Abdelmoteleb et al., 2021). However, the rules of timing for consumption in the United States and EU differ, and peer reviewed, verifiable use is important. Protein sequence comparisons to known allergens are difficult to interpret as there are many evolutionarily related species expressing some proteins with up to 70% overall identity to known minor allergens

Fourteen common food allergens sources that
must be labeled in europe

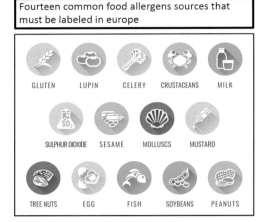

New food sources
must be evaluated for allergy
including: Algae or seaweed,
or insects

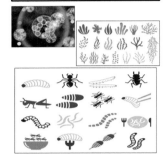

Fig. 2 Evaluating new food sources that are not recognized as GRAS must be evaluated, possibly using a similar process as for new GM proteins.

in databases such as www.AllergenOnline.org (Abdelmoteleb et al., 2021). That includes cyclophilins, heat shock proteins, profilins, and conserved enzymes. The abundance of the proteins and stability in pepsin may be useful in considering risk, but do not provide perfect correlations with risk.

Foods made from the cultured fungal mycoprotein called Quorn have been consumed for more than 30 years in the United Kingdom. The source species is *Fusarium venenatum*. There have been some consumer complaints as self-reported with 312 of 1752 judged as realistic and one was a fatal reaction described in one paper (Jacobson and DePorter, 2018). A recently described potential food product from a different species of the same genus (*Fusarium* strain flavolapis) is being developed using a different culture system. The developers have considered potential risks of allergenicity based on bioinformatics comparisons that show moderate sequence identity matches to a number of allergenic proteins of uncertain potency (Abdelmoteleb et al., 2021). Clearly, foods that contain species of these fungal lines must be labeled in the United States to enable those with an allergy to the fungus to avoid future consumption and reactions. However, as described, the bioinformatics findings were overpredictive of allergy (Abdelmoteleb et al., 2021).

The use of cultured insects such as cricket or mealworm for food products brings up the potential for broad cross-reactivity to shrimp and other important crustacean allergens (de Gier and Verhoeckx, 2018). Yet, insects of a wide variety of species have been consumed in many countries for centuries. Until recently the countries in the EU and United States have not used insects as a major protein or nutrient source. A company in the Netherlands has developed cultivation practices and food preparation for mealworms. Therefore scientists in the Netherlands have evaluated the potential risks of food allergy based on the assumption that some proteins in the mealworm are highly identical to shrimp tropomyosin and a few other allergens and that risks of food allergy could arise due to cross-reactivity. The subjects who were most at risk worked in the facility and had developed airway allergies to this species. Additionally, a few subjects with shrimp allergy shared IgE binding with the mealworm proteins and may have potential risks of allergy if they consume the mealworm in food. The source of feed for the insects may also present risks of allergy if the digestive tract of the insects is included in food and if they retain dietary proteins. Similar considerations should be evaluated for foods that would be made from crickets and other insects, but the primary risks are always to those with allergies to the source material. Risks of potential cross-reactivity are harder to judge accurately except for extremely high identity amino acid sequence matches, usually in evolutionarily related sources.

GM events should be considered along with questions of the safety of new products produced by other methods, and without demonstrated scientific evidence of increased food allergy, food toxicity, or environmental damage (Anderson et al., 2021). There are many differences of minor components in foods from the wide diversity of seed types used for all major crops in any country. Some are caused by random mutations or by hybrids of varieties that are distinct. Those varieties do not go through the same food safety evaluation process that is outlined by CODEX (2003, 2009). As the agronomic properties are judged acceptable by plant breeders, farmers, and food companies, they are generally accepted.

Conclusions

The need for innovation in agriculture is great. We are experiencing climate change and a growing population that is shrinking the available farmland. We have seen, in recent years, a steady decline in farmworkers in most countries. Many processed food companies are developing new and interesting ways to present and package foods. In general, food safety has improved markedly in the past 200 years, mostly due to sanitation and cooking practices. Because of global trade and global communications, the diversity of foods we eat in most countries has increased rapidly. Since agricultural production has become more industrialized and often more uniform across countries, the benefits are there and major risks are reduced, but the risks that are individualized such as food allergy and celiac disease have risen to capture the attention of most consumers. Part of that may be due to reduced exposure of individuals to some allergenic foods at an early age or due to exposure through the skin (Abrams et al., 2020). But those notions are hypothetical (Schroer et al., 2021). Importantly, the food safety evaluation process for GMOs and novel foods seems to be working in preventing epidemics of allergy and celiac disease.

Additional information

Additional information on genetic engineering, gene editing, and food safety can be viewed in references included at as Further Reading (Akhter et al., 2013; Chuanxu et al., 2020; da Graca, 1991; Davidson, 2008; El-Mounadi et al., 2020; FAO/WHO, 2001; Ferreira et al., 2002; Fu et al., 2017; Halbert and Manjunath, 2004; Islam et al., 2019; Joint FAO/WHO Expert Consultation, 1996; Kazan and Gardiner, 2018; Kumar et al., 2020; McCollum et al., 2016; Nester et al., 2002; Padgette et al., 1995, 1996; Palma et al., 2014; Peterson et al., 2018; Raybourne et al., 2003; Reddy and Nandula, 2012; Sidhu et al., 2000; Sun et al., 2019; Wang et al., 2020; Donnolly, 2020; Diaz et al., 2002).

References

Abdelmoteleb, M., Zhang, C., Furey, B., Kozubal, M., Griffiths, H., Champeaud, M., Goodman, R.E., 2021. Evaluating potential risks of food allergy of novel food sources based on comparison of proteins predicted from genomes compared to www.AllergenOnline.org. Food Chem. Toxicol. 147, 111888. https://doi.org/10.1016/j.fct.2020.111888.

Abrams, E.M., Chan, E.S., Sicherer, S., 2020. Peanut allergy: new advances and ongoing controversies. Pediatrics 145 (5). https://doi.org/10.1542/peds.2019-2102.

Anderson, J.A., Herman, R.A., Carlson, A., Mathesius, C., et al., 2021. Hypothesis-based food, feed and environmental safety assessment of GM crops: a case study using maize event DP-2-2216-6. GM Crops Food 12 (1), 282–291.

Assou, J., Zhang, D., Roth, K.D.R., Steinks, S., Hust, M., Reinard, T., Winkelmann, T., Boch, J., 2021. Removing the major allergen Bra j 1 from brown mustard (*Brassica juncea*) by CRISPR/Cas9. Plant J. https://doi.org/10.1111/tpj.15584.

Astwood, J.D., Leach, J.N., Fuchs, R.L., 1996. Stability of food allergens to digestion in vitro. Nat. Biotechnol. 14, 1269–1273.

Beyer, P., Al-Babili, S., Ye, X., Lucca, P., Scshaub, P., Welsch, R., Potrykus, I., 2002. Golden Rice: introducing the beta-carotene biosynthesis pathway into rice endosperm by genetic engineering to defeat vitamin A deficiency. J. Nutr. 132 (3), 506S–510S.

Biswas, P.S., Swamy, B.P.M., Kader, M.A., Hossain, M.A., Boncodin, R., Samia, M., Hassan, M.L., Wazuddin, M., MacKenzie, D., Reinke, R., 2021. Development and field evaluation of near-isogenic lines of GR2-EBRRI dhan29 Golden Rice. Front. Plant Sci. 12, 619739. https://doi.org/10.3389/fpls.2021.619739.eCollection.

Bleakley, S., Hayes, M., 2017. Algal proteins: extraction, application, and challenges concerning production. Foods 6 (5), 33. https://doi.org/10.3390/foods6050033.

Bogh, K.L., Madsen, C.B., 2016. Food allergens: is there a correlation between stability to digestion and allergenicity? Crit. Rev. Food Sci. Nutr. 56 (9), 1545–1567.

Burkhardt, P.K., Beyer, P., Wunn, J., Kloti, A., Armstrong, G.A., Schledz, M., von Lintig, J., Potrykus, I., 1997. Transgenic rice (*Orzyza sativa*) endosperm expressing daffodil (*Narcissus psedonarcissus*) phytoene synthase accumulates phytoene, a key intermediate of provitamin A biosynthesis. Plant J. 11 (5), 1071–1078.

CODEX Alimentarius, 2009. Foods Derived from Modern Biotechnology. World Health Organization and Food and Agriculture Organization of the United Nations, Rome, Italy.

CODEX CAC/GL 46-2003, 2003. Guideline for the Conduct of Food Safety Assessment of Foods Produced using Recombinant-DNA microorganisms.

De Gier, S., Verhoeckx, K., 2018. Insect (food) allergy and allergens. Mol. Immunol. 100, 82–106.

Delaney, B., Goodman, R.E., Ladics, G.S., 2018. Food and feed safety of genetically engineered food crops. Toxicol. Sci. 162 (2), 361–371.

Eiwegger, T., Hung, L., San Diego, K.E., O'Mahoney, L., Upton, J., 2019. Recent developments and highlights in food allergy. Allergy 74 (12), 2355–2367.

EPA, U.S, 1998. Reregistration Eligibility Decision (RED): Bacillus thuringiensis. U.S. Environmental Protection Agency, Washington, DC.

FDA, 1992. Federal Register Policy Statement on Foods Derived from New Plant Varieties. vol. 57. no. 104, May 29, 1992.

Federal Register volume 81, No. 159, August 17, 2016. Substances Generally Recognized as Safe.

Fu, T.J., Abbott, U.R., Hatzos, C., 2002. Digestibility of food allergens and nonallergenic proteins in simulated gastric and simulated intestinal fluid-a comparative study. J. Agric. Food Chem. 50 (24), 7154–7160.

Ghislain, M., Byarugaba, A.A., Magembe, E., Njoroge, A., Riverra, C., et al., 2019. Stacking three late blight resistance genes from wild species directly into African highland potato varieties confers complete field resistance to local blight races. Plant Biotechnol. J. 17 (6), 1119–1129.

Gonsalves, D., 1998. Control of papaya ringspot virus in papaya: a case study. Annu. Rev. Phytopathol. 36, 415–437.

Goodman, R.E., 2021. Allergen Databases for Food Safety of GMOs and Novel Foods. OpenAccessGovernment. https://edition.pagesuite-professional.co.uk/html5/reader/production/default.aspx?pubname=&edid=4349e4ed-4dd6-42e2-8cb8-e6b9bf436e0e.

Goodman, R.E., Vieths, S., Sampson, H.A., Hill, D., Ebisawa, M., Taylor, S.L., van Ree, R., 2008. Allergenicity assessment of genetically modified crops—what makes sense? Nat. Biotechnol. 26 (1), 73–81.

Goodman, R.E., Panda, R., Ariyarathna, H., 2013. Evaluation of endogenous allergens for the safety evaluation of genetically engineered food crops: review of potential risks, test methods, examples and relevance. J. Agric. Food Chem. 61, 8317–8332. https://doi.org/10.1021/jf400952y.

Goodman, R.E., Ebisawa, M., Ferreira, F., Sampson, H.A., van Ree, R., Vieths, S., Baumert, J.L., Bohle, B., Lalithambika, S., Wise, J., Taylor, S.L., 2016. AllergenOnline: a peer-reviewed, curated allergen database to assess novel food proteins for potential cross-reactivity. Mol. Nutr. Food Res. 60 (5), 1183–1198.

Habig, J.W., Rowland, A., Pence, M.G., Zhong, C.X., 2018. Food safety evaluation for R-proteins introduced by biotechnology: a case study of VNT1 in late blight protected potatoes. Reg. Toxicol. Pharmacol. 95, 66–74.

Hamim, I., Rwahnih, M.A., Borth, W.B., Suzuki, J.Y., Melzer, M.J., Wall, M.M., Green, J.C., Hu, J.S., 2019. Papaya ringspot virus isolates from papaya in Bangladesh: detection, characterization, and distribution. Plant Dis. 103 (11), 2920–2924.

Harlander, S.K., 2002. Safety assessments and public concern for genetically modified food products: the American view. Toxicol. Pathol. 30 (1), 132–134.

Herman, R.A., Price, W.D., 2013. Unintended compositional changes in genetically modified (GM) crops: 20 years of research. J. Agric. Food Chem. 61, 11695–11701.

Herman, R.A., Woolhiser, M.M., Ladics, G.S., Korjagin, V.A., Schafer, B.W., Storer, N.P., Green, S.B., Kan, L., 2007. Stability of a set of allergens and non-allergens in simulated gastric fluid. Int. J. Food Sci. Nutr. 58 (2), 125–141.

Hileman, R.E., Silvanovich, A., Goodman, R.E., Rice, E.A., Holleschak, G., Astwood, J.D., Hefle, S.L., 2002. Bioinformatics methods for allergenicity assessment using a comprehensive allergen database. Int. Arch. Allergy Immunol. 128 (4), 280–291.

Jacobson, M.F., DePorter, J., 2018. Self-reported adverse reactions associated with mycoprotein (Quorin-brand) containing foods. Ann. Allergy Asthma Immunol. 120 (6), 626–630.

Jin, Y., Goodman, R.E., Tetteh, A.O., Lu, M., Tripathi, L., 2017. Bioinformatics analysis to assess potential risks of allergenicity and toxicity of HRAP and PFLP proteins in genetically modified bananas resistant to Xanthomonas wilt disease. Food Chem. Toxicol. 109 (Pt. 1), 81–89. https://doi.org/10.1016/j.fct.2017.08.024.

Jouanin, A., Boyd, L., Visser, R.G.F., Smulders, M.J.M., 2018. Development of wheat with hypoimmunogenic gluten obstructed by the gene editing policy in Europe. Front. Plant Sci. 9, 1523. https://doi.org/10.3389/fpls/2018.01523.

Kotsonis, F.N., Mackey, M.A. (Eds.), 2002. Nutritional Toxicology, second ed. Taylor and Francis, London and New York.

Luthi, C., Alvarez-Alfageme, F., Ehlers, J.D., Higgins, T.J.V., Romeis, J., 2013. Resistance of αAI-1 transgenic chicpea (Cicer aretinum) and cowpea (Vigna uncuiculata) dry grains to bruchid beetles (Coleoptera: Chrysomelidae). Bull. Entomol. Res. 103 (4), 373–381.

McClintock, J.T., Schaffer, C.R., Sjoblad, R.D., 1995. A comparative review of the mammalian toxicity of Bacillus thuringiensis-based pesticides. Pestic. Sci. 45, 95–105.

NAS (National Academy of Sciences), 2018. A Review of the Citrus Greening Research and Development Efforts Supported by the Citrus Research and Development Foundation: Fighting a Ravaging Disease., https://doi.org/10.17226/25026. http://nap.edu/25026.

Nordlee, J.A., Taylor, S.L., Townsend, J.A., Thomas, L.A., Bush, R.K., 1996. Identification of a Brazil-nut allergen in transgenic soybeans. N. Engl. J. Med. 334 (11), 688–692. https://doi.org/10.1056/NEJM199603143341103.

Ofori-Anti, A.O., Ariyarathna, H., Chen, L., Lee, H.L., Pramod, S.N., Goodman, R.E., 2008. Establishing objective detection limits for the pepsin digestion assay used in the assessment of genetically modified foods. Regul. Toxicol. Pharmacol. 52 (2), 94–203.

Paine, J.A., Shipton, C.A., Chaggar, S., Howells, R.M., Kennedy, M.J., Vernon, G., Wright, S.Y., Hinchliffe, E., Adams, J.L., Silverstone, A.L., Drake, R., 2005. Improving the nutritional value of Golden Rice through increased pro-vitamin a content. Nat. Biotechnol. 23, 482–487.

Palazzola, L., Gianazza, E., Eberini, I., 2020. Literature Search—Exploring in Silico Protein Toxicity Prediction Methods to Support the Food and Feed Risk Assessment. EFSA Supporting Publication 2020: EN-1875. 89 pp, https://doi.org/10.2903/sp.efsa.2020.EN-1875.

Panda, R., Ariyarathna, H., Amnuaycheewa, P., Tetteh, A., Pramod, S.N., Taylor, S.L., Ballmer-Weber, B.K., Goodman, R.E., 2013. Challenges in testing genetically modified crops for potential increases in endogenous allergen expression for safety. Allergy 68 (2), 142–151. https://doi.org/10.1111/all.12076.

Peprah, B.B., Parkes, E., Manu-Aduening, J., Kulakow, P., van Biljon, A., Labuschagne, M., 2020. Genetic variability, stability and heritability for quality and yield to improve yield characteristics in provitamin A cassava varieties. Euphytica 216 (2), 31. https://doi. org/10.1007/s10681-020-2562-7.

Petrick, J.S., Bell, E., Koch, M.S., 2020. Weight of the evidence: independent research projects confirm industry conclusions on the safety of insect-protected maize MON 810. GM Crops Food 11 (1), 30–46.

Pinotti, L., Ottoboni, M., Giromini, C., Dell'Orto, V., Cheli, F., 2016. Mycotoxin contamination in the EU feed supply chain: a focus on cereal byproducts. Toxins 8, 45. https:// doi.org/10.3390/toxins8020045.

Retraction, 2015. Retraction of Tang G, Hu Y, Yin S-a, Wang Y, Dallal GE, Grusak MA, and Russell RM. β-Carotene in Golden Rice is as good as β-carotene in oil at providing vitamin A to children. Am J Clin Nutr 2012;96:658–64. American Journal of Clinical Nutrition 102 (3). https://doi.org/10.3945/ajcn.114.093229. 715-715.

Saleem, A.S., Ali, Z., Yeh, S.D., Saeed, W., Binat Imdad, A., Akbar, M.F., Goodman, R.E., Naseem, S., 2021. Genetic variability and evolutionary dynamics of atypical papaya ringspot virus infecting papaya. PLoS One 16 (10), e0258298. https://doi.org/10.1371/ journal.pone.o258298.

Sanders, P.R., Lee, T.C., Growth, M.E., Astwood, J.D., Fuchs, R.L., 1998. Safety assessment of insect-rotected corn. In: Thomas, J.A. (Ed.), Biotechnology and Safety Assessment. Taylor and Francis, New York, NY, pp. 241–256.

Santos, A.F., Alpan, O., Hoffmann, H.-J., 2021. Basophil activation tests: mechanisms and consideration for use in clinical trials and clinical practice. Allergy 76 (8), 2420–2432.

Schroer, B., Groetch, M., Mack, D.P., Venter, C., 2021. Practical challenges and considerations for early introduction of potential allergens for prevention of food allergy. J Allergy Clin Immunol Pract 9 (1), 44–56. https://doi.org/10.1016/j.jaip.2020.10.031.

Silvanovich, A., Bannon, G., McClain, S., 2009. The use of E-scores to determine the quality of protein alignments. Regul. Toxicol. Pharmacol. 54, S26–S31.

Singerman, Ariel, Rogers, M, 2020. The Economic Challenges of Dealing with Citrus Greening: The Case of Florida. Journal of Pest Management 11 (1), 1–7. https://doi. org/10.1093/jipm/pmz037.

Siruguri, V., Bharatraj, D.K., Vankudavath, R.N., Mendu, V.V., Gupta, V., Goodman, R.E., 2015. Evaluation of Bar, Barnase, and Barstar recombinant proteins expressed in genetically engineered Brassica juncea (Indian mustard) for potential risks of food allergy using bioinformatics and literature searches. Food Chem. Toxicol. 83, 93–102.

Swamy, B.P.M., Samia, M., Boncodin, R., Marundan, S., Rebong, D.B., Ordonio, R.L., Miranda, R.T., Rebong, A.T.O., Alibuyog, A.Y., Adeva, C.C., Reinke, R., MacKenzie, D.J., 2019. Compositional analysis of genetically engineered GR2E "Goden Rice" in comparison to that of conventional rice. J. Agric. Food Chem. 67 (28), 7986–7994.

Swamy, M.B.P., Maundan, S., Samia, M., Ordonio, R.L., Rebong, D.B., Miranda, R., Alibuyog, A., Rebong, A.T., Tabil, M.A., Suralta, R.R., Alfonso, A.A., Biswas, P.S., Kader, M.A., Reinke, R.F., Boncodin, R., MacKenzie, D.J., 2021. Development and characterization of GR2E Golden rice introgression lines. Sci. Rep. 11 (1), 2496. https://doi. org/10.1038/s41598-021-82001-0.

Tang, G, Qin, J, Dolnikowski, GG, Russell, RM, Grusak, MA, 2009. Golden Rice is an effective source of vitamin A. Am J Clin Nutr 89 (6), 1776–1783. https://doi.org/10.3945/ ajcn.2008.27119.

Tang, G., et al., 2012. Retraction of β-Carotene in Golden Rice is as good as β-carotene in oil at providing vitamin A to children. Am. J. Nutr. 102, 715.

Taylor, M.L., Hartnell, G.F., Riordan, S.G., Nemeth, M.A., Karuanandaa, K., George, B., Astood, J.D., 2003. Comparison of broiler performance when fed diets containing grain from YieldGard (MON810), YieldGard x roundup ready (GA21), nontransgenic control or commercial corn. Poult. Sci. 82, 823–830.

The European Parliament and the Council of the European Union, 2015. Regulation (EU) 2015/2283 of the European Parliament and of the Council of 25 November 2015. https://eur-lex.europa.eu/legal-content/EN/TXT/PDF/?uri=CELEX:32015R2283. (Accessed 25 November 2015).

Thomas, K., Aalbers, M., Bannon, G.A., Bartels, M., Dearman, R.J., Esdaile, D.J., Fu, T.J., Glatt, C.M., Hadfield, N., Hatzos, C., Hefle, S.L., Heylings, J.R., Goodman, R.E., Henry, B., Herouet, C., Holsapple, M., Ladics, G.S., Landry, T.D., MacIntosh, S.C., Rice, E.A., Privalle, L.S., Steiner, H.Y., Teshima, R., van Ree, R., Woolhiser, M., Zawodny, J., 2004. A multi-laboratory evaluation of a common in vitro pepsin digestion assay protocol used in assessing the safety of novel proteins. Regul. Toxicol. Pharmacol. 39 (2), 87–98. https://doi.org/10.1016/j.yrtph.2003.11.003.

van Hage, M., Hamsten, C., Valenta, R., 2017. ImmunoCAP assays: pros and cons in allergology. J. Allergy Clin. Immunol. 140 (4), 974–977.

Verhoeckx, K., Bogh, K.L., Dupont, D., Egger, L., Gadermaier, G., Larre, C., Mackie, A., Menard, O., Adel-Patient, K., Picariello, G., Portmann, R., Smit, J., Turner, P., Untersmayr, E., Epstein, M.M., 2019. The relevance of a digestibility evaluation in the allergenicity risk assessment of novel proteins. Opinion of a joint initiative of COST action ImpARAS and COST action INFOGEST. Food Chem. Toxicol. 129, 405–423.

Wang, N., Stelinski, L.L., Pez-Stelinski, K.S., Graham, J.H., Zhang, Y., 2017. Tale of the huanglongbing disease pyramid in the context of the citrus microbiome. Phytopathology 107 (4), 380–387. https://doi.org/10.1094/PHYTO-12-16-0426-RVW.

WHO Fumonisins, 2018. Food Safety Digest. https://www.who.int/foodsafety/FSDigest_Fumonisins_EN.pdf.

Wu, Z., Mo, C., Zhang, S., Li, H., 2018. Characterization of papaya ringspot virus isolates infecting transgenic papaya 'Huanong no. 1' in South China. Sci. Rep. 8 (1), 8206. https://doi.org/10.1038/s41598-018-26596-x.

Further reading

Akhter, M.S., Basavaraj, Y.B., Akanda, A.M., Mandal, B., Jain, R.K., 2013. Genetic diversity based on coat protein of papaya ringspot virus (Pathotype P) isolates from Bangladesh. Indian J. Virol. 24 (1), 70–73.

Chuanxu, L., Zhang, J., Ren, Z., Xie, R., et al., 2020. Development of multiresistance rice by an assembly of herbicide, insect and disease resistance genes with transgene stacking system. Pest Manag. Sci. 77 (3), 1536–1547.

da Graca, J.V., 1991. Citrus greening disease. Annu. Rev. Phytopathol. 29, 109–136.

Davidson, S.N., 2008. Forbidden fruit: transgenic papaya in Thailand. Plant Physiol. 147 (2), 487–493.

Diaz, C., Fernandez, C., McDonald, R., Yeung, J.M., 2002. Determination of cry 9C protein in processed foods made with StarLink corn. J. AOAC Int. 85 (5), 1070–1076.

Donnolly, J., 2020. The Great Irish Famine. https://learningintheopen.org/2020/11/12/the-great-famine-jim-donnelly/.

El-Mounadi, K., Morales-Floriano, M.L., Garcia-Ruiz, H., 2020. Principles, applications, and biosafety of plant genome editing using CRISPR-Cas9. Front. Plant Sci. https://doi.org/10.3389/fpls.2020.00056.

FAO/WHO, 2001. Evaluation of Allergenicity of Genetically Modified Foods. Report of a Joint FAO/WHO Expert Consultation on Allergenicity of Foods Derived from Biotechnology. 22–25 January 2001. Rome, Italy.

Ferreira, S.A., Pitz, K.Y., Manshardt, R., Zee, F., et al., 2002. Virus coat protein transgenic papaya provides practical control of papaya ringspot virus in Hawaii. Plant Dis. 86 (2), 101–105.

Fu, Y., Wu, Y., Yuan, Y., Gao, M., 2017. Complete genome sequence of bacillus thuringiensis Serovar rongseni reference strain SCG04-02, a strain toxic to *Plutella xylostella*. Am. Soc. Microbiol. 5 (39), e00691-17.

Halbert, S.E., Manjunath, K.L., 2004. Asian citrus psyllids (Sternorrhyncha: Psyllidae) and greening disease of citrus: a literature review and assessment of risk in Florida. Fla. Entomol. 87 (3), 330–353.

Islam, M.N., Ali, M.S., Choi, S.-J., Hyun, J.-W., Baek, K.-H., 2019. Biocontrol of citrus canker disease caused by *Xanthomonas citri* subsp. *citri* using an endophytic Bacillus thuringiensis. Plant Pathol. J. 35 (5), 486–497.

Joint FAO/WHO Expert Consultation, 1996. Joint FAO/WHO Expert Consultation on Biotechnology and Food Safety, Rome, Italy, 30 Sept to 4 October.

Kazan, K., Gardiner, D.M., 2018. Transcriptomics of cereal-*Fusarium graminearum* interactions: what we have learned so far. Mol. Plant Pathol. 19 (3), 764–778.

Kumar, K., Gambhir, G., Dass, A., Tripathi, A.K., Singh, A., Jha, A.K., et al., 2020. Genetically modified crops: current status and future prospects. Planta 251, 91. https://doi.org/10.1007/soo425-020-03372-8.

McCollum, G., Hilf, M., Irey, M., Luo, W., Gottwald, T., 2016. Susceptibility of sixteen citrus genotypes to 'Candidatus Liberibacter *asiaticus*'. Plant Dis. 100 (6), 1080–1086.

Nester, E.W., Thomashow, L.S., Metz, M., Gordon, M., 2002. 100 Years of *Bacillus thuringiensis*: A Critical Scientific Assessment. American Society for Microbiology, Washington, DC.

Padgette, S.R., Kolacz, K.H., Delannay, D.B., Re, J.B., et al., 1995. Development, identification and characterization of glyphosate-tolerant soybean line. Crop Sci. 35, 1451–1461.

Padgette, S.R., Taylor, N.B., Nida, D.L., Bailey, M.R., et al., 1996. The composition of glyphosate-tolerant soybean seeds is equivalent to that of conventional soybeans. J. Nutr. 126, 702–716.

Palma, L., Munoz, D., Berry, C., Murillo, J., Caballero, P., 2014. Bacillus thuringiensis toxins: an overview of their biocidal activity. Toxins 6 (12), 3296–32325.

Peterson, M.A., Collavo, A., Overjero, R., Shivram, V., Walsh, M., 2018. The challenge of herbicide resistance around the world. Current summary. Pest Manag. Sci. 74 (10), 2246–2259.

Raybourne, R.B., Williams, K.M., Vogt, R., Reissman, D.B., Winterton, B.S., Rubin, C., 2003. Development and use of an ELISA test to detect IgE antibody to Cry9C following possible exposure to bioengineered corn. Int. Arch. Allergy Immunol. 132 (4), 322–328.

Reddy, K.N., Nandula, V.K., 2012. Herbicide resistant crops: history, development and current technologies. Indian J. Agron. 57 (1), 1–7.

Sidhu, R.S., Hammond, B.G., Fuchs, R.L., Mutz, J., et al., 2000. Glyphosate-tolerant corn: the composition and feeding value of grain from glyphosate-tolerant corn is equivalent to that of conventional corn (Zea mays L.). J. Agric. Food Chem. 48, 2305–2312.

Sun, L., Nasrullah, K.F., Nie, Z., Wang, P., Xu, J., 2019. Citrus genetic engineering for disease resistance: past, present and future. Int. J. Mol. Sci. 20, 5256. https://doi.org/10.3390/ijms20215256.

Wang, H., Sun, S., Ge, W., Zhao, L., Hou, B., Wang, K., Lyu, Z., et al., 2020. Horizontal gene transfer of Fhb7 from fungus underlies fusarium head blight resistance in wheat. Science 368 (6493). https://doi.org/10.1126/science.aba5435.

CHAPTER 13

History of global food safety, foodborne illness, and risk assessment

Benjamin M. Liu[a,b,c,d]

[a]Division of Pathology and Laboratory Medicine, Children's National Hospital, Washington, DC, United States
[b]Departments of Pediatrics, Pathology, and Microbiology, Immunology & Tropical Medicine, George Washington University School of Medicine and Health Sciences, Washington, DC, United States
[c]The Center for Genetic Medicine Research, Children's National Research Institute, Washington, DC, United States
[d]The District of Columbia Center for AIDS Research, Washington, DC, United States

Brief history of food, foodborne illness, and toxicology

Generally speaking, food is any substance that can be consumed to provide nutritional sustenance for a living organism (Abuajah et al., 2015). Food is usually of plant, animal, or fungal origin and possesses essential nutrients, for instance, carbohydrates, fats, proteins, vitamins, and/or minerals. The substance/food is ingested and assimilated to provide energy, maintain life, and/or stimulate growth. Nutritional sustenance is common and necessary for the survival of all living organisms. Human history is full of interesting examples of poisoning by ingestion, both intentional and unintentional. For instance, the Chinese Emperor Qin Shi Huang died from ingesting mercury pills in an attempt to make himself immortal (Wexler, 2015). History is also full of examples of the use of knowledge of toxic effects for murder, aphrodisiac, or narcotic effects. Thus there has long been some sense of risk with "Don't eat that, or …."

In contrast, food, throughout human history, has also been reported to have medical properties (Estes, 1996). A variety of foodstuffs were believed, for many centuries, to have specific therapeutic or healing attributes. The application of functional components of food in the treatment and prevention of diseases has been documented in written form dating back to biblical times and even earlier (Abuajah et al., 2015; Greenway, 2020). These functional components have shown the potential to provide physiological

History of Food and Nutrition Toxicology
https://doi.org/10.1016/B978-0-12-821261-5.00013-1

benefits and promote well-being via acting simultaneously at different or identical target sites. Reported effects include reducing the risk of cancer, cardiovascular disease, osteoporosis, inflammation, type II diabetes, and other chronic degenerative diseases, lowering blood cholesterol, neutralization of reactive oxygen species and charged radicals, anticarcinogenic effect, and low-glycemic response (Abuajah et al., 2015).

Consuming foods contaminated with disease-causing pathogens, such as bacteria, fungi, viruses, or even parasites, can cause foodborne illnesses, which is referred to as food poisoning (Parmet et al., 2003). Although reported worldwide but more commonly found in developing countries, foodborne illnesses are also an issue adversely affecting the health and life quality in developed countries. For example, in 1999 it was estimated that there were 5000 deaths in the United States related to foodborne pathogens (Morris, 2011). The organisms that most commonly cause foodborne illnesses include *Campylobacter*, *Clostridium perfringens*, *Escherichia coli*, *Listeria*, Norovirus, and *Salmonella* (Foodsafety.gov, n.d.). Among those issues responsible for food poisoning, raw, unwashed, or undercooked foods being contaminated with pathogens have the greatest risk. Foodborne illnesses may manifest with typical symptoms, including nausea, vomiting, diarrhea, abdominal cramps, and even fever. All populations are vulnerable to foodborne illnesses. However, infants, the elderly, and immunocompromised people with diabetes, cancer, or AIDS are some of the most susceptible. In some cases, foodborne illness may lead to severe complications, such as hemolytic uremic syndrome, a combination of anemia, profuse bleeding, and kidney failure (Parmet et al., 2003). However, most foodborne illnesses are preventable if the food is processed and washed properly to remove disease-causing pathogens.

With the advent of new technologies commonly used in biological and medical research (Liu et al., 2018, 2019, 2020; CDC, n.d.; LeMessurier et al., 2020; Peng et al., 2015; Liu, 2017), especially molecular methods, a variety of novel assays have been employed to investigate foodborne disease outbreaks. PulseNet USA is the molecular surveillance network for foodborne disease in the United States, which consists of state and local public health laboratories, as well as food regulatory agencies (Tolar et al., 2019). PulseNet has standardized protocols to perform pulsed-field gel electrophoresis (PFGE) and whole genome sequencing (WGS) and to analyze the results using standardized software. The Center for Disease Control and Prevention (CDC) and its public health partners in all 50 states have implemented PFGE and now WGS to detect, investigate, and stop outbreaks and combat drug-resistant bacteria (CDC, n.d.). The PulseNet's organism-specific databases provide a central storage location for molecular and demographic data related to an isolate. Sequences from investigations are obtained and compared in the databases, thereby facilitating the rapid detection of clusters of foodborne diseases that may represent widespread outbreaks. WGS information has been used to investigate and solve outbreaks caused by *Listeria*, *Salmonella*, *Campylobacter*, and disease-causing *E. coli* (CDC, n.d.). WGS genotyping data also allow for analysis of antibiotic resistance and virulence profiles after being uploaded in real time to the PulseNet databases, which will continue to be beneficial to the improvement of food safety surveillance activities (Tolar et al., 2019).

Food toxicology has a long history and its origins may trace back to primitive humans (Ybañez and Montoro, 1996). Food toxicology copes with the substances that can be detected in food that, when consumed, may cause harm to the consumers (Tsatsakis et al., 2018; Choudhuri et al., 2019). Toxic substances can be naturally occurring ingredients (toxins) that are added when the food is prepared, any chemical substance (toxicant) that is formed during cooking, man-made additives that are added directly to food, or any components that come from the immediate environment, such as packaging (Lane, 2014; Kruger et al., 2014). The practice of food toxicology covers the detection of toxic substances in food, characterization of their physical and chemical properties, the study of their fate in the body (absorption, distribution, metabolism, and excretion), and the investigation of their adverse health effects (Choudhuri et al., 2019). Food toxicology has a variety of subdisciplines and has received increasing public attention in recent years as the demand for food safety increases with greater public awareness. This is especially true with worldwide web-based media coverage of food safety issues, foodborne illness, and increased awareness of the health benefits of foods, as well as the rapid availability of information to consumers.

Food safety regulations in selected global regions

Food is a complex mixture, including animals, plants, and microorganisms. Industrially processed foods include these basic materials with additional ingredients added to the food for a specific effect or enhancement of the material, including coloring. Advances in food science and technology have given the global food industry the tools needed to substantially increase food production. However, with a projected global population approaching

10 billion by 2050, even more advanced technology will be needed to keep pace. Food safety is a major public health issue, especially in heavily populated countries (Hayes et al., 2016; Beck et al., 2014; He and Shi, 2021). In developed countries, there are established standards for food handling, preparation, storage, and delivery. In contrast, however, in some developing countries, such standards may be limited often with less enforcement. The following section discusses food safety regulations in several countries and regions.

Food safety regulation in the United States

Food systems in the 1900s were rapidly changing as the US population grew, increasing urbanization occurred, large-scale food production increased, and food imports and exports grew in volume and value. In 1906 Harvey Wiley of the US Department of Agriculture influenced the passing of the Pure Food and Drug Act, the first US food regulation to address adulteration of food (Gad, n.d.). Although this legislation had the burden to prove adulteration, it did not have the intended effect of stopping the unsafe manufacturing and sale of food with impure or deleterious ingredients. In 1908 shortly after the passage of the Pure Food and Drug Act, the Agriculture and Food Chemistry Division (AGFD) within the Department of Agriculture was formed under the leadership of Dr. Wiley (Armstrong, 2009).

In 1938 the US Congress passed the Federal Food, Drug, and Cosmetic Act (FDCA), which was the beginning of modern food regulations in the United States (Armstrong, 2009). FDCA established that manufacturers must prove the safety of their products with a clear definition of the identity (ingredients) of the product, standards of quality of the product, and standards of the container. Food additives were organized under the act into three main categories: (1) direct or indirect additives, (2) natural components, and (3) potential contaminants. This act has been amended multiple times to keep pace with developments in the food industry. For example, the Food Additives Amendment was enacted in 1958 to further control substances added to food (Armstrong, 2009), and the Food Safety Modernization Act (FSMA) in 2011 enables the US Food and Drug Administration (US FDA) to better protect public health by strengthening the food safety system from farm to table.

In the United States, different federal government agencies play different roles in ensuring food safety. For example, the US FDA oversees federal requirements to prohibit false or misleading food labels. The Federal Trade Commission enforces the prohibition against false or misleading advertising. USDA Food Safety and Inspection Service regulates aspects of the safety and labeling of poultry, certain egg products, and traditional meats. Environmental Protection Agency (EPA) ensures the safety of drinking water and regulates the use of pesticides that can contaminate drinking water and/or leave pesticide residue on food.

Food safety regulation in Canada

A range of regulations is set out in Canada to ensure health and safety, which include the Food and Drug Act (FDA), Safe Food for Canadians Act, and Consumer Packaging and Labelling Act (chfa, n.d.). As the primary legislation for food in Canada, the FDA regulates laws on food labeling, advertising, and claims, and set up food standards and compositional requirements for foods for special dietary uses, food additives, chemical and microbial hazards, veterinary drug residues, packaging material, and pesticides. The FDA enforces honest food labeling, advertising, and claims and adherence to regulations on food labeling. The FDA ensures that truthful but not misleading information is presented to Canadians who may make informed food decisions. Nutrition and health claims must be scientifically validated and constructed to provide the consumer with meaningful information for a purchase decision (https://chfa.ca/en/Regulatory/Food-Regulations).

Three federal government departments—Health Canada, the Canadian Food Inspection Agency (CFIA), and Agriculture and Agri-Food Canada (AAFC)—play complementary roles in developing, enforcing, and interpreting policies and guidance stemming from the FDA and its Food and Drug Regulations (FDR). Health Canada (https://www.canada.ca/en/health-canada.html) is the agency that sets up standards for the nutritional quality and safety of all foods sold in Canada. The Food Directorate, within the Health Products and Food Branch, is responsible for managing the health benefits and risks of food products by evaluating scientific evidence and developing and implementing requirements under the FDA and its associated policies and standards. This mandate is exercised under the authority of the FDA, whose regulatory mandate is enforced under the FDR. The function of CFIA is to enforce health and safety standards outlined in the FDA and its associated regulations; mitigate risks to food safety; and administer non-health and safety regulations regarding packaging, labeling, and advertising (https://inspection.canada.ca). AAFC is responsible for ensuring innovative food products are safely integrated into the marketplace, and for providing information and support, and helping the industry understand regulatory requirements associated with the FDA (https://agriculture.canada.ca).

Food safety regulation in the European Union

The European Food Safety Authority (EFSA) was established in 2002 and is the European Union (EU) agency that provides advice on safety and risks associated with food (EU, n.d.). EFSA cooperates with the national food safety authorities of the 28 member states, Iceland and Norway, as well as observers from Switzerland and EU candidate countries. Food legislation mandated by the EU parliament must be incorporated into individual countries' national legislation within a certain period of time. Individual member states may also have other laws, regulations, and controls concerning food safety if these laws do not prevent trade with other member states. For example, there is the Beer Purity Law of 1516 that is still in force but only in Germany.

Examples of member country food safety agency include Agence nationale de sécurité sanitaire de l'alimentation, de l'environnement et du travail (ANSES), the French governmental agency that deals with food safety. ANSES was created in 2010 with the merger of the French Food Safety Agency and the French Agency for Environmental and Occupational Health Safety. Another example is the Federal Ministry of Food and Agriculture (BMEL) of the Federal Republic of Germany (German Federal Ministry of Food, Agriculture and Consumer Protection, n.d.). It was founded as the Federal Ministry of Food, Agriculture, and Foresting in 1949.

Since December 13, 2014, based on the EU Food Information for Consumers Regulation 1169/2011, food businesses have been required to provide allergy information on food sold unpackaged, in catering outlets, deli counters, bakeries, and sandwich bars (Food Standards Agency, n.d.). The so-called Natasha's Law was added to the 2014 legislation and came into force on October 1 of that year, following the death of Natasha Ednan-Laperouse who tragically died after eating a sandwich containing the allergen sesame. As a result of this legislation, individual ingredient labeling is required for foods prepacked on the premise for direct sale (thesaferfoodgroup, n.d.).

Food safety regulation in Australia and New Zealand

Food Standards Australia New Zealand (FSANZ) develops food standards for Australia and New Zealand. The food standards are enforced by state and territory departments, agencies, and local councils. The Ministry for Primary Industries in New Zealand and the Australian Department of Agriculture and Water Resources regulate imported foods. FSANZ requires food safety systems to be implemented in all food businesses (https://www.foodstandards.gov.au). The food safety systems are adopted to ensure food safety for consumers and to decrease the incidence of food poisoning, which includes basic food safety training for at least one person in each business.

The Council of Australian Governments (COAG) Industry and Skills Council agreed to new regulatory standards for training providers and regulators—the Standards for Registered Training Organizations (RTOs) 2015. Food safety training can be delivered in various forms by different organizations, for instance, RTOs. After the food safety training, staff in food businesses are issued a nationally recognized certificate containing competency codes (https://www.foodstandards.gov.au).

Basic food safety training covers the following items (https://www.foodstandards.gov.au): (1) recognition of the hazards that are associated with the main types of food and the procedures that can be implemented to prevent the growth of bacteria that can cause food poisoning and to prevent foodborne illness; (2) addressing potential problems that can be linked with food product packaging such as leaks and damage to vacuum packs, compromised packaging, pest infestation, as well as any pest-associated problems and disease spread; (3) safe food handling and processing, which includes safe procedures for each process in the food production, for instance, receiving, cooking, cooling, reheating, food storage, preparation, repacking, displaying products, handling products when serving customers, packaging, cleaning and sanitizing, pest control, transport, and delivery. Safe food handling and processing also cover potential causes of cross-contamination; (4) special attention is paid to customers who are particularly at risk of foodborne illness, as well as those who have allergies or intolerance; (5) correct cleaning and sanitizing procedures, cleaning products, and their correct use, and the storage of cleaning items such as brushes, mops, and cloths; (6) personal hygiene, hand washing, illness, and protective clothing.

Food safety regulation in selected Asian countries and regions

Foodborne diseases caused by microbial pathogens are believed to be the predominant food safety issues in China. The management of microbial food safety in China can be divided into three stages: before 2000, 2000–09, and from 2010 to the present (He and Shi, 2021). Before 2000, China's main food concern was focused on food security and then gradually shifted to food safety. After that, food safety gained increasing attention since several foodborne outbreaks were identified. Most of the steps involved with food production are overseen by the Chinese government, including agricultural production, the manufacture of food packaging, containers, chemical additives, drug production, and business regulation. From 2000 to 2009, although chemical food safety was considered a priority issue during this stage, the initiation of foodborne pathogen surveillance highlighted the significance of microbial food safety, followed by the establishment of a national food contamination monitoring system in 2000 and the promulgation of the China Food Safety Law in 2009. Food quality, safety, and integrity are governed by the People's Republic of China (PRC) Food Safety Law (2015) and its implementing regulations (gov.cn, n.d.).

Microbial food safety has been listed as a high priority supported by many national food safety policies. A national foodborne disease molecular tracing network was launched accordingly. Comprehensive statutory requirements are set out by the PRC Food Safety Law, which governs the production, circulation, recall, and import/export of food products in China. Since the creation of the State Food and Drug Administration in 2003, the Chinese government has attempted to consolidate food regulation to reduce food safety problems. At the same time, media coverage and advancement in food safety education and research supported by central and local governments play important roles in addressing and solving microbial food safety problems in China (He and Shi, 2021).

In Hong Kong Special Administrative Regions (SAR) of China, the Food and Environmental Hygiene Department (FEHD) is responsible for food hygiene and environmental hygiene, and for ensuring safe and fit food is sold for consumption (www.fehd.gov.hk). It replaced part of the role of the Urban Council and the Urban Services Department, and the Regional Council and the Regional Services Department. The Centre for Food Safety is the food safety authority under FEHD, whose mission is to ensure that food is safe and fit for consumption through tripartite collaboration among the government, food trade, and consumers (https://www.fehd.gov.hk/english/food_safety/index.html).

The basic food law in Hong Kong SAR is laid down in Part V of the Public Health and Municipal Services Ordinance (Cap. 132). The main provisions cover general protection for food purchasers, offenses in connection with the sale of unfit food and adulterated food, composition, labeling of food, food hygiene, and seizure and destruction of unfit food. As a food law in Hong Kong, the Food Safety Ordinance (Cap. 612) provides new food safety control measures, including a registration scheme for food importers and food distributors and a requirement for food traders to maintain proper records of the movements of food to enhance food traceability. The Food Safety Ordinance (Cap. 612) empowers the authorities to set out regulations to tighten import control on specific food types and prohibit the import and supply of problem food and order the recall of such food (https://www.cfs.gov.hk/english/food_leg/food_leg.html).

In South Korea, the Korea Food and Drug Administration (KFDA) has been working for food safety since 1945. It has been renamed the Ministry of Food and Drug Safety (MFDS; https://www.mfds.go.kr/eng/index.do) and is the government agency that is responsible for ensuring the safety and efficiency of foods; offering people safe drugs, medical devices, and cosmetics; and supporting the development of the food and pharmaceutical industries, thereby promoting public health (https://www.mfds.go.kr/). MFDS has a series of procedures to ensure food safety, including the Food Safety Management System, Safety Management of Health Functional Food, and Management of Standards and Criteria. In South Korea, food contact materials and articles are regulated under the Food Sanitation Act. The regulation of food contact materials and articles is carried out under the Food Sanitation Act, which prohibits the use or presence of toxic and/or harmful chemicals in food contact containers, utensils, and packaging materials that could endanger human health.

The Food Safety and Standards Authority of India (FSSAI) is a statutory body established under the Ministry of Health & Family Welfare, Government of India and was established under the Food Safety and Standards Act, 2006, a consolidating statute related to food safety and regulation in India (https://www.fssai.gov.in). This agency is the regulating body that is responsible for developing the standards of food and other issues related to food safety and protecting and promoting public health through the regulation and supervision of food safety. The FSSAI has its headquarters in New Delhi and 6 regional offices located in Delhi, Guwahati, Mumbai, Kolkata, Cochin, and Chennai; 14 referral laboratories notified by FSSAI; 72 State/UT laboratories located throughout India; and 112 accredited private laboratories notified by FSSAI. FSSAI follows a dynamic process to develop standards based on the latest developments in food science, food consumption patterns, new food products, and additives. Changes in processing technology have led to changed specifications, advancements in food analytical methods, and the identification of new risks or other regulatory options (Nuffoods Spectrum, n.d.).

History of risk assessment in food safety

The concept of risk and risk assessments has a long history, possibly originating more than 2400 years ago when the Athenians offered their concept of assessing risk before making decisions (Bernstein, 1996). However, risk assessment and risk management as a scientific field is a young discipline with no more than a few decades of history (Aven, 2016). Risk assessment is a process with the combined effort to identify and analyze potential events that may adversely impact individuals, populations, assets, and/or the environment (i.e., hazard analysis) and make judgments on the tolerability of the risk based on a risk analysis while considering influencing factors (i.e., risk evaluation) (Rausand, 2013; Manuele, 2016). By performing a risk assessment, one can determine possible mishaps, their likelihood and consequences, and the tolerances for such events, which can be developed into a broader risk management strategy to help reduce potential risk-related consequences.

Food safety in the United States has long been a concern (Lehman and Fitzhugh, 1954; Dorne and Renwick, 2005; Dourson and Stara, 1983; Jiang et al., 2022; National Research Council, 1983). The assessment of the safety of foods traces back to the first comprehensive regulations for the control of food safety in the 1906 Food, Drug and Cosmetic (FD&C) Act (US FDA) (Brock et al., 2003). The US Congress passed, and President Roosevelt signed, the Pure Food and Drug Act and the Meat Inspection Act to regulate food safety at the federal level (Wu and Rodricks, 2020). Modern agricultural and other practices continue to increase the risk of chemical exposures, which has resulted in major amendments to federal food laws, one of the most controversial being the Delaney Clause aimed specifically at cancer-causing chemicals (Wu and Rodricks, 2020).

Moreover, the publication of Rachel Carson's *Silent Spring* in 1962 documented the environmental harm caused by the indiscriminate use of pesticides and brought environmental concerns to the American public (en.wikipedia, n.d.). Following the publication of *Silent Spring*, a decade of political activism in the United States resulted in the enactment of major laws to set legally enforceable limits on human exposure to chemicals in the workplace and contaminating the general environment (National Research Council, 1983; Rodricks, 2013; Merrill, 2001). These laws added to a host of laws that had been enacted in the pre-*Silent Spring* era that enforced the regulation of chemicals used in foods, drugs, and consumer products (Rodricks, 2013; Merrill, 2001). Increasing public attention was attracted to the problems that public health and regulatory officials had been struggling with since the passage of the first federal law mandating the protection of people from unsafe exposures to the products of the chemical industry: the Pure Food and Drug Act of 1906 (Rodricks, 2013; Merrill, 2001). The new environmental and occupational health laws of the 1970s and 1980s set out the requirements for food, drug, consumer product, and pesticide regulators (Rodricks, 2013; Merrill, 2001).

The appreciation of the importance of doses can be traced back to at least the 16th century, when the Swiss pharmacologist, Paracelsus, made the famous insight of that "all substances are poisons: only the dose separates a poison from a remedy." But little attention was paid to the problem of identifying safe doses without toxic effects in a large human population with highly diverse genetic backgrounds until at least the 1950s (Rodricks, 2013). For instance, in the 1940s and 1950s, much effort was made to control certain air emissions so that human health would not be put at risk of significant air pollution problems. Similarly, public health officials endeavored to impose exposure limits on newly discovered contaminants in drinking water and foods, and recommendations for workplace exposure limits during the first half of the 20th century (National Research Council, 1977). But none of these efforts was based on an explicitly described methodology that allowed for establishing safe levels of exposure to chemicals (Rodricks, 2013). These problems started to be addressed after new laws relating to substances added to foods were passed in the 1950s, which required the FDA to decide whether substances could be considered safe if added to food.

In 1954 Lehman and Fitzhugh proposed a 100-fold margin of safety for food additives, based on a factor of 10 to account for high- to low-dose extrapolation and a factor of 10 to account for variability in the human population in early attempts to predict the safety of a food additive (Lehman and Fitzhugh, 1954). Following this, in the mid-1950s came the Acceptable Daily Intake (ADI), a safe dose for humans that was established at 1/100 the maximum dose that leads to no adverse effect observed in animal testing (Rodricks, 2007). If the human intake of a food additive present in food, when the food was consumed, is less than the ADI, the level of the additive could be considered safe and approved for use (Rodricks, 2013). Additional factors (safety factors or uncertainty factors) have been proposed to account for the lack of long-term studies, reproductive and developmental studies, and insufficient or poor data. Of note, instead of ADI, the US EPA has chosen to use the term Toxicity Reference Dose (RfD).

The primary aim of predictive toxicology is to improve risk assessment (Committee on Applications of Toxicogenomic Technologies to Predictive Toxicology, 2007). The application of toxicogenomic technologies to risk assessment can potentially improve the understanding of dose–response relationships, cross-species extrapolations, exposure quantification, the underlying mechanisms of toxicity, and the basis of individual susceptibilities to particular compounds. In the 1970s risk analysis and risk-based decision-making were introduced into the area of chemical toxicity as several authors began to emphasize the concept that safety is not an absolute (Lowrance, 1976). They reasoned that in most cases there are no distinct cutoffs between safe and unsafe exposures to a food additive. This was further promoted by the problem of carcinogenic chemicals (National Research Council, 1983). To address carcinogenic risk, the US Congress enacted statutes in the 1950s and early 1960s that required the FDA to ban the use of food and color additives shown to be carcinogenic (National Research Council, 1983). For example, the Delaney Amendment required a strict prohibition on the intentional addition to food of any substance shown to be a carcinogen. Lehman and Fitzhugh asserted that ADIs should not be developed for carcinogens in animals or humans (Rodricks, 2013). In the mid-1970s, with a large number of chemical contaminants in the environment found to have carcinogenic properties, different guidelines have been developed for risk assessment which plays an important role in food safety. Both the EPA and FDA adopted several proposals of methods from the scientific literature to estimate low-dose risks for carcinogens. These methods assumed that there were no identifiable threshold doses for carcinogens and established there was a linear relationship between dose and risk (Rodricks, 2007). The magnitude of carcinogenic risk to be tolerated should be considered in the decision-making process in different circumstances (Rodricks, 2013). The Food Protection Committee of the National Research Council (NRC/NAS, 1970) recommended the use of safety factors or uncertainty to establish acceptable intakes, which were subsequently adopted by the Joint Food and Agricultural Organization and World Health Organization Expert Committees on Food Additives (1972) and Pesticide Residues (1965) of the World Health Organization. This approach has been applied to noncarcinogenic food additives and pesticides and, in slightly modified form, for acceptable exposures to occupational and various environmental pollutants.

Later in the 20th century, food safety risk assessment became more systematized when quantitative risk assessment methods were given greater scientific status in a seminal National Research Council report (National

Research Council, 1983). In 1983, as requested by the US Congress, a committee of the National Academy of Sciences (NAS) issued a report (Risk Assessment in the Federal Government: Managing the Process—the "Red Book"). The NAS committee reviewed and endorsed the new risk-based approaches and offered perspective and guidance on risk assessment and management (National Research Council, 1983). In this report, risk assessments were divided into four basic steps: (i) hazard identification to determine the link between a particular chemical and particular health effects; (ii) dose–response assessment to determine the relationship between the magnitude of exposure and the probability of occurrence of the health effects in question; (iii) exposure assessment to determine and compare the extent of human exposure before or after application of regulatory controls; and (iv) risk characterization to describe the nature and often the magnitude of human risk, including attendant uncertainty (National Research Council, 1983). As pointed out by Rodricks (2013), the report had a far-reaching impact on food safety and risk assessment as it set the stage for chemical regulation, with its recommendations in effect today. Since the issuance of the Red Book, the science of risk assessment has taken on greater rigor and incorporated methods based on a better understanding of carcinogenicity or other forms of toxicity and the biological processes of carcinogenesis and toxicology. The risk assessment/management distinction has emerged with greater clarity. The application of these principles described in the Red Book has expanded from chemical to other types of hazards, including microbial pathogens and nutrients (Rodricks, 2007, 2013; Merrill, 2001).

The risk assessment paradigm is continually being altered and for the most part, improved. FDA is one of the first federal health regulatory agencies to apply quantitative risk assessment methodology to policy analysis and cancer risk assessment (Merrill, 1997). FDA regulates food safety through the risk assessment process, while EFSA performs similar risk assessments in the EU (Merrill, 1997). The nature and likelihood of a harmful effect are assessed to characterize the level of risks and the necessary strategies to mitigate the adverse effect on individuals or at the population level. Health risk assessments are too often qualitative but should include statistical estimates of probabilities for specific populations. In 2009 the National Research Council issued another study titled *Science and Decisions: Advancing Risk Assessment* (National Research Council, 2009) that offers many recommendations on applications of risk assessment and a new framework for decision-making. This report is comprehensive in terms of both the science and utility of risk assessment and points the way to the future (Rodricks, 2013).

References

Abuajah, C.I., Ogbonna, A.C., Osuji, C.M., 2015. Functional components and medicinal properties of food: a review. J. Food Sci. Technol. 52, 2522–2529. https://doi.org/10.1007/s13197-014-1396-5. Epub 2014 May 16 25892752. PMCID: PMC4397330.

Armstrong, D.J., 2009. Food chemistry and U.S. food regulations. J. Agric. Food Chem. 57, 8180–8186. https://doi.org/10.1021/jf900014h.

Aven, T., 2016. Risk assessment and risk management: review of recent advances on their foundation. Eur. J. Oper. Res. 253, 1–13.

Beck, B.D., Seeley, M., Calabrese, E.J., 2014. Use of toxicology in the regulatory process. In: Hayes' Principles and Methods of Toxicology, sixth ed.

Bernstein, P.L., 1996. Against the Gods: The Remarkable Story of Risk. John Wiley & Sons, New York.

Brock, W.J., Rodricks, J.V., Rulis, A., Dellarco, V.L., Gray, G.M., Lane, R.W., 2003. Food safety: risk assessment methodology and decision-making criteria. Int. J. Toxicol. 22 (6), 435–451. https://doi.org/10.1177/109158180302200605. 14680991.

CDC. https://www.cdc.gov/foodsafety/newsletter/technology-detect-outbreaks-7-18-19.html.

chfa. https://chfa.ca/en/Regulatory/Food-Regulations.

Choudhuri, S., Chanderbhan, R.F., Mattia, A., 2019. Chapter 27: Food toxicology: fundamental and regulatory aspects. In: Casarett & Doull's Toxicology: The Basic Science of Poisons, ninth ed.

Committee on Applications of Toxicogenomic Technologies to Predictive Toxicology, 2007. Applications of Toxicogenomic Technologies to Predictive Toxicology and Risk Assessment. National Academies Press.

Dorne, J.L.C.M., Renwick, A.G., 2005. The refinement of uncertainty/safety factors in risk assessment by the incorporation of data on toxicokinetic variability in humans. Toxicol. Sci. 86, 20–26.

Dourson, M.L., Stara, J.F., 1983. Regulatory history and experimental support of uncertainty (safety) factors. Regul. Toxicol. Pharmacol. 3, 224–238.

en.wikipedia. https://en.wikipedia.org/wiki/Silent_Spring.

Estes, J.W., 1996. The medical properties of food in the eighteenth century. J. Hist. Med. Allied Sci. 51, 127–154. https://doi.org/10.1093/jhmas/51.2.127.

EU. https://european-union.europa.eu/priorities-and-actions/actions-topic/food-safety_en.

Food Standards Agency "Allergy and Intolerance: Guidance for Businesses—Food Standards Agency". www.food.gov.uk. Food Standards Agency.

Foodsafety.gov, Bacteria and Viruses. www.foodsafety.gov.

Gad, S.C., Toxicology, third ed., CRC Press Boca Raton, FL, pp. 113–149.

German Federal Ministry of Food, Agriculture and Consumer Protection. n.d. Bundesministerium für Ernährung, Landwirtschaft und Verbraucherschutz.

gov.cn. http://www.gov.cn/zhengce/2015-04/25.

Greenway, F.L., 2020. Food as medicine for chronic disease: a strategy to address noncompliance. J. Med. Food 23 (9), 903–904. https://doi.org/10.1089/jmf.2020.29007.flg.

Hayes, A.W., Kruger, C.L., Clemens, R.A., 2016. Whom should we trust? Case in point: red and processed meats. Food Safety August/September, 63–66.

He, S., Shi, X., 2021. Microbial food safety in China: past, present, and future. Foodborne Pathog. Dis. 18 (8), 510–518. https://doi.org/10.1089/fpd.2021.0009. Epub 2021 Jul 8 34242111.

Jiang, X., Zhao, Y., Tang, C., Appelbaum, M., Rao, Q., 2022. Aquatic food animals in the United States: status quo and challenges. Compr. Rev. Food Sci. Food Saf. 21 (2), 1336–1382. https://doi.org/10.1111/1541-4337.12923. Epub 2022 Feb 12 35150203.

Kruger, C.L., Reddy, C.S., Conze, D.B., Hayes, A.W., 2014. Food safety and foodborne toxicants. In: Hayes' Principles and Methods of Toxicology, sixth ed.

Lane, R.W., 2014. The Wissenschaften of toxicology: harming and helping through time. In: Hayes' Principles and Methods of Toxicology, sixth ed.

Lehman, A.J., Fitzhugh, O.F., 1954. 100-fold margin of safety. Assoc. Food Drug Off. U.S.Q Bull. 18, 33–35.

LeMessurier, K.S., Rooney, R., Ghoneim, H.E., Liu, B., Li, K., Smallwood, H.S., Samarasinghe, A.E., 2020. Influenza A virus directly modulates mouse eosinophil responses. J. Leukoc. Biol. 108 (1), 151–168.

Liu, B., 2017. Universal PCR primers are critical for direct sequencing-based enterovirus genotyping. J. Clin. Microbiol. 55, 339–340.

Liu, B., Yang, J.X., Yan, L., Zhuang, H., Li, T., 2018. Novel HBV recombinants between genotypes B and C in 3'-terminal reverse transcriptase (RT) sequences are associated with enhanced viral DNA load, higher RT point mutation rates and place of birth among Chinese patients. Infect. Genet. Evol. 57, 26–35.

Liu, B., Forman, M., Valsamakis, A., 2019. Optimization and evaluation of a novel real-time RT-PCR test for detection of parechovirus in cerebrospinal fluid. J. Virol. Methods 272, 113690. https://doi.org/10.1016/j.jviromet.2019.113690. Epub 2019 Jul 5 31283959.

Liu, B., Totten, M., Nematollahi, S., Datta, K., Memon, W., Marimuthu, S., Wolf, L.A., Carroll, K.C., Zhang, S.X., 2020. Development and evaluation of a fully automated molecular assay targeting the mitochondrial small subunit rRNA gene for the detection of Pneumocystis jirovecii in Bronchoalveolar lavage fluid specimens. J. Mol. Diagn. 22 (12), 1482–1493. https://doi.org/10.1016/j.jmoldx.2020.10.003.

Lowrance, W.W., 1976. Of Acceptable Risk: Science and the Determination of Safety. William Kaufmann, Inc, Altos, GA.

Manuele, F.A., 2016. Chapter 1: Risk assessments: their significance and the role of the safety professional. In: Popov, G., Lyon, B.K., Hollcraft, B. (Eds.), Risk Assessment: A Practical Guide to Assessing Operational Risks. John Wiley & Sons, ISBN: 9781118911044, pp. 1–22.

Merrill, R.A., 1997. Food safety regulation: reforming the Delaney Clause. Annu. Rev. Public Health 18, 313–340. https://doi.org/10.1146/annurev.publhealth.18.1.313. 9143722.

Merrill, R., 2001. Regulatory toxicology. In: Casarett & Doull's Toxicology, sixth ed. McGraw Hill, New York.

Morris, G., 2011. How safe is our food? Emerg. Infect. Dis. 17, 126–128. https://doi.org/10.3201/eid1701.101821.

National Research Council, 1977. Drinking Water and Health. vol. 1 National Academy Press, Washington, DC.

National Research Council, 1983. Risk Assessment in the Federal Government: Managing the Process. The National Academies Press, Washington, DC, https://doi.org/10.17226/366.

National Research Council, 2009. Science and Decisions: Advancing Risk Assessment. National Academy Press, Washington, DC.

Nuffoods Spectrum n.d. "FSSAI Appoints New Members for Scientific Panels". Nuffoods Spectrum. Retrieved 13 February 2015.

Parmet, S., Lynm, C., Glass, R.M., 2003. Food-borne illnesses. JAMA 290 (10), 1408. https://doi.org/10.1001/jama.290.10.1285.

Peng, Y., Liu, B., Hou, J., Sun, J., Hao, R., Xiang, K., Yan, L., Zhang, J., Zhuang, H., Li, T., 2015. Naturally occurring deletions/insertions in HBV core promoter tend to decrease in HBeAg positive chronic hepatitis B patients during antiviral therapy. Antivir. Ther. 20, 623–632.

Rausand, M., 2013. Chapter 1: Introduction. In: Risk Assessment: Theory, Methods, and Applications. John Wiley & Sons, ISBN: 9780470637647, pp. 1–28.

Rodricks, J.V., 2007. Calculated Risks. The Toxicity and Human Health Risks of Chemicals in our Environment, second ed. Cambridge University Press, Cambridge.

Rodricks, J.V., 2013. One-hundred years of toxicological risk assessment. ECG Bull. February. https://www.envchemgroup.com/one-hundred-years-of-toxicological-risk-assessment.html.

thesaferfoodgroup. https://www.thesaferfoodgroup.com/knowledge/natashas-law-are-you-ready/.

Tolar, B., Joseph, L.A., Schroeder, M.N., Stroika, S., Ribot, E.M., Hise, K.B., Gerner-Smidt, P., 2019. An overview of PulseNet USA databases. Foodborne Pathog. Dis. 16 (7), 457–462. https://doi.org/10.1089/fpd.2019.2637.

Tsatsakis, A., Vassilopoulou, M.L., Kovatsi, L., Tsitsimpikou, C., Karamanou, M., Leon, G., Liesivuori, J., Hayes, A.W., Spandidos, D.A., 2018. The dose response principle from philosophy to modern toxicology: the impact of ancient philosophy and medicine in modern toxicology science. Toxicol. Rep. 5, 1107–1113. https://doi.org/10.1016/j.toxrep.2018.10.001.

Wexler, 2015. History of Toxicology and Environmental Health, Toxicology in Antiquity, Volume II. Academic Press, Elsevier, Amsterdam, ISBN: 978-0-12-801506-3.

Wu, F., Rodricks, J.V., 2020. Forty years of food safety risk assessment: a history and analysis. Risk Anal. 40 (S1), 2218–2230. https://doi.org/10.1111/risa.13624. Epub 2020 Nov 1 33135225.

Ybañez, N., Montoro, R., 1996. Trace element food toxicology: an old and ever-growing discipline. Crit. Rev. Food Sci. Nutr. 36 (4), 299–320. https://doi.org/10.1080/10408399609527727.

Index

Note: Page numbers followed by *f* indicate figures and *t* indicate tables.

H

Hazard Analysis and Critical Control Point (HACCP) plan, 195
Hazard identification/characterization, for food allergy, 131–132
Health claims, 163–164
  nutrition and, 305
  qualified, 164
Heavy metals
  contamination, 110–111
  and dietary metal intake, 110–111
Hepatotoxicity, weight loss supplement, 170–172
Herbal dietary supplements, 160
Herbicide-tolerant (HT) crops, 146–148, 285–286
Hippocrates, 3
History of Food Adulteration and Analysis (Filby), 258–259
Huanglongbing, 149–150, 287
Human diet minerals, 69–70, 71*t*. *See also* Minerals
Humane Methods of Slaughter Act (HMSA), 199–200
Human leukocyte antigen (HLA), 48
Hydroxycut, 170–171
5-Hydroxytryptamine (5-HT), 44
Hypericum perforatum (St. John's Wort), 176
Hyperkinesis, and food additives, 92
Hypersensitivity, 124–127, 240
Hypervitaminosis D, 61–62
Hypoglycin A, 11–14*t*
Hyponatremia, 77

I

ImmunoCAPs, 281
Immunoglobulin E (IgE)-mediated food allergies, 22, 124, 126, 129–130
Inherent foodborne toxicants, 33–34
  mycotoxins, 41–46
  plant toxins, 34–49, 36*f*
  seafood toxins, 46–49
Inherent food constituents, 18
Inheritance powders, 5
Insects
  as food sources, 291–293, 292*f*
  insect-resistant crops, 144–146, 289–290
Institute of Food Technologists, 89, 93

Insulin-like Growth Factor Acid-Labile Subunit (IGFALS), 44
Intentional adulteration, of food, 196
Interim period, GRAS, 241
International Agency for Research and Cancer (IARC), 285–286
International Food Biotechnology Council (IFBC), 142
International Life Sciences Institute (ILSI), 110–111
International Potato Center, 151
Iron, 80–81
  deficiency symptoms, 81, 81*f*
  food sources, 81
  iron-deficiency anemia, 81
  toxicity/upper limits, 82

J

Japonica rice, 287–288
Joint FAO/WHO Expert Committee on Food Additives (JECFA), 9, 27, 89, 93, 106, 110–111, 228, 312
Joint Institute for Food Safety and Applied Nutrition (JIFAN), 110–111
The Jungle (Sinclair), 9, 198, 263–264, 265*f*, 269

K

Keratinocyte-neuron coculture model, 48
Korea Food and Drug Administration (KFDA), 309
Krebs cycle, 66–67

L

Labeling requirements, 162
Lactobacillus sp.
  L. acidophilus, 161
  L. casei, 161
  L. fermentum, 161
Lactose intolerance, 124–125
Lakes, food colors, 91
The Lancet, 259–260
La Voisin, 5
Lead, 6
  in drinking water, 112
Leafy vegetables, vitamin K in, 62–63, 63*f*
LEAP Study (Learning Early About Peanut allergy), 123
Learning disabilities, and food additives, 92

Printed in the United States
by Baker & Taylor Publisher Services